C000045703

The Actor's Brain
Exploring the cognitive
neuroscience of free will

The Actor's Brain
Exploring the cognitive neuroscience of free will

Sean A Spence

Professor of General Adult Psychiatry,
University of Sheffield

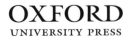

OXFORD
UNIVERSITY PRESS

OXFORD
UNIVERSITY PRESS

Great Clarendon Street, Oxford, OX2 6DP,
United Kingdom

Oxford University Press is a department of the University of Oxford.
It furthers the University's objective of excellence in research, scholarship,
and education by publishing worldwide. Oxford is a registered trade mark of
Oxford University Press in the UK and in certain other countries

© Oxford University Press, 2009

The moral rights of the author have been asserted

First published 2009

All rights reserved. No part of this publication may be reproduced, stored in
a retrieval system, or transmitted, in any form or by any means, without the
prior permission in writing of Oxford University Press, or as expressly permitted
by law, by licence or under terms agreed with the appropriate reprographics
rights organization. Enquiries concerning reproduction outside the scope of the
above should be sent to the Rights Department, Oxford University Press, at the
address above

You must not circulate this work in any other form
and you must impose this same condition on any acquirer

Published in the United States of America by Oxford University Press
198 Madison Avenue, New York, NY 10016, United States of America

British Library Cataloguing in Publication Data
Data available

Library of Congress Cataloguing in Publication Data
Data Available

ISBN 978-0-19-852666-7

Oxford University Press makes no representation, express or implied, that the
drug dosages in this book are correct. Readers must therefore always check
the product information and clinical procedures with the most up-to-date
published product information and data sheets provided by the manufacturers
and the most recent codes of conduct and safety regulations. The authors and
the publishers do not accept responsibility or legal liability for any errors in the
text or for the misuse or misapplication of material in this work. Except where
otherwise stated, drug dosages and recommendations are for the non-pregnant
adult who is not breast-feeding

'Man is an animal that stands up. He is not very big
and he has to work for a living.'[1]

'Laborare est orare'[2]

---

1   One of a series of nineteenth century children's exam answers, cited in Herzog D.
    Cunning. Princeton: Princeton University Press, 2006, 127.
2   The Benedictine concept, 'To work is to pray', cited in Hendra T. *Father Joe: The man
    who saved my soul*. New York: Random House, 2005, 45.

To my mother, Mary, without whom there would have been no 'actions'.

Contents

Acknowledgements

First of all, my sincere thanks to Mr. Richard Marley, Professor Bill Fulford, and the anonymous reviewers at Oxford University Press for their comments on this book during its earliest gestation and to Mr. Martin Baum and Ms. Carol Maxwell for their continued patience as it has neared its (eventual!) delivery date.

During the preparation of this manuscript, I have received immense help from my assistant, Mrs. Jean Woodhead, and my colleagues and students at the Sheffield Cognition and Neuroimaging Laboratory (SCANLab), especially Dr. Tom Farrow, Dr. Mike Hunter, Dr. Cath Kaylor-Hughes, Dr. Sudheer Lankappa, Dr. Sarah Jones, Dr. Robert Fung, Ms. Alex Hope-Urwin, Ms. Diana Ward, Ms. Alice Mackay, Mr. Martin Brook, Mr. Chris Hobbs, and our ever-kind and resourceful departmental manager, Ms. Beverley Nesbitt.

The content of this text, with its emphasis on human beings' voluntary behaviours and their trajectories through time, has served to remind me of the debts of gratitude that I owe to many people who have impacted upon my own development over many years. Medicine has been a factor in my existence from the very start; being the product of a Caesarean section, neither my mother nor I might have survived had it not been for equitable access to modern health care in the 1960s. I thank whoever it was that saved us. I give thanks for the British NHS. I have also been fortunate enough to have encountered some inspirational teachers along the way: 'Mr. Daly', who read *The Hobbit* aloud in the afternoons and played Holst's *The Planets* suite to us at primary school in Ruislip, in the early 1970s; Dr. Carol Lyons, who helped me to understand chemistry, as a teenager in Bromley, later in that decade; Mr. Dermot McMahon, who really cared whether or not his students got from school to university; Father Greystone, who 'went the extra mile'; Dr. Jessica Kirker, who inculcated a 'toolbox' of psychodynamic skills into our cohort of raw psychiatric trainees, at the Gordon Hospital in the early 1990s; and Father Charles Farrell, who posed the question 'What would the brain of a moral person look like?', in New York City in 1999. I thank the jazz musicians who have patiently answered my impromptu questions about the nature of improvization (especially Peter King and the late Steve Lacy). I owe Professor Alwyn Lishman many thanks for much informal advice over the years. I owe Professor Steven Hirsch an appreciation of rigour, and unflinching honesty. I am very grateful to you all.

Prologue: Against freedom

Much of the inspiration for writing this book, and for attempting to articulate the questions that it concerns, stems from my reading of a series of experiments conducted by Benjamin Libet and his colleagues in the United States in the early 1980s. Professor Libet worked at the University of California and his studies concerned the novel application of electroencephalography (EEG), a means via which the brain's electrical activity may be detected and measured, by using electrodes applied to the surface of the scalp. Such apparatus allows investigators to record electrical activity in 'real time', its trace emerging as the jittery signatures of multiple needles translating brain signals into static readout. The non-clinical reader of this book may have seen the frantic movement of such needles in movies or in television programmes when the emergence of an epileptic seizure within a person's brain is associated with increased electrical activity distributed across its entire surface: many needles zigzagging in unison (Fig. 1). By looking at the shape and position of the traces that emerge, via such needles, investigators can estimate where a seizure might have arisen: they can attempt to 'localize' its 'focus'. Hence, EEG can be very useful in providing knowledge about what it is that is happening inside the brain, over the course of milliseconds; it can also say something about where such activity originates.

However, another way of using EEG is to collect recordings while a person (a 'subject') experiences the same events over and over again, repeatedly. For instance, if we want to find out *when* it is that a subject's brain changes its pattern of electrical activity immediately *before* she moves her right index finger, then we could ask her to perform this action on multiple occasions (perhaps as many as 40 'trials'), each time collecting an electrical trace of what her brain activity looks like, at both the moment when her finger actually moves and over the seconds preceding that movement. Then, if we can combine these traces (by using the moment of verifiable movement as a common reference point: i.e. 'time-locking' the EEG traces to this event), we can obtain a mathematical average, a trace that shows us, in the form of a wavy line, *when* the change in brain activity began, relative to the ensuing movement (of the right index finger). How many milliseconds went by between our subject's brain activity changing and her finger moving? In Figure 2, we see the sort of signal that may be obtained in this way. Notice how it seems to rise over the hundreds

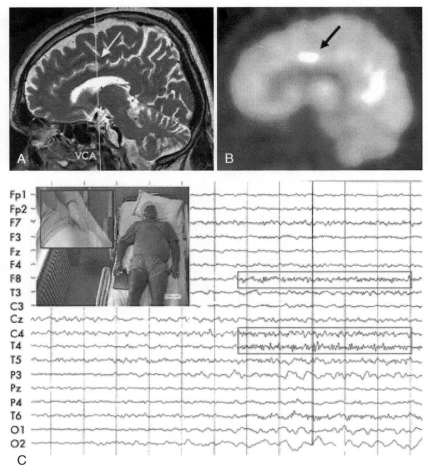

Fig. 1 Images showing the brain of a man who exhibited a lesion of the right medial frontal lobe, giving rise to focal epilepsy, which was manifest through the movements of an anarchic left hand (active during epilepsy in the contralateral frontal lobe). (A) The structural MRI scan, (B) the PET scan (the arrow indicates the active focus of this man's epilepsy), and (C) the EEG trace (enclosed in a box) coinciding with the onset of his focal epilepsy. (From Brazdil et al., *Journal of Neurology, Neurosurgery and Psychiatry* 2006; 77: 992–993, with permission from the BMJ Publishing Group Ltd.)

of milliseconds prior to the act, followed by a tapering off when the action finally occurs. Actually, this electrical signal constitutes a 'negative' value, a *reduction* in the electrical potential prior to the onset of the movement, but the convention is to display it on an inverted graph, where 'negative' is pointing 'up'; hence, the EEG signal is seen to 'increase' towards the moment of action.

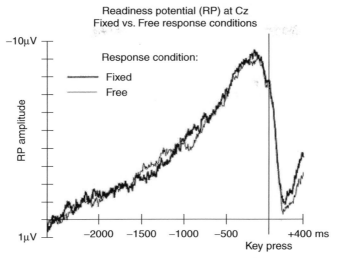

Fig. 2 EEG data summated to show the readiness potential (RP) arising immediately prior to a voluntary act (the key press indicated on the horizontal axis). Note that the signal appears to increase but is actually an increasing negative potential, seen over the vertex of the skull, at EEG position Cz (see Fig. 1). The signal is already decreasing by the time of the key press. (From Haggard and Eimer, Experimental Brain Research 1999; 126: 128–133. Such signals may be fractionated into 'early' and 'late' RPs; see Fig. 5 and Chapter 3, with kind permission from Springer Science and Business Media).

What did Benjamin Libet do that was so interesting?

As the reader may have guessed from the title of this prologue, and indeed from the title of this book, the question that Libet posed, which was particularly interesting, concerned the antecedents of voluntary action. In other words, what happens in the brain just *before* a person makes a 'freely chosen' voluntary movement?

Libet's subjects were asked to flex either their right index fingers or their wrists rapidly, 'whenever they felt like it'. In other words, they were invited to behave 'spontaneously', to act only when they wished to act. Libet's team collected the EEG signals occurring before and after such movements, and found that signals arose over the midline of the skull (in a region called the 'vertex') that preceded the emergence of voluntary behaviours by some hundreds of milliseconds (as in Fig. 2).

This was interesting, but it wasn't surprising. Such signals have been detected and reported by other investigators since the 1960s (Kornhuber and Deecke [1965] in particular, but see also Walter et al. [1964] and Gilden et al. [1966]). However, Libet discovered that the *shape* of the signal detected prior to a

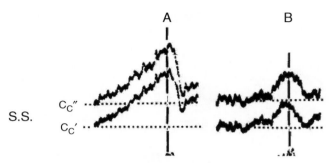

Fig. 3 Readiness potential (RP) recorded over the vertex of the skull in a volunteer (S.S.) studied by Libet and colleagues. (A) Slow increase in the RP prior to a planned act and (B) later emergence of this signal prior to a 'spontaneous' act. (From Libet et al., *Electroencephalograph and Clinical Neurophysiology* 1982; 54: 332–335; with permission from Elsevier Ltd.)

movement varied according to whether his subjects felt that they had spent some time 'planning' their movement or had, instead, acted truly 'spontaneously'. Where there was an element of planning, the signal was *slower* to emerge but began much *earlier* (i.e. it sometimes started over a second before the subject's movement finally materialized, rising as a shallow gradient in the electrical trace; see Fig. 3). In contrast, when the subject acted suddenly, truly 'spontaneously', the signal was *sharper*, arising *later*, and closer to the act in terms of time; however, it still arose *prior* to the act (Libet et al., 1982).

So, the degree of planning or spontaneity affording an action is reflected in the electrical signal detectable (over the midline of the skull) just prior to its execution. The implication is that if we act truly 'spontaneously', then the change in signal emerges later; it arises closer in time to the action itself.

However, there was more to come. For, through an ingenious experimental variation upon the everyday use of a clock face, Libet and colleagues went further. They asked their subjects to estimate *when* they had become aware of their own *urge* to act. In other words, when was it that they formed an 'intention' to move? Now, in order to understand how the investigators addressed this question, we need to look a little more closely at how they performed their experiment (Fig. 4).

Libet's subjects reportedly sat in a comfortable chair, and were attached to all the EEG equipment required to detect their brains' electrical activity. They also wore electrodes on their right forearms, designed to record electrical activity emerging from the muscles responsible for finger and wrist movements (resulting in an electromyogram or EMG). This arrangement enabled the investigators to calculate the temporal interval (i.e. the time lag) between

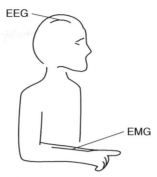

Fig. 4 Cartoon showing the experimental arrangement throughout Libet's experiments (Libet et al. 1983). An electroencephalograph (EEG) signal was detected over the scalp of the volunteers while an electromyograph signal was detected over the muscles of the right forearm.

the movement-related signal developing in their subject's brain, just prior to the movement (as detected on the EEG), and the onset of that movement, in their muscles (as detected on the EMG). Furthermore, the subjects were asked to look straight ahead at a simulated clock face, a clock on which the 'second hand' (in this case, a dot of light) moved faster than on a conventional clock face and where each '2.5 s' on its surface actually corresponded to 106 ms of real time (Libet et al., 1983).

Therefore, if the subjects were able to note the time at which their urge to move their fingers surfaced within their minds (or at least did so 'consciously'), and they were able to report this 'time of intention' to the investigators after each movement, then the latter could potentially calculate the relative timing of three events:

1) The 'arrival' of the *urge* to move in the subject's consciousness (as indicated by the clock face time at which the subjects felt their intentions form),

2) The onset of the change in *electrical activity* in their brain preceding the associated movement (as recorded on the EEG), and

3) The time of the resulting *movement* executed (as measured on the EMG).

What is surprising in any of this? Well, perhaps the result is because the sequence of events that Libet discovered was *not* the sequence that I have just outlined (i.e. '1', '2', and '3' in the preceding list). Instead, it was the following: the brain's change in EEG signal ('2') came first, followed by the subject's recognition of the urge to act ('1'), and then followed by the action itself ('3'). In other words, the intention to act occurred *later* in time than the change in brain activity predictive of that same act.

Or, to put things in another way, the sequence of events was not the one that we should have expected from our experience of everyday life (and classical philosophy, where thought is said to lead to action [e.g. Macmurray, 1991]):

INTENTION → BRAIN EVENT → MOVEMENT

Rather, it was the following:

BRAIN EVENT → INTENTION → MOVEMENT

Libet and his colleagues summarized their findings in the following way:

> It is concluded that [the] cerebral initiation of a spontaneous, freely [chosen] voluntary act can begin unconsciously, that is, before there is any (at least recallable) subjective awareness that a 'decision' to act has already been initiated cerebrally. This introduces certain constraints on the potentiality for conscious initiation and control of voluntary acts.
>
> (Libet et al., 1983, p. 623).

So, albeit conveyed through the careful language of science, Libet and his colleagues appear to be saying that a voluntary act may emerge unconsciously, that is, before the 'author' of that act has 'decided' to act. Now, if this is the case, then what space is left for freedom?

Questions and assumptions

When one first learns of Libet's experiments (which remain the subject of recurrent heated debates [e.g. Young, 2006; Spence, 2006]), one may feel

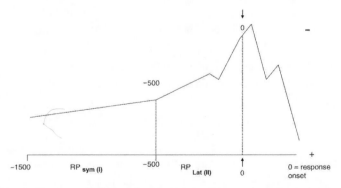

Fig. 5 Cartoon showing the fractionation of the readiness potential (RP) into two parts (i.e. early, before −500 ms, and late, after −500 ms, relative to the point of action, indicated at 0). RP(I) is maximal over the midline, and hence symmetrical, RP(II) is lateralised to the motor and premotor cortex involved in the ensuing action. There is a clear increase in the electroencephalograph (EEG) signal (RP gradient) over the last 500 ms before the act.

rather shocked, as if something long cherished has suddenly been taken away. Can it possibly be true that the thought that I think when I decide to make a movement is *not* the true originator of that movement? Is it likely that it *really* constitutes the late corollary of an earlier choice, a choice that 'I' did not make (consciously) but which was made by 'my brain' (in advance of 'my' awareness of it)? Is this credible? Should we even be talking about ourselves in this way, as dual entities possessing 'minds' and 'brains'? It seems as if this may be part of our problem: the Libet findings rankle so long as we identify solely with our 'conscious' minds, while we ascribe 'responsibility' to our consciousness rather than our 'brain' and all that arises there (conscious and unconscious alike). Indeed, as we shall see later in this book, we, as a community of sentient beings (organisms, persons), seem to have a lot invested in maintaining such a distinction; there are numerous inconvenient ramifications that accrue once we start to question some of our most cherished assumptions in this area. Not least is the following: if intentions are illusory (i.e. non-causal), then does the legal distinction between murder and manslaughter remain coherent? Does it matter? Is it important? Well, we shall return to this question towards the end of this book (especially in Chapter 9), but the point is this: these issues that we raise are not trivial.

Crucially, the controversy caused by Libet's work concerns its apparent undermining of our notions of 'freedom of the will': it is as if the choices made within our minds have their own inner determinants, as if the decisions that we make have 'already' been made ('somewhere else', out of consciousness). Are human choices predetermined? This is a very old question. Indeed, philosophers and theologians have probably sparred over this topic for thousands of years. However, following Libet, this problem begins to resemble a scientific question rather than a philosophical or theological point of debate. The 'determinism' that we contest, here, is one that is extended over hundreds of milliseconds (not the years of a life, the aeons of an evolutionary 'descent', or the age of the universe).

Nevertheless, before we proceed further, I need to mention a number of caveats and riders to the conclusions drawn from Libet's work. Indeed, I shall return to some of the more technical, experimental, details in Chapter 3. For now, though, I shall dwell upon what it is that Libet thought he'd found, what the constraints of his experiments were, and what they add to some of the assumptions and beliefs that humans have long held about themselves and the choices that they make. I should also state, explicitly, that (in my opinion) this whole field of inquiry owes an immense debt of gratitude to Benjamin Libet for his truly pioneering work; so, where I critique his conclusions, this is meant with respect, and very much in the spirit of open and honest debate.

This critique does not seek to lessen his contribution in any way; indeed, it relies upon a great deal of pioneering work performed by Libet and others (some of these scientists will be mentioned in Chapter 3.)

Deconstructing Libet

To begin with, it is clear that Libet's work was conducted under quite specific and exacting circumstances. His subjects were being investigated experimentally, in a laboratory, and asked to introspect in quite unusual ways. Moreover, they had to perform arbitrary and meaningless activities: the rapid flexion of a finger or a wrist. This is all reasonable of course because this was an experimental study and the investigators needed to control the environment and the task as much as possible in order to be able to focus upon their scientific questions; nevertheless, this procedure is not very close to what we might call 'everyday, real life'. [Indeed, if you read the recurrent debates about Libet's work, you will come across those activities that philosophers routinely identify as exemplars of everyday, real-life pursuits: going for a beer, driving in a car, riding on a bike, going to the fridge, taking out a beer, going for a walk, entering a bar, or ordering a beer. Could there be an emergent pattern here? Maybe, it tells us more about philosophers than it does about real life, but the point is that all 'neat' examples are inherently problematic—we spend much our time multitasking, carrying out rather mundane tasks while 'thinking of something else'; in other words, we're not necessarily concentrating on what it is that we're doing.]

Furthermore, Libet's subjects were, by definition, highly compliant. They were prepared to sit for many sessions, performing rather pointless activities and reporting to the experimenters when it was that they felt as if they had experienced an 'urge' to act. We are rarely called upon to do this sort of thing in everyday life, so we have to remain cautious when interpreting what it is that Libet found. Actually, his technique is reminiscent of what it might be like to begin to learn certain forms of meditation or to sit in silence during a session of psychotherapy (or indeed, confession), introspecting, or studying one's own thoughts and internal processes. Nevertheless, for the closely monitored, simple actions that he was interested in, it does seem clear that Benjamin Libet demonstrated that the brain began to change its activity patterns prior to each act, and that the change in activity arose *prior to* the subjective awareness of an intention (to act) being experienced (consciously) by his subjects.

Indeed, given the degree of introspection required of Libet's subjects, one might even speculate that they were in a *better* position than most of us to truly deliberate about their intentions because they were solely required to do this (they were not multitasking in the office or at the supermarket, and not driving on the motorway while conversing at the same time.) So, if anyone should have been in a position to act 'truly spontaneously', with their thoughts constituting the origins of their actions, then these subjects should have been the ones for whom it worked. And yet it didn't. Their intentions arose 'too late'. Thought did not lead to action (apparently).

Libet's paradox

One way of responding to Libet's work is to say that his findings are valid (i.e. they accurately describe what they purport to describe) but that they 'only' describe a special case: they apply solely to the performance of spontaneous acts, which are arbitrary and unimportant. This line of argument holds that in real life when we need to perform a complex task or something that is truly important to us, we don't just do the first thing that comes into our minds. Instead, we deliberate and think things over. So, even if the action that eventually emerges is itself initiated by something that 'goes on' in our brains, something that occurs prior to our awareness, this is not the challenge to freedom that it might at first have seemed because *really* we had made up our minds already, during all of those earlier periods of deliberation. On this reading of Libet, his work reveals only a very short-term determinism, literally the trigger signal to perform a prespecified act, whereas over the longer term, the validity of human agency (our 'choice' and 'responsibility') is preserved (and justified) by the existence of deliberation and planning. This is a view with which I have a certain amount of sympathy, but I have to be honest and state that I think there is a problem in this account of freedom and it is one that is readily apparent within Libet's own body of work. Indeed, ironically, it is an aspect of that work which Libet himself does not seem to have fully integrated into his thesis (Libet, 2004).

Now, I should justify what I have just said. The 'problem' I am referring to emerges in an earlier body of Libet's work, and it is a problem, once again, not because of any weakness in the execution of that work but because of the very profound conclusions it foists upon us.

In that earlier series of experiments, concerning the subjective timing of sensory experiences (rather than motor acts), Libet and his colleagues had obtained access to patients who were undergoing neurosurgery for the treatment of epilepsy and other serious neurological conditions. Such patients would receive local anaesthesia, to enable the neurosurgeon to open up their skulls; yet, they remained awake throughout the procedures (this is often necessary if the surgeon requires 'live' feedback from the patient regarding the effect of a surgical intervention.) Libet and his group used this opportunity to investigate the characteristics of sensory experiences occurring in these conscious human subjects. One line of work involved stimulating the sensory areas of the brain to discover 'how long' such stimulation would need to last before the subject (patient) experienced a sensation attributable to that stimulus. *When* did they become aware of an experience corresponding to the direct stimulation of the surface of their brain? Libet found that such stimulation needed to last for approximately 500 ms before his subjects reported an ensuing experience.

Indeed, he also tried the experiment 'in reverse'. He stimulated the skin on a distant part of the body and then considered how long such stimulation might be required to last before it gave rise to an experience (a sensation within the subject's 'awareness'). Furthermore, was there a temporal 'window', a space in time, during which subsequent (direct) stimulation of the brain might disrupt awareness of that incoming signal (sensation)? Libet found that such a temporal window did exist. If stimulation of the sensory cortex occurred within 500 ms of an initial (incoming) skin stimulus, then it could abolish or amplify the perception of that stimulus (i.e. the subject's experience of the 'true', veridical, external stimulus; Libet et al., 1964; Libet et al., 1979; the rationale and development of this work is also clearly described in Chapter 2 of Libet's book *Mind Time* [2004, pp. 33–122].)

Therefore, a period of 'neuronal adequacy' seemed to be required in order for a subject to become aware of (i.e. to experience) a sensory event (Libet, 2004). The duration of that period was approximately 500 ms. In other words, one needs to stimulate the cortex for this long before a human subject experiences corresponding conscious phenomena, and following peripheral skin stimulation, there is a 'window' of a similar duration during which direct stimulation of the brain may 'delete' such an incoming signal. Hence, there is a finite temporal delay between the onset of neural activity and our consciousness of that activity (and that finite delay is on the order of 500 ms).

Now, one can interpret these data as demonstrating something that one must already have assumed if one is a 'materialist': in order for a conscious physical being to experience consciousness of specific items of subjective data ('qualia', in the language of philosophy), a minimum, finite period of neuronal activity must have occurred. Hence, whenever one is aware of anything—the sight of a bird, the taste of honey, the sound of Charlie Parker's alto saxophone—one is experiencing the consequences of *preceding* periods of neuronal activity. Note, also, that for our present purposes, the absolute duration of that period of activity or 'adequacy' is unimportant. What *is* important is that there is a *finite delay* between neural onset and conscious awareness (Spence, 1996). This 'delay' is crucial.

So, if we return to Libet's later experiments concerning voluntary behaviour (ca. 1983), where his subjects experienced their intentions to act some hundreds of milliseconds *after* the onset of a (predictive) change in their EEG signal

(Fig. 4), we find Libet arguing that, despite the subject becoming aware of the intention to act only *after* the onset of electrical activity predictive of that ensuing act, there might, nevertheless, still be a role for their subjective, conscious, awareness if it contributed to a potential power of 'veto'. Hence, he argued, awareness is not totally vestigial. The subjects might become aware of their intentions but then refrain from acting; they might 'decide' against it, 'delete it', and stop themselves, so that the 'intended' action would not follow. To Libet, this suggested that while conscious intentions to act might not constitute the *initiators* of voluntary actions, they might nevertheless serve a proscriptive role: they might *veto* actions that were contextually inappropriate. In this way, he argued for our retention of the concept of 'free will', albeit free will that is essentially negative (because, ultimately, it is solely a means of suppressing actions not generating them; Libet, 2004). Indeed, some have even called this version of free will 'free won't'!

Again, this is a view with which it is easy to sympathize. We have probably all had the experience of 'changing our minds' about an action and feeling as if we had literally blocked the movement that might have emerged: we suddenly decide not to change lanes on the motorway, even though we have prepared to indicate our intentions; we choose the white cup not the blue, though we had reached for the latter while making coffee; we put the phone down, despite having picked it up while we intended to make a call, because we have 'changed our minds'. Hence, Libet's interpretation seems phenomenologically sound: we often have the *experience* of 'changing our minds'. However, there is a problem with this line of argument, and it is one that also undermines the dismissal of Libet's work, as solely applying to arbitrary, spontaneous acts.

The problem for long-term freedom

It strikes me that all of Libet's work informs our understanding of what we might call the 'processing constraints' of the human nervous system. Simply stated, it takes a certain period of time for subjective phenomena to arise out of material biology, physical matter. Of course, this is essentially a recapitulation of the problem of consciousness, albeit in another guise: here, we are not attempting to address the 'hard problem' ('How does consciousness arise from matter?'); instead, we are acknowledging one of its implications (i.e. 'We don't know how consciousness arises from matter, but we do know that it takes a certain period of time to do so.') Hence, an 'intention to act' is the *late* corollary of emergent brain activity. Furthermore, a sensory stimulus also requires a finite period of neuronal activity ('adequacy') for a human subject to become aware of it, to experience it. In other words, a *temporal delay is inherent in human mental life: we are always experiencing the 'past'*.

However, if this is true, then Libet's conscious 'veto' is not what he thinks it is, for the awareness that we have of vetoing an action, if we are to be consistent, is itself likely to be the *late* corollary of earlier (unconscious) brain activity. So, although we may feel, at times, as if conscious awareness is responsible for our 'changing our minds', it is actually likely to be only as causally effective as the intention to act (above; Spence, 1996). In other words, the veto itself is likely to be the late phenomenological correlate of earlier neural activity (arising some hundreds of milliseconds beforehand). It is not likely to be *causally* effective at all.

Furthermore, this is not the end of the matter. For, if the same principle applies to *all* conscious awareness, if my thoughts are *always* the late phenomenological consequence of foregoing neural activity (and this is already inherent in the assumptions of materialism), then this set of circumstances will also apply to those deliberations that I undertake when I have a problem to resolve, when I have 'time to think'. Each of the putative solutions 'entering' my (conscious) mind will itself constitute a consequence (a result) of earlier brain activity. Hence, even when I am 'thinking' through a problem, at length, the solution 'exists' *before* I am aware of thinking it. For, in order for my conscious mind to recognize the solution, surfacing within it, there must have (already) passed a period of neuronal adequacy. So, now it seems that the Libet experiments *have* changed the ground for freedom after all, not only with respect to our arbitrary, spontaneous, and 'freely' chosen acts but also for all the acts that we might think about or 'premeditate' within our 'minds'.

Hence, the problem remains for those who wish to defend freedom: who is it or what is it that is 'free'? It seems as if freedom is exerted outside of, or *prior to*, our conscious awareness. Freedom, if it exists, may be *unconscious* (Spence, 1996). And what kind of freedom is that?

In search of the 'it'

Faced with these conclusions (i.e. the emergence of intentions into our minds, which we now believe to be the consequences of earlier, unconscious processes), there are two scientific questions that we might address:

1) If we imagine ourselves walking 'backwards' in time, from the point at which an 'intention' coheres within our conscious awareness, then we might wish to discover what it is that initiates an action that to us, the subject, seems so 'purposeful'. In other words, we might be interested in examining the biology of volition (voluntary behaviour). This will form the topic of our first two chapters.

2) Alternatively, if we turn to face in the opposite direction, and allow ourselves to walk 'forward' in time, then we might choose to chase that

experience of 'intending', that sense of 'owning our actions' (i.e. our 'agency'), in order to see what it is that constitutes this illusory state. I use the word 'illusory' because although an intention *feels* decisive and veridical, it seems actually to imply a causality which consciousness itself does not contribute. What we experience ourselves as 'intending' has (in some sense) already been 'intended' (albeit unconsciously). We shall address this problem in the third chapter of this book.

Whatever we do 'choose' to do, it is interesting to ponder what it is that we think lies 'beneath' or 'behind' our choices, especially if the latter are *not* the products of our conscious minds. Is there 'something' there that initiates behaviour? Does 'it' have a purpose? If so, it can seem rather mysterious. One is reminded of a passage from Bernhard Schlink's *The Reader* (first published in 1997):

> Often enough in my life I have done things I had not decided to do. Something—whoever that may be—goes into action; 'it' goes to the woman I don't want to see anymore; 'it' makes the remark to the boss that costs me my head; 'it' keeps on smoking although I have decided to quit, and then quits smoking just when I've accepted the fact that I'm a smoker and always will be. I don't mean to say that thinking and reaching decisions have no influence on behaviour. But behaviour does not merely enact whatever has already been thought through and decided. It has its own sources … (p. 18)

Is this 'it' the same 'it' that initiates those behaviours that we experience (albeit belatedly) as being under 'our' control? Is this an 'it' that we should anticipate encountering as we walk 'backwards' in time from the moment of our conscious intentions? If it is, then this is an 'it' that we might all try to identify, and understand, within ourselves. Is 'it' the author of 'our' actions?

Chapter 1

Moving a finger

From the short-term point of view, human structure makes human behaviour possible.[3]

Wood Jones (1941) wrote: 'We shall look in vain if we seek for movements that man can do and a monkey cannot, but we shall find much if we seek for purposive actions that man can do and a monkey cannot.' The heart of the matter lies in the term 'purposive actions', for it is in the elaboration of the central nervous system and not in the specialisation of the hand that we find the basis of human skill.[4]

This chapter is concerned with understanding some of the structures and processes that support human beings' freedom of movement, their volition, their voluntary behaviour. However, such are the controversies surrounding the nature and possibility of such 'freedom' that half of the words comprising my first sentence may have already invited closer, critical scrutiny. What do I mean by 'structures' and 'processes', and what is the nature of their 'support'? Furthermore, what do I now mean by the word 'freedom'? Haven't we just disposed of freedom, in the Prologue? I shall respond by proposing that in order to *fully* understand our condition, a condition which we shall tease apart over the ensuing chapters of this book, we need to start with some very basic anatomy (structures) and then consider local physiology (processes). If we can describe these adequately, then we shall have delineated the basis of what it is that is necessary (though not necessarily sufficient) for a human being to be 'able' to produce a voluntary act: a movement in the world that did not exist

---

[3] Anthropologist Sherwood Washburn, cited by: Wilson FR. *The Hand: How its use shapes the brain, language, and human culture.* New York: Pantheon Books, 1998: p. 16.

[4] From J.R. Napier. The prehensile movements of the human hand. *Journal of Bone and Joint Surgery* 1956; 38B: 902–913.

prior to that human subject's 'choosing' to perform it. Hence, I propose that structures and processes support such an action; they facilitate its emergence.

However, when it comes to 'freedom', I hope that the reader may bear with me for several chapters. For, only when we have dealt with what it is that is 'necessary' for 'actions' to be permissible shall we be in a position to consider whether freedom is at all defensible. Thankfully, that challenge is still some way off!

A simple question

Thus, to begin with, let us consider a deceptively simple question: *How do I make my finger move*? Indeed, for the sake of argument, let us imagine that I wish to understand the basic 'wiring' and 'signalling' that specifically allow my *right index finger* to move, just as it might have moved had I been a volunteer in one of Benjamin Libet's experiments (described in our Prologue; see Fig. 4).

So, here I am: I sit in a comfortable chair, I am relaxed and not distracted, the room is quiet and warm, and all I need to do is to move this single finger, my right index finger, 'spontaneously', at 'freely chosen' intervals. What is it that allows me to do this? What does my body have to have inside it for 'me' to be 'free' to do such a thing? What is necessary for such a 'purpose' to be achieved?

Well, to explain this situation adequately, I need to take the reader from the 'motor' regions in the grey matter of the human brain down into, and through, the white matter of the brain and spinal cord, through the grey matter of the latter and on into the nerves that communicate with the muscles that make each finger move. I shall try to clarify what it is that is known and useful to us at each stage along this journey (while recognizing that I am only describing the most salient features; I cannot compete with, nor shall I merely recapitulate, the vast resources of *Gray's Anatomy*, though these volumes shall be foremost among my guides [Standring, 2005; Williams and Warwick, 1980]). Where possible, I shall present data that are reported in more than one source (much of our anatomical data may now be regarded as 'canonical', but please consult the References section at the end of the book). If there is debate or disagreement about certain features, then I shall state the range of opposing views and values. Finally, when we have arrived at the innervation of the musculature of the right index finger, I shall retrace my steps and provide an account of the 'higher' centres of the human brain (in Chapter 2, where we shall focus on the premotor and prefrontal cortices in particular), those that are implicated in choosing the 'moment' of such a finger movement.

The actor's brain

The human brain weighs approximately 1400 g in adult men (within a range of 1100–1700 g) and slightly less in adult women (women having, on average, smaller bodies than men). This amounts to roughly 2% of the total adult body weight. Such an adult brain contains approximately 10 billion (10^{10}) neurons communicating with each other via junctions called 'synapses', of which there may be approximately 10^{12} (Mountcastle, 1997). Whereas the passage of signals within neurons relies on electrical conductance (the propagation of 'action potentials' along their length), communication at synapses is largely neurochemical, reliant upon neurotransmitters being released into the spaces between cells (neurons). Neurotransmitters can bind at synaptic 'receptors' and thereby evoke effects on their target neurons.

The brain is housed within a protective shell of bone, the skull, and receives its nutrition via the major blood vessels of the neck, arising ultimately from the heart, within the chest (or 'thorax'). Glucose (in the blood) and oxygen (carried by the red blood corpuscles, the 'erythrocytes') are vital for the brain's survival. The latter receives approximately 15% of the cardiac output (the volume of circulation emerging from the heart) and accounts for approximately 20–25% of the body's oxygen consumption. It extracts glucose at a rate of 5.5 mg/100 g of brain tissue/min, thereby averaging a total consumption of approximately 77 mg/min (Ganong, 1979). Hence, in purely metabolic terms, the brain is an expensive organ to 'support'.

What would we do without glucose? Well, the impact of a sudden fall in glucose supply on brain function is readily apparent when a person suffering from diabetes mellitus experiences a 'hypo'. This usually occurs as a consequence of an imbalance between food intake (too little) and medically prescribed insulin (too much); the latter drives down the serum glucose concentration, with obvious results. Hypoglycaemia rapidly, and radically, impacts speech, coordination, consciousness, and ultimately life itself. Without glucose, we would die; without oxygen, the results are similar. We have a very narrow temporal window, literally a few minutes, during which we might recover from an interruption of our brain's oxygen supply (as might occur following a cardiac arrest, when the heart stops), but irreversible loss of neural function may occur even then (i.e. we may 'live', but with substantial neurological impairment). At high altitudes, falling oxygen pressure may similarly disrupt cognitive function: disorientation and confusion may arise among mountain climbers who eschew the use of oxygen cylinders and other modern technical equipment, and also among aircraft personnel following in-flight power failures.

If we could remove the roof of the skull and examine the brain's surface anatomy, what should we find? Well, at first, we would see an apparently symmetrical organ (though this is somewhat misleading), comprising, most prominently, two mounds of tissue: the left and right cerebral hemispheres, collectively termed the cerebrum (Fig. 6a and 6b; see Table 1 for some commonly used descriptive anatomical terms). If we were to be standing in front of our subject, then his or her left hemisphere would be to our right, and his or her right hemisphere to our left (Fig. 6a). If we approached our subject face-to-face, then above his or her eyes we should see the frontal lobes (Fig. 6b). These comprise approximately 31–37% of the total cerebral hemispheric volume (Semendeferi et al., 1997). Furthermore, if we could part the two cerebral hemispheres, and look down between them, then we should find that they are connected via a thick bundle of white matter fibres—the corpus callosum. This is a major conduit for information transfer between the two sides of the brain (Fig. 7).

The surface of each cerebral hemisphere exhibits a mass of waxy-looking convolutions, ridges (gyri) and the clefts (sulci) between them, sheathed in protective, connective tissue (the *pia mater*) and laced with fine blood vessels. The brain tissue that we can see, the outer surface, is the cerebral cortex, a thin but widely distributed layer of 'grey matter', approximately 1.5–4.5 mm in thickness, which follows the prominent folds of the cerebrum, being somewhat thicker over the gyri and thinner within the sulci. If the whole of this cortical mantle were to be laid out flat, rather than folded and enveloped within the skull, then it would extend over some 2200–2600 cm^2.

As a rule of thumb, nervous system grey matter contains the cell bodies of neurons and white matter contains their 'wiring'—the 'axons', through which they send their signals to other nerve cells at a distance (i.e. the conduits via which they convey information *away* from their own cell bodies). Neurons also possess 'dendrites', processes via which they receive messages from other nerve cells (i.e. essentially, the dendrites convey those signals that are 'incoming'). So, whereas the grey matter of the cortex is a ribbon of nerve cells, the white matter below it comprises a vast array of communication networks, all insulated within fatty, myelin sheaths (indeed, it is these sheaths that make the 'white matter' white).

Cortical laminae

The cerebral cortex contains the outermost components of the central nervous system and situates them within six distinct layers, or laminae, of varying structure, the precise appearances of which vary according to the region of

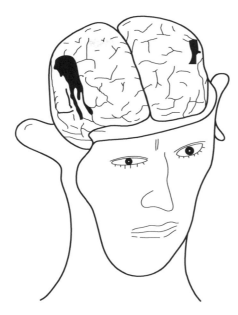

Fig. 6a Cartoon demonstrating the appearance of the frontal lobes when the skull of the subject is opened. The orbitofrontal cortices lie above the subject's eyes. The prominent black shadows on either side of the cortex illustrate the region where the insulae would become visible were the frontal and temporal lobes to be partially excised.

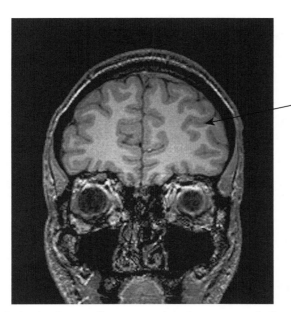

Fig. 6b A structural magnetic resonance imaging scan seen in the coronal plane. The arrow indicates the left frontal lobe, as the subject is looking towards the viewer.

Table 1 Anatomical terms

Terms	Meaning
Anterior/ Posterior	In front of (anterior to) or behind (posterior to) a given reference point. The body is usually assumed to be standing erect, facing forwards, with the arms outstretched, and the palms of the hands also facing to the front. Hence, the frontal lobes are anterior, and the parietal lobes posterior, to the central sulcus. The reference plane is often a vertical, 'coronal', plane passing through the subject's body from left to right.
Medial/ Lateral	Towards (medial) or away from (lateral to) the midline of the body (assumed to be a vertical, 'sagittal', plane bisecting the body into right and left halves). Again, the body is usually assumed to be erect. In the spinal cord, the grey matter is medial to the lateral corticospinal tract. In the homunculus of the cortical motor strip, the 'foot area' is medial to the 'face area' (hence, the latter is lateral to the former).
Superior/ Inferior	Above and below a reference plane, which is usually a transverse ('axial') plane, perpendicular to the coronal and sagittal planes, and parallel to the ground. The brain is superior to the spinal cord.
Dorsal/ Ventral	The back or 'above' (dorsal) compared with the front or 'below' (ventral). Useful when describing quadruped animals or bipedal apes that use their arms to support themselves. Their backs are 'dorsal', their fronts 'ventral'. In the brain, the upper, outer surfaces (e.g. of the prefrontal cortex [PFC]) are dorsal and the lower, inner surfaces (e.g. of the orbitofrontal cortex, over the eyes) are ventral.
Rostral/ Caudal	Within the brain, those regions that are furthermost forwards, towards the frontal pole (at the very front of the frontal lobes), are 'rostral' to those areas closer to the spinal cord (and the latter are 'caudal' to the former).
Proximal/ Distal	In terms of body parts being closer (proximal) to or further away from (distal to) the trunk, the elbow is proximal to the hand but distal to the shoulder.
Ipsilateral/ Contralateral	The right hand is on the same side of the body as the right cerebral hemisphere (i.e. they are 'ipsilateral' to each other) but is normally 'controlled' by the left hemisphere (to which it is 'contralateral').
Afferent/ Efferent	Incoming pathways are 'afferent' whereas departing (effector) pathways are 'efferent'. In many (but not all) contexts, the afferent conveys sensory information whereas the efferent carries motor information, for example, in the dorsal (afferent) and ventral (efferent) nerve roots of the spinal cord.
Agonist/ Antagonist	In anatomy, the agonist muscle is the one contracting to perform a given movement while its antagonist relaxes (e.g. in the case of the biceps and triceps during upper limb movement). Other meanings apply in pharmacology (and these are dealt with in Chapter 4).
Adduction/ Abduction	Referring to movements towards (adduction) and away from (abduction) the midline. A man throwing a spear first abducts his arm (as he draws the spear back) and then adducts it (as the spear is brought across the body in order to be propelled at a distance). When we cross our arms, we are 'adducting' at the elbows.

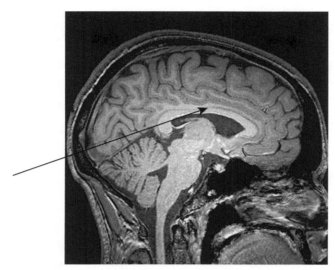

Fig. 7 Structural magnetic resonance imaging scan of a healthy subject, seen in the sagittal plane, with the arrow indicating the position of the corpus callosum.

cortex being examined. It is worth spending some time on what there is to be found here.

The cortical laminae are conventionally numbered I to VI, from the outermost to the innermost, and their constituents vary:

I   The outermost lamina has been called the *plexiform* or *molecular layer* and, when stained (with specific pigments) and viewed in cross-section, appears to comprise a narrow band of fibres, most of which run horizontally. It is a place where nerve projections meet. It receives 'afferent' (incoming) fibres from outside (beneath) the cortex; it contains 'apical dendrites', the receptive extensions of cortical neurons (their cell bodies being located lower down, within the deeper laminae); and it also contains intrinsic fibres from cortical 'interneurons' (these are nerves, the extensions of which are confined to the cortical laminae themselves—i.e. they do not send messages beyond the cortex; they tend to serve 'inhibitory' functions within it).

II The *outer (or external) granular layer* is named so because of its appearance, attributable to the many smaller neuronal cell bodies situated at this level of the cortex. Some of these are described as 'stellate' and they may predominate in certain cortical areas (recall that the laminae vary in their appearance, according to where they are, throughout the cortex). Stellate cells are interneurons and they can inhibit other interneurons (which are themselves inhibitory). There may also be some 'pyramidal' neurons

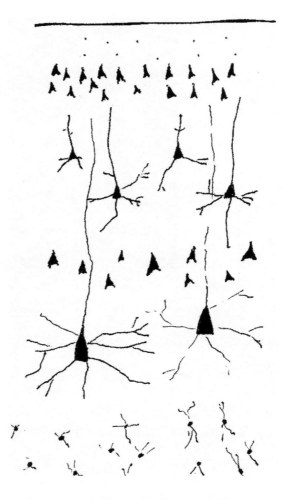

Fig. 8 Diagrammatic representation of the cytoarchitectural structure of the human cerebral cortex grey matter. Lamina I is the most superficial level and Lamina VI is the deepest level of grey matter. The prominent large cells seen in Lamina V (the inner pyramidal cell layer) are Betz cells, which are characteristic to the human motor cortex (Brodmann area 4). Similar, though smaller, cells are seen in the outer pyramidal cell layer (Lamina III).

present (called so because of their shape), projecting beyond the cortex (down into and through the white matter). At level II, nerve fibres are mostly seen to run vertically throughout the lamina.

III The *outer (or external) pyramidal layer* contains many large pyramidal neurons. As elsewhere, these project beyond the cortex. Fibres are vertically oriented, and the prevalent pyramidal cells tend to be smaller towards the top of this level and larger lower down.

IV The *inner granular layer* also contains stellate cells. The interneurons at this level receive projections from the underlying thalamus (the major information-relay station in the brain; it also comprises grey matter but is set deep down within the cerebral white matter; see Fig. 11). Inhibitory interneurons project to layers II and III (above). Lamina IV contains many neuronal projections.

V   The *inner pyramidal layer* contains large pyramidal cells, the axons from which project subcortically, through and beneath the white matter. It is lamina V that is particularly important when we come to consider the motor cortex of the human brain, for at this level in the motor cortex such cells have extremely large bodies (up to 80 μm in diameter), attracting the name 'Betz cells'. These neurons contain the 'excitatory' neurotransmitter chemicals glutamate and aspartate; because their nerve fibres reach down to communicate with the neurons of the spinal cord, and also the brain stem (or 'bulb', containing the nuclei of cranial nerves), these emerging pathways are called the 'corticospinal' and 'corticobulbar' (or alternatively, 'corticonuclear') tracts, respectively. The corticospinal tracts are pivotal to the control of the body's movement, and the corticobulbar (corticonuclear) tracts are central to those movements executed via the cranial nerves (their nuclei located in the brainstem, their axons communicating with the muscles that act on the eyes, jaws, face, tongue, larynx, and diaphragm; see Table 2). When stained with appropriate pigments, level V is seen to contain many vertically orientated, ascending and descending, fibres (though it also contains a band of horizontal fibres called the 'inner band of Baillarger').

VI The innermost cortical layer lies at the boundary with the underlying white matter. It has been called the *polymorphic layer* because its cells are of many different shapes. It too receives input from neurons in the underlying thalamus, and it also receives 'collaterals', branches arising from the axonal projections of neurons located higher up in the cortex (in laminae II, III, and V). It is not always possible to define a clear boundary between this lamina and the underlying white matter; they may 'blend' into one another.

Locating the motor cortex

Now, if we return to the surface of our subject's brain, then we find that it may be described in terms of relatively large, discrete regions, demarcated by the larger sulci—the clefts between the 'lobes' of the brain. For example, the Rolandic fissures, also known as the 'central sulci', run across the top of brain, from right to left (in the 'coronal' plane, akin to a backwardly displaced 'crown'; Fig. 9); they separate the frontal lobes (anteriorly) from the parietal lobes (posteriorly; Table 1). The latter elements are of course bilateral structures: we have left and right frontal lobes (anterior to the sulci), and left and right parietal lobes (posterior to them).

Table 2 Identity and contribution of the cranial nerves in the modern human

Cranial nerve	Functional contribution
1. Olfactory nerve	Olfactory receptors are located in the nasal mucosae and their axons ascend through the cribriform plate to reach the olfactory bulbs, located on the undersurface of the frontal lobes (one on either side). From each bulb, an olfactory tract passes posteriorly along the inferior surface of the frontal lobe before dividing into medial and lateral striae. The latter terminates in the uncus (of the temporal lobe), the former in the paraolfactory area of the frontal lobe itself. Hence, the sense of smell, olfaction, may be disturbed by trauma to the frontal regions and lesions of the temporal lobe. Unusual smells may form part of the 'aura' or warning symptoms associated with the onset of a temporal lobe epileptic seizure. 'Anosmia' denotes a lack of smell sensation.
2. Optic nerve	The photoreceptors of the eye (located in the retina) project to the brain via the optic nerve. Information from the lateral (temporal) half of each retina is conveyed via the lateral fibres of the optic nerve, and information from the medial (nasal) half of the retina passes through its medial fibres. The optic nerve itself passes along the optic canal (at the back of the eye) before joining its counterpart (from the contralateral eye) and forming the optic chiasm (an X-shaped structure, lying between the internal carotid arteries and just anterior to and above the pituitary gland; this becomes salient when a pituitary tumour arises, because the latter may compress the chiasm, from below and behind, leading to 'tunnel vision', a consequence of its exerting pressure on medial optic tract fibres [carrying information from the medial retinal regions] and hence affecting the lateral visual fields). Next, the fibres continue posteriorly on either side as the optic tracts. Each contains information arising from the temporal half of its ipsilateral retina and 'crossed' fibres originating in the nasal half of the contralateral retina. Hence, each tract carries data concerning the *opposite* half of the visual space (i.e. the contralateral visual hemi-field). These tracts communicate with the lateral geniculate bodies, from where they form the optic radiations that project to the 'higher' visual centres (located in occipital cortices). There are projections to the midbrain (to the superior colliculi, involved in the pupillary reflexive responses to light: the pupils dilate in the dark and constrict in the light) and projections to the hypothalamus, which are implicated in maintaining circadian rhythms (i.e. the timing of 'the body clock').
3. Oculomotor nerve	This nerve originates in the midbrain, at the same level as the superior colliculi, and innervates all the muscles of the eye *except* the lateral rectus and superior oblique (which are innervated by the abducens and trochlear nerves, respectively). Hence, if the oculomotor nerve were to be lesioned, the ipsilateral eye would rotate inferolaterally (i.e. 'down and out').

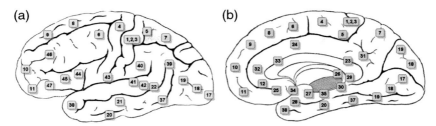

Fig. 9 Diagrammatic representation of the lateral (a) and medial (b) surfaces of the human cerebral cortex, showing the approximate positions of Brodmann areas (BAs). Notice that BAs 4 (motor cortex) and 6 (premotor cortex) are represented on both surfaces of the cortex. On its medial surface, BA 6 constitutes the supplementary motor area (SMA) (Reproduction of lithograph plate from 20th U.S. edition of Gray's Anatomy of the Human Body, originally published in 1918). From Wikimedia. See p. 27.

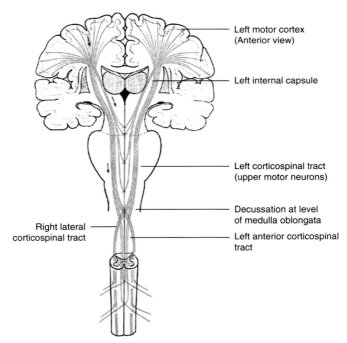

Fig. 12 Diagrammatic representation of the path of the corticospinal tracts from the human motor cortex to the spinal cord, in the longitudinal axis. Upper motor neurons in the left motor cortex pass via the left internal capsule and eventually reach the medulla oblongata where they decussate. Most of their fibres pass over the midline and thereafter constitute the right lateral corticospinal tract. A smaller number of fibres carry on as the left anterior corticospinal tract before crossing the midline closer to their termination in the ventral horn of the spinal cord (on the right side). From Wikimedia. See p. 34.

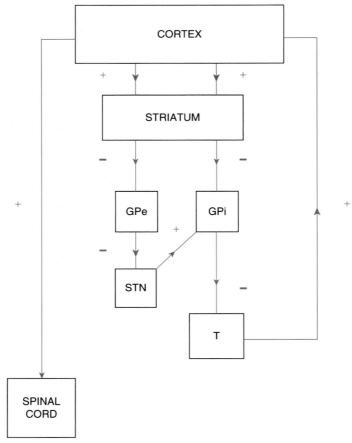

Fig. 11 Schematic showing the components of the human motor system distributed across the cortex, striatum, basal ganglia, thalamus, and spinal cord. The red (+) projections represent excitatory neurotransmitter activity whereas the green (–) represent inhibitory neurotransmitter activity. The human motor cortex projects directly to the spinal cord and also to the striatum. From the striatum, there are inhibitory relays to the globus pallidum externa (GPe) and interna (GPi). The former constitutes the first limb of the indirect pathway and the latter the first limb of the direct pathway. In the indirect pathway, there is a further inhibitory relay to the subthalamic nucleus (STN) followed by an excitatory projection to the GPi. Both pathways are then completed by a further inhibitory relay between the GPi and thalamus (T). A further excitatory projection leaves the motor thalamus for the cortex. See p. 31.

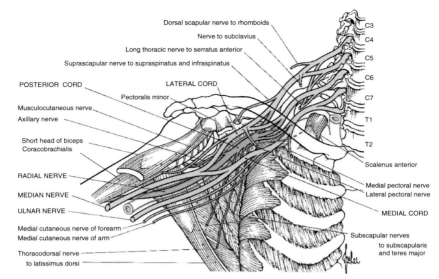

Fig. 18 Diagram showing the structures comprising the right brachial plexus. The radial and median nerves are particularly implicated in the extension and flexion of the right index finger. (Diagram reprinted with permission from Medical Research Council's 'Aids to the examination of the peripheral nervous system' Memorandum No. 45). From HMSO. See p. 48.

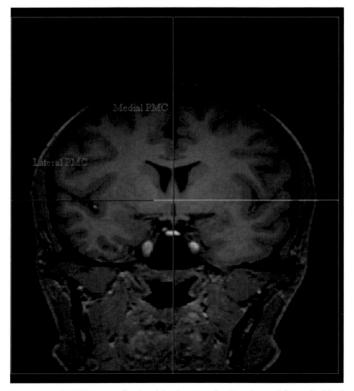

Fig. 23 A structural MRI scan of a healthy human brain, viewed from behind in the coronal plane, showing the medial and lateral premotor cortices of the left hemisphere. See p. 70.

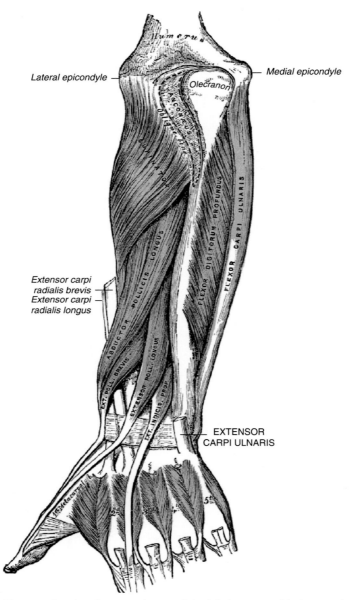

Fig. 20 Diagram showing the musculature of the left forearm, with the extensor indicis projecting to the left index finger. Extensor indicis supports the extension of the index finger. See p. 51.

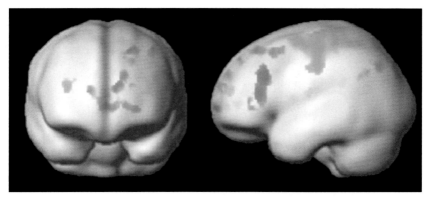

Fig. 24b Statistical parametric maps represented on a smooth brain template. The areas in red show activity during the second when normal healthy males moved their right index finger 'spontaneously'. The areas in blue demonstrate areas that have previously been activated and are relatively 'deactivated' at the moment of spontaneous action. There is prominent deactivation in the left dorsolateral prefrontal cortex (seen in the lateral view on the right). These data reprinted from *Neuroimage, 23: Hunter* et al. *Spatial and temporal dissociation in prefrontal cortex during action execution.*© *2004,* with permission from Elsevier Ltd. See p. 72.

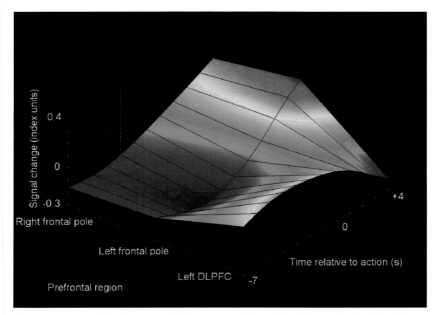

Fig. 24c Cartoon showing a graphic representation of the changes in focal activity in prefrontal regions immediately prior to a spontaneous act (in healthy human males). Seven seconds before the act (at minus seven) there is increasing activity within the left dorsolateral prefrontal cortex (DLPFC). This reaches a peak and then declines over the course of the action. In contrast, focal activity is decreased at the frontal poles prior to the action but gradually increases towards the point of activity itself. These data reprinted from *Neuroimage, 23: Hunter et al. Spatial and temporal dissociation in prefrontal cortex during action execution.*© *2004,* with permission from Elsevier Ltd. See p. 73.

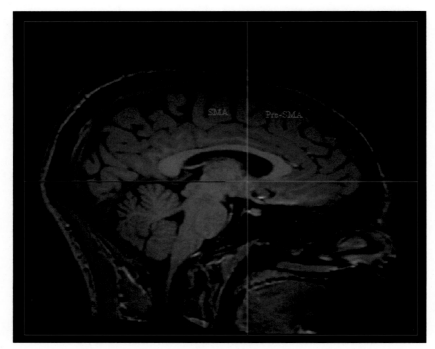

Fig. 26 Structural MRI scan of a healthy human brain showing the approximate position of the supplementary motor area on the medial surface of the frontal lobe (viewed in the sagittal plane). The ascending (green) line shows the plane passing through the anterior commissure. The SMA 'proper' lies behind this line while the so-called pre-SMA lies anterior to it. The pre-SMA exhibits executive properties while the SMA proper is a motor output region, connected to the primary motor cortices. See p. 78.

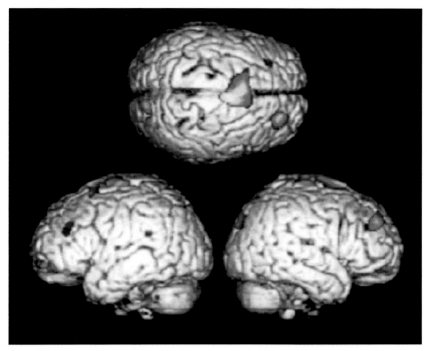

Fig. 30 Data showing those areas of the brain where there is greater activity during 'inner prayer'. Most prominent is the bilateral activation of the supplementary motor area (Brodmann area 6). Taken from *Azari* et al, *'Short Communication. Neural Correlates of religious experience', European Journal of Neuroscience* with permission of Blackwell Publishing. See p. 91.

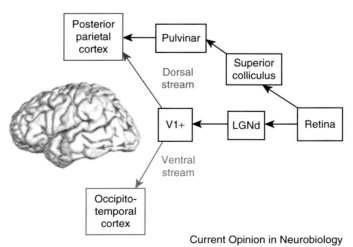

Fig. 32 Cartoon showing the organization of the dorsal 'where is it' and ventral 'what is it' pathways of the visual system. The 'where is it' pathway utilizes structures within the parietal cortex to localize a perceived object. The 'what is it' pathway utilizes structures in the temporal lobe to identify the object seen. *Reprinted from Current Opinion in Neurobiology, 14;(2), Goodale & Westwood, An evolving view of duplex vision: separate but interacting cortical pathways for perception and action. 203–211,* © *2004, with permission from Elsevier Ltd.* See p. 94.

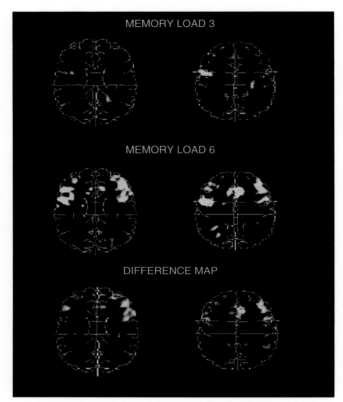

Fig. 33 Data taken from a study by Rypma & colleagues showing that activation within dorsolateral prefrontal cortex increases as working memory load is increased. When subjects are required to recall 6 as opposed to 3 items of information (in working memory) there is greater activity in bilateral dorsolateral prefrontal cortex and also the anterior cingulate cortex (close to the midline). *Reprinted from NeuroImage, 9 (2), Rypma et al. Load-dependent rules of frontal brain regions in the maintenance of working memory, 216–226.* © *1999* with permission from Elsevier Ltd. See p. 96.

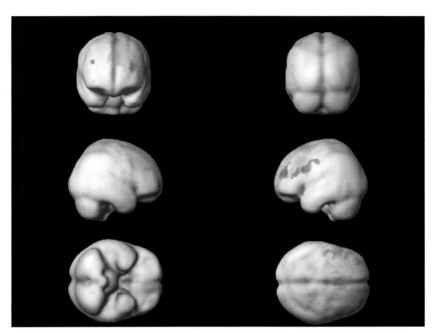

Fig. 34 Data taken from a paper by Spence & colleagues (in press) showing those areas of the brain activated during multiple verbal fluency paradigms. These data were obtained using functional magnetic resonance imaging. Most prominent among the activations are those seen in the left dorsolateral prefrontal cortex, the supplementary motor area and anterior cingulate cortex of the medial prefrontal region and also some activity within the left inferior frontal region. See p. 98.

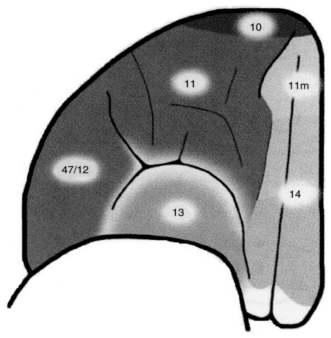

Fig. 38 Cartoon showing the approximate distribution of Brodmann areas on the inferior surface of the right orbitofrontal cortex in humans. Brodmann area 10 is located anteriorally at the frontal pole. Brodmann area 47 is located laterally on the inferior surface of the frontal lobe. Taken from Petrides and Makey (2006; see refs) with permission from Oxford University Press. See p. 113.

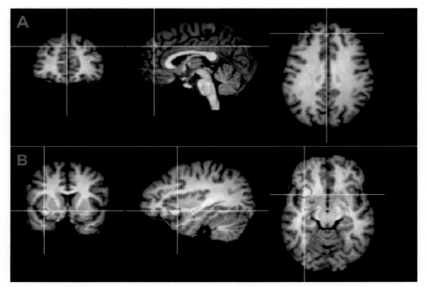

Fig. 47 Data showing those areas of the brain exhibiting greater activity when subjects cancelled their intentions to act. 'A' shows brain slices through dorsomedial frontal cortex; 'B' shows slices through anterior insula. (From Brass and Haggard, *Journal of Neuroscience* 2007; 27: 9141–9145). See p. 148.

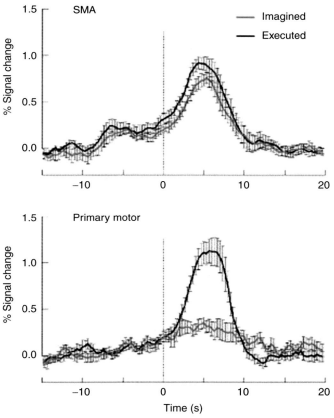

Fig. 42 Graphs showing a blood oxygen level-dependant response in the primary motor cortex and supplementary motor areas (SMAs) during motor activity in healthy humans, acquired using functional magnetic resonance imaging. Note that activity increases in the primary motor cortex during executed movements but not during imagined movements. In contrast, activity in the SMA increases during executed and also imagined movements. Hence, the SMA appears to be involved in the planning of movements whereas the involvement of the primary motor cortex is restricted to the final execution of an explicit movement. (From Cunnington et al., *Human Movement Science* 2005; 24: 644–656 with permission from Elsevier Ltd.) See p. 131.

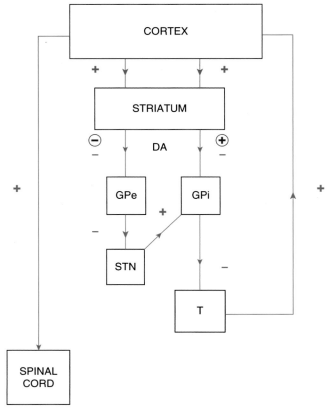

Fig. 50 Cartoon demonstrating the organization of basal ganglia-thalamo-cortical loops in relation to the motor system and also the influence of the neurotransmitter dopamine. Within each loop there is a direct and indirect pathway. The direct pathway facilitates cortical activation via excitatory projections between the thalamus and cortex. Dopamine (DA) facilitates the functioning of the direct pathway (as indicated by the + in the figure). Meanwhile, the indirect pathway reduces output to the cortex. The indirect pathway is inhibited by dopamine (as indicated by the minus sign shown in the figure). See p. 158.

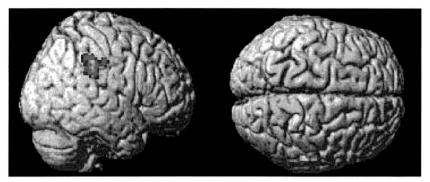

Fig. 73 Images of a magnetic resonance imaging scan showing areas of increased activation in patients with schizophrenia while moving their right index finger 'spontaneously'. The area of activation lies in the right parietal cortex. Activity is greater in those patients who experience the first rank symptoms (FRSs) of schizophrenia (including alien control). (From Ganesan et al., American Journal of Psychiatry 2005; 162(8):1545). See p. 236.

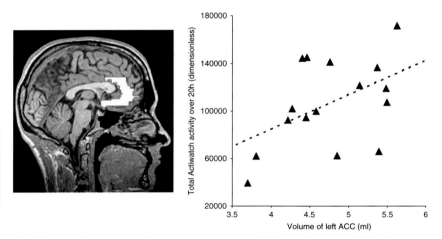

Fig. 76 Data from a magnetic resonance imaging (MRI) study showing that in people with chronic schizophrenia the volume of daytime activity is positively correlated with the volume of their left anterior cingulate cortex (ACC). Reprinted from the *British Journal of Psychiatry*. Structural brain correlates of unconstrained motor activity in people with schizophrenia, Farrow T, F et al, 2005, 187 pp 481–482, with permission from The Royal College of Psychiatrists. See p. 248.

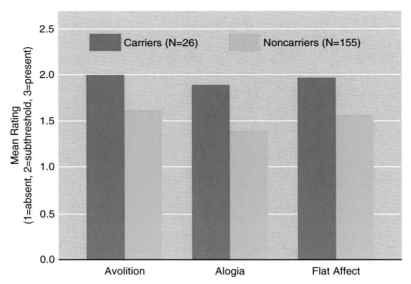

Fig. 77 Graph showing that carriers of the index dyspindin genotype exhibit more severe negative symptoms of schizophrenia than those patients who do not carry the index genotype. (From DeRosse et al., *American Journal of Psychiatry* 2006; 163: 532–534). See p. 252.

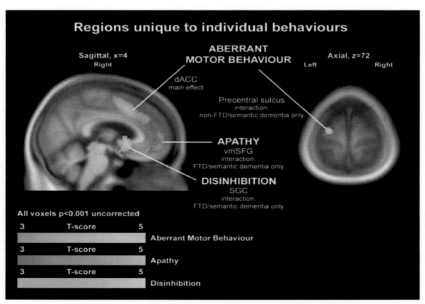

Fig. 79 Image showing the structural brain correlates of abnormal behaviours in people with different forms of dementia. Note that apathy is associated with grey matter deficits within the ventromedial superior frontal gyrus, as indicated in blue. (Rosen et al, *Brain* 2005; 128: 2612–2625) with permission from Oxford University Press. See p. 257.

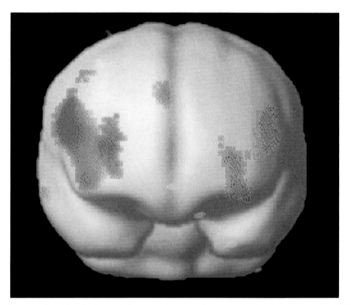

Fig. 87 A smoothed brain template showing positron-emission tomography (PET) data obtained from patients with hysteria, healthy controls feigning motor abnormality, and healthy controls performing motor tasks normally. Patients exhibiting hysterical motor phenomena had reduced prefrontal activation in the left dorsolateral and ventrolateral prefrontal regions (red). In contrast, healthy subjects who are asked to deliberately feign motor impairment had reduced activity in the right prefrontal regions (green). Reprinted from *The Lancet* 355/9211. Discrete neuropsychological correlates in prefrontal cortex during hysterical and feigned disorder of movement. Spence SA et al (2000) with permission from Elsevier Ltd. See p. 277.

Accused's
Version

Accusers'
Version

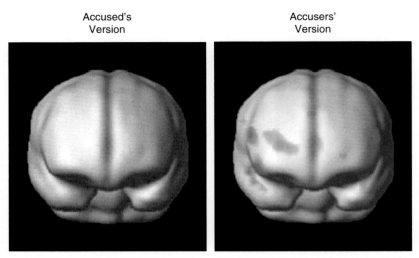

Fig. 93 Data derived from a single subject who was accused and convicted of harming a child. When the subject endorsed her accusers' versions of events (image on right), she exhibited increased activation of prefrontal regions relative to those scans in which she provided her own account of events. Although they do not prove that she is innocent, these data are consistent with her version of events. Reprinted from *European Psychiatry* 23. Munchausen syndrome by proxy or miscarriage of justice: an initial application of functional neuroimaging to the question of guilt versus innocense. Spence SA et al (2008) with permission from Elsevier Ltd. See p. 303.

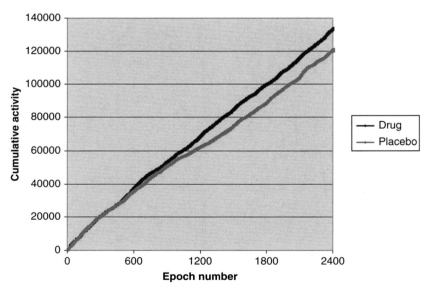

Fig. 99 Graph demonstrating daytime activity in a group of people with chronic schizophrenia. In the course of a randomized double-blind placebo-controlled trial, patients exhibited greater activity on the day that they received the drug modafanil than on the day that they received the placebo. Reprinted from the *British Journal of Psychiatry*; 189: 461–462. Farrow TFD et al, 2006, with permission from The Royal College of Psychiatrists. See p. 369.

Table 2 (continued) Identity and contribution of the cranial nerves in the modern human

Cranial nerve	Functional contribution
	This nerve also innervates the levator palpebrae superioris muscle (therefore, a lesion would also leave a drooping eyelid: 'ptosis'.) Furthermore, the oculomotor nerve carries 'parasympathetic' autonomic innervation to the eye, the substrate for pupillary constriction. Hence, a fixed dilated pupil is another consequence of an oculomotor lesion. The latter is especially associated with aneurysms of the posterior communicating artery or microvascular disease (e.g. consequent upon diabetes mellitus).
4. Trochlear nerve	This nerve originates in the midbrain at the level of the inferior colliculi. It passes through the brainstem to supply the superior oblique muscle of the eye. Hence, a lesion would precipitate double vision (diplopia) on looking downwards (as the affected eye cannot move in that direction while the unaffected eye can; therefore, there are two, discrepant, visual images).
5. Trigeminal nerve	This nerve provides motor innervation to the muscles of mastication (eating) and also sensory supply to the whole of the facial region (including the cornea; hence, it is implicated in the 'blink' reflex that follows on stimulation of the eye's surface). Its motor nucleus is located at the mid-pontine level and receives innervation from the motor cortex. There are three sensory branches conveying information from the face to the brain stem: the *ophthalmic* division supplies the forehead, the *maxillary* division supplies the cheek, and the *mandibular* division supplies the jaw. A lesion of the trigeminal nerve produces jaw weakness (on opening and chewing), facial sensory loss, and loss of the corneal ('blink') reflex.
6. Abducens nerve	Originating in the lower pons, this nerve supplies the lateral rectus muscle of the eye. Hence, a lesion will produce diplopia in the lateral dimension (as the affected eye cannot 'abduct' [laterally] while the unaffected eye 'adducts' [medially]; thus, there emerge two, discrepant, visual images).
7. Facial nerve	Predominantly a motor nerve supplying all the muscles of the facial area except those involved in mastication (which are supplied by the trigeminal nerve). The motor nucleus of the facial nerve is located in the pons. However, the nerve also subserves some specific sensory functions (taste sensation over the anterior two-thirds of the tongue) and provides parasympathetic supply to the lacrimal and salivary glands. The facial nerve is commonly affected in a condition called 'Bell's palsy', characterized by unilateral facial weakness and impaired taste sensation over the anterior tongue. One of the distinctions elicited on classical neurological examination is that between lower motor neuron paralysis of the facial area, such as that occurring in Bell's palsy, and upper motor neuron paralysis consequent upon a 'higher' lesion (e.g. following a stroke that affects the motor cortex or internal capsule).

Table 2 (continued) Identity and contribution of the cranial nerves in the modern human

Cranial nerve	Functional contribution
	Because the upper third of the face is 'represented' across the motor regions of both hemispheres, an upper motor neuron lesion precipitates facial weakness confined to the lower two-thirds of the face (contralaterally), whereas a lower motor neuron lesion affects all ('three-thirds') of the facial muscles (ipsilaterally). Hence, in the case of a unilateral upper motor neuron lesion, the contralateral lower face is paralyzed, but the patient can still 'wrinkle' their forehead (bilaterally).
8. Vestibulocochlear nerve	This nerve conveys auditory information from the cochlea and 'balance'-related data from the semicircular canals and otolith organs of the ear. Hence, a lesion of this nerve, such as an 'acoustic neuroma', causes deafness, tinnitus (ringing in the ear), and loss of balance. Entry to the brain is at the level of the cerebellopontine angle.
9. Glossopharnygeal nerve	This nerve carries motor, sensory, and parasympathetic information and is particularly implicated in supplying taste sensation to the posterior third of the tongue. Its motor fibres originate at the rostral nucleus ambiguus and supply the stylopharnygeus muscle; sensory fibres access the tractus solitarius, and parasympathetic fibres originate in the inferior salivatory nucleus (from where they innervate the parotid salivary gland). A lesion of this nerve would implicate the lower brain stem.
10. Vagus nerve	Again, a nerve with mixed contributions: the motor element is involved in the control of the soft palate, palate, and laryngeal movement; its sensory role involves taste sensation, conveyed from the epiglottis, and tactile sensation from the pinna of the ear. The parasympathetic role is, however, very significant and impacts many structures (e.g. it conveys parasympathetic tone to the heart: vagal nerve stimulation slows the heart rate). Damage to the vagus precipitates a loss of gag reflex, dysphagia (difficulty in swallowing), and dysarthria (difficulty in speaking).
11. Spinal accessory nerve	A motor nerve that originates in the medulla and spinal cord and supplies those muscles involved in turning the head and 'shrugging' the shoulders: the sternocleidomastoid and trapezius muscles.
12. Hypoglossal nerve	This nerve supplies the motor innervation of the tongue. It originates in the hypoglossal nucleus of the posterior medulla. Lesions of the nerve, which are 'lower motor neuron' in character, produce a flaccid, wasted, and weakened tongue. This can be found in motor neuron disease. Dysphagia and dysarthria result. A 'spastic' tongue, rigid and paralyzed, is associated with 'upper motor neuron' lesions (e.g. following strokes in motor areas). The lower motor picture is termed 'bulbar' palsy (reflecting the involvement of the medulla) whereas the upper motor neuron picture is termed 'pseudo-bulbar' palsy.

Source: Adapted from Barker and Barasi (2003) and Mitchell and Mayor (1977).

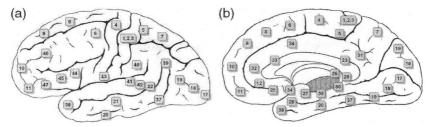

Fig. 9 Diagrammatic representation of the lateral (a) and medial (b) surfaces of the human cerebral cortex, showing the approximate positions of Brodmann areas (BAs). Notice that BAs 4 (motor cortex) and 6 (premotor cortex) are represented on both surfaces of the cortex. On its medial surface, BA 6 constitutes the supplementary motor area (SMA) (Reproduction of lithograph plate from 20th U.S. edition of Gray's Anatomy of the Human Body, originally published in 1918). From Wikimedia. (See colour plate section).

As I am interested in what allows me to make my *right* index finger move, deliberately, I shall be especially concerned with the *left* frontal lobe, for it is the left motor cortex that exerts particular control over my right hand (as the right motor cortex exerts greater control over my left). Indeed, as I am right-handed (in common with the majority, ~90%, of the population), my left hemisphere's motor cortex will also be *larger* than its neighbour, on the right (hence, the human brain is *not* perfectly symmetrical; see Amunts et al., 1996; Volkmann et al., 1998). Furthermore, the left motor strip plays an additional role in modulating (i.e. influencing) the contralateral ('non-dominant', right) motor strip.

Now, the primary motor cortex constitutes the most posterior region of the frontal lobe, on either side of the brain. It occupies the precentral gyrus (i.e. the gyrus lying directly anterior to the central sulcus). In the language of neuroanatomy, the primary motor cortex is also known as 'Brodmann area 4' (BA 4; Fig. 9). Such terminology is derived from the anatomist Korbinian Brodmann's seminal attempts to differentiate the various regions of the cortex on the basis of their microscopic ('cytoarchitectural') anatomy. Thus, cytoarchitecturally, Brodmann area 4, the primary motor cortex, is characterized by its exhibiting a high density of very large pyramidal cells in lamina V (the Betz cells we alluded to earlier) and relatively few granular cells in lamina IV (hence, it is said to be 'agranular'). Furthermore, the pyramidal neurons in lamina V are clustered into groups (of ~300 μm in width) that are themselves distributed at intervals (of ~100 μm) in the horizontal dimension (Mountcastle, 1997). Forty percent of the neurons in each of these clusters project to a *single* ('lower') motor neuron pool in the spinal cord (thereby conveying impulses to relatively discrete distal structures—i.e. the muscles), whereas the remainder project to the motor neuron pools of *groups* of muscles that are active during similar movements. The pyramidal cells in lamina V also send collateral axons upwards (vertically) into a 300–500 μm zone extending through the adjacent laminae. This provides an excitatory drive to adjacent neurons and, via inhibitory interneurons, a 'surround inhibition' of other, neighbouring structures. (This would seem to imply a biological facilitation of distal movement specificity— i.e. fine motor control).

Of special importance in BA 4 is the 'representation' of the movements of the voluntary musculature of the *contralateral* side of the body throughout the motor cortex, in the form of a so-called 'homunculus' (an image of a half-body; see Fig. 10). Moreover, this homunculus' musculature appears rather distorted: it exhibits an exaggerated representation of the face and hand muscles, whereas those of the leg and foot are far less prominent. This 'distortion'

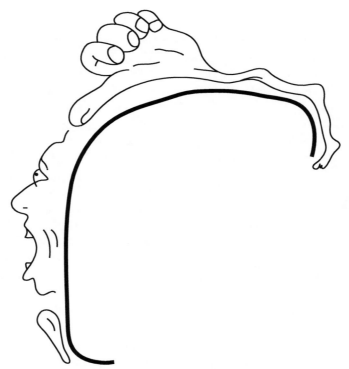

Fig. 10 Cartoon showing the homunculus of the left motor cortex (Brodmann area 4) of the human brain. Notice that the representation of the muscles of the face (on the lateral surface of the cortex) and the hand (over the apex of the cortex) is much larger than that of other body areas (e.g. the lower limb represented over the medial cortex). This difference in representation is indicative of the greater precision required for the muscles of the face and hand to move and function efficiently. The muscles of the tongue are represented further inferiorly to the face area.

is thought to reflect the central importance of face and hand movements to human communication and dexterity, and the variety and subtlety of actions that may be performed using these 'effectors'. Hence, we 'should' expect to find that my right index finger is relatively widely represented in the motor cortex on the left side of my brain, and that its 'field' of representation will be located towards the lateral aspect, the apex or crown, of the homunculus, as it 'arches' out across the cortex and just before it descends along the vertical limit of my left hemisphere (Fig. 10).

When microelectrodes are used to directly stimulate the primary motor cortex, the latter exhibits a relatively low threshold for the production of movements, compared with other cortical regions. This is thought to reflect the relatively high concentration of Betz cells in BA 4 (Passingham, 1993). At approximately 40% of the sites, low-level stimulation results in the contraction of a single muscle (in a corresponding, contralateral body structure). At other sites, and at increasing magnitudes of stimulation, the primary motor cortex elicits contraction of small *groups* of muscles (Mountcastle, 1997). As expected, the movements elicited are manifested on the opposite (contralateral) side of the body and, crucially, do not have to be solely confined to simple muscle twitches; rather, they can resemble coherent, recognizable responses, having an 'aspect of purpose or volition . . . of the same nature as those which the animal makes in its ordinary intelligent action' (Ferrier [1876], as cited in Jeannerod [1997]). Hence, it appears that the motor cortex is not solely concerned with representing muscles per se but with the forms of movement (the combined responses) that groups of muscles may execute, together, during the performance of a coherent act. Indeed, as the evolutionary scale is ascended, so does the discreteness of such movements, elicited through electrical stimulation, increase. In other words, the 'actions' observed (following stimulation) become more refined, better 'sculpted', as we ascend the primate kingdom. This is thought to reflect the 'degree of selectivity of. . . neuronal connections in higher primates' (Jeannerod, 1997; see also the section 'A finger moves, discretely').

Of course, as well as sending signals 'out', the motor cortex also receives 'incoming' signals from a variety of other structures in the brain. These signals reach the motor cortex via 'afferent' projections arising from several key structures:

Thalamic projections

The thalamus sends efferent (outgoing) projections to BA 4 from its 'ventral posterolateral' (VPL) nucleus, which itself receives afferent (incoming) projections from deep cerebellar nuclei (the cerebellum is a structure lying beneath the cerebral hemispheres and comprises paired hemispheric lobes; it is involved in the regulation of movement and cognition.) Furthermore, the VPL nucleus provides us with another example of a brain region that carries a topographic map (a representation) of the contralateral side of the body (akin to the homunculus of the motor cortex and other, comparable fields located within the cerebellum and premotor cortex). Indeed, there is a point-to-point projection from these VPL representations to those of BA 4 (targeted on lamina IV, the inner granular layer).

The motor cortex also receives other thalamic projections from the centro-median and parafascicular nuclei; these relay signals to BA 4 that have originated within the basal ganglia (which are relatively large grey matter nuclei, located close to the thalamus, and are also of immense importance in the genesis of movement; Fig. 11; see also Chapter 4).

Parietal lobe projections

The parietal cortex lies posterior to the central sulcus (Fig. 9). Its first gyrus, the 'postcentral gyrus', contains the primary somatosensory cortex ('S1'), and again, this cortical strip carries a homunculus, comprising a map of the contralateral half of the subject's body. However, in this case, the map comprises a *sensory* representation of that hemi-body (with greater coverage devoted to those areas of the skin and mucous membranes that are more sensitive to touch). Hence, we encounter yet another distorted map of a 'half-body', one possessing exaggerated fingers and lips; again, we move from the lower limb, represented medially through an upper 'half-torso', towards the hemi-face, represented outermost (on the lateral aspect of the hemisphere). The primary motor cortex receives topographically (i.e. spatially) organized projections from its 'ipsilateral' primary somatosensory cortex (i.e. from S1 of the parietal lobe lying on its own side of the brain). Hence, in the language of neuroanatomy, BA 4 receives projections from BAs 1 and 2 (both located within the postcentral gyrus), and these afferents terminate within layers II and III of BA 4 (where they mainly contact pyramidal cell neurons). Neurons from S1 also synapse on (i.e. communicate with) the Betz cells in lamina V of the motor cortex (the origins of the corticomotor neurons pivotally involved in motor control). Hence, through the latter route, sensory information may, potentially, influence motor signalling (thereby modifying movements) during the execution of an explicit motor act.

The motor cortex receives additional inputs from the 'secondary' somatosensory cortex (S2; also within the parietal cortex but lying posterior to S1). Furthermore, there is evidence that some neurons in the motor cortex are not solely 'motor' in their response characteristics: they can respond to peripheral

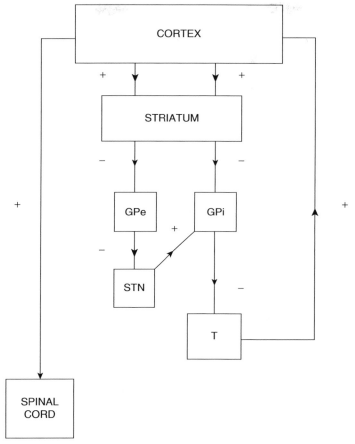

Fig. 11 Schematic showing the components of the human motor system distributed across the cortex, striatum, basal ganglia, thalamus, and spinal cord. The red (+) projections represent excitatory neurotransmitter activity whereas the green (−) represent inhibitory neurotransmitter activity. The human motor cortex projects directly to the spinal cord and also to the striatum. From the striatum, there are inhibitory relays to the globus pallidum externa (GPe) and interna (GPi). The former constitutes the first limb of the indirect pathway and the latter the first limb of the direct pathway. In the indirect pathway, there is a further inhibitory relay to the subthalamic nucleus (STN) followed by an excitatory projection to the GPi. Both pathways are then completed by a further inhibitory relay between the GPi and thalamus (T). A further excitatory projection leaves the motor thalamus for the cortex. (See colour plate section).

nerve stimulation (i.e. incoming sensory information), exhibiting a topographic representation similar to that seen in S1. Hence, relatively superficial, cutaneous, stimulation elicits responses in the more posterior motor cortex, adjacent to the central sulcus, whereas deeper, visceral, stimulation elicits responses in the more anterior motor cortex (BA 4).

Frontal projections

The motor cortex receives projections from several other frontal regions, both ipsilaterally and from the contralateral frontal lobe. Although BA 4 is very much construed as the 'output' region of the motor system, projecting to the brain stem and spinal cord in order to 'effect' movement (of the face and limbs, respectively; Figs. 10 and 11), there are 'higher' centres (supervening within a functional hierarchy) that play pivotal roles in the planning and programming of such movement (see Chapter 2). Thus, the 'premotor' cortices, BA 6, lie on the lateral surfaces of the frontal lobes (Fig. 9), and arch over towards their medial (inner) surfaces (where they attract the description 'supplementary motor areas' [SMAs] though they are still located within BA 6). These regions project backwards, into the primary motor cortex (BA 4). In turn, BA 4 sends its own projections to ipsilateral and contralateral SMAs, and has reciprocal connections with its counterpart in the other hemisphere (i.e. the contralateral BA 4).

The motor cortex also receives projections from the insula, an area of the cortex so enveloped within the convolutions of the frontal and temporal lobes (see Fig. 6a) that it may not be visible upon initial opening of the skull. (However, in the dissected brain displayed in Fig. 6a, the overlying tissue of the frontal and temporal lobes has been removed, dissected away, so that the insulae are visible on both sides of the brain). The insula serves a great many functions, some of which are concerned with subjective awareness of the body, its autonomic responses (e.g. heart or pulse rate), and visceral sensations.

Thus, the motor cortex enjoys connections and (hence, by implication) relationships with many of its cortical neighbours, and these seem (from a 'teleological', functional point of view) to serve to integrate information over discrete areas of the brain concerned with the movement of the body, its position in space, and the monitoring of its organs throughout action performance.

However, the motor cortex also projects to a variety of 'subcortical' structures (those regions lying beneath the cortex), such as the striatum (areas of the basal ganglia pivotal to action; Fig. 11), pontine and subthalamic nuclei (further examples of subcortical islands of grey matter), and in the brain stem, a number of nuclei serving a great many different functions (e.g. the reticular formation, superior colliculi, and the red, vestibular, and inferior olivary nuclei). Indeed, to understand the role of the motor cortex in action, we really need to go *beneath* the cortex, to examine its contribution to the corticospinal tract.

The corticospinal tract

The corticospinal (also known as the 'pyramidal') tract is the conduit via which the pyramidal neurons in the motor cortex (BA 4) exert their influence over the motor centres of the spinal cord, thereby modulating voluntary behaviour. However, despite its alternative title (a reference not to the pyramidal cells of BA 4 but to the pyramidal *shape* of its massed fibres as they traverse the medulla oblongata of the brain stem), it is important to note that this tract receives only about 30% of its fibres from the primary motor cortex. Additional contributions arise from the SMAs, and premotor and parietal cortices. Nevertheless, the corticomotor (or 'upper motor neuron') axons emerging from the motor cortex (i.e. from the cell bodies of lamina V pyramidal neurons located in BA 4) do comprise the tract's largest diameter fibres. Many will eventually terminate within the ventral horn of the spinal cord (see Figs. 12 and 15) and, at those cord levels where the segment concerned mediates dexterous movements of the hands and fingers, most of them will terminate in the *lateral* ventral horn, near the relevant 'lower' motor neurons (i.e. those motor neurons whose cell bodies are located in the grey matter of the spinal cord, from where their axons extend to eventually communicate with the voluntary musculature beyond the spinal column; see Fig. 15). Indeed, it is the *lateral* ventral horn that is particularly involved in the emergence of finely controlled movements, those executed by the 'distal' musculature (i.e. the muscles lying furthest from the trunk, such as those controlling the movements of the fingers).

Hence, when we come to consider how my right index finger moves, we necessarily invoke a transmission of information, all along an extensive neural pathway, stretching from the left motor cortex (BA 4) above, through specific regions of the midbrain and spinal cord below, and on into the lower motor neuron units that communicate with the peripheral musculature.

However, as we have already noted, not all the axons running within the corticospinal tract originate within the motor cortex. Around 40–60% of the corticospinal axons emerge from the parietal cortices, including BAs 3a and 5, and S2. The majority of such parietal corticospinal fibres terminate within the deep layers of the *dorsal* horn of the spinal cord (where they serve sensory functions). Hence, there is an apparent circularity to the flow of information between the parietal (sensory) systems and those more obviously 'motor' systems located within the motor cortex and the spinal cord. At the level of the motor cortex, parietal regions project to their related primary motor cortical targets, so that sensory information reaching one parietal cortex, from the

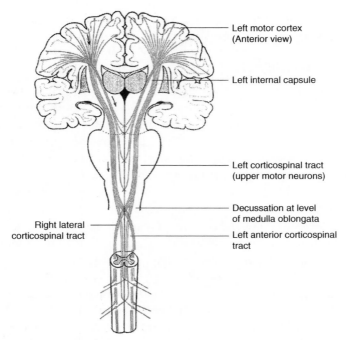

Left motor cortex
(Anterior view)

Left internal capsule

Left corticospinal tract
(upper motor neurons)

Right lateral
corticospinal tract

Decussation at level
of medulla oblongata

Left anterior corticospinal
tract

Fig. 12 Diagrammatic representation of the path of the corticospinal tracts from the human motor cortex to the spinal cord, in the longitudinal axis. Upper motor neurons in the left motor cortex pass via the left internal capsule and eventually reach the medulla oblongata where they decussate. Most of their fibres pass over the midline and thereafter constitute the right lateral corticospinal tract. A smaller number of fibres carry on as the left anterior corticospinal tract before crossing the midline closer to their termination in the ventral horn of the spinal cord (on the right side). From Wikimedia. (See colour plate section).

spinal cord, may subsequently influence the course of actions initiated in its neighbouring, ipsilateral BA 4. However, motor and sensory fibres also lie in close proximity to each other throughout the length of the spinal cord. Hence, there is an open circuit of neuronal influence modifying ongoing action. I say 'open circuit' because the flow of information from the spinal cord to the parietal cortex and from there to the motor cortex does not comprise a 'closed loop'; as we have already seen, there are multiple contributions to motor control, emerging from many levels within the nervous system (e.g. the premotor and subcortical centres). Nevertheless, what is remarkable is the obvious potential provided within the human sensorimotor system for information to reverberate throughout its related networks.

To return to the specifically motor corticospinal neurons (i.e. the 'cortico-motor' axons arising from the pyramidal cells in BA 4), these will exert their influence on the contracting (i.e. 'agonist') muscles involved in a specific voluntary act (they modulate the force of such a movement, though not necessarily its amplitude). Indeed, their activity can be shown to precede that seen in the distal musculature. In electromyographic recordings obtained from contracting muscles, the latter's (agonist) activity is seen to arise approximately 50–100 ms *after* the electrical activity recorded from the related motor neurons. Hence, we may conclude that motor neurons are involved in the generation (initiation) of action rather than the 'simple' monitoring of its progress (in which case their activity 'should' have occurred after, rather than prior to, muscular contraction). Therefore, electrical activity arising in corticomotor neurons, themselves lying in the 'finger' area of my left motor cortex (BA 4), can be predicted to exhibit a causal relationship with (i.e. arise temporally antecedent to) the voluntary movements of my right index finger. It is this neural signal that (ultimately) causes the finger to move. But how does this 'signal' get there? How does it complete its journey? To understand this, we need to consider how the corticospinal tract makes its way as far as the spinal cord—that is, what happens on its journey between the motor cortex and the spinal cord.

When viewed in the coronal plane (Fig. 12), the corticospinal tract rather resembles a river, with its many tributaries emerging among the cortical folds of the primary motor, parietal, and premotor cortices (the latter lying relatively anterior, further forward within the frontal lobes; Fig. 9). These tributaries converge as they descend within the cerebral white matter (comprising a narrowing funnel of fibres called the 'corona radiata'), eventually entering the confined channels of the 'internal capsule', the white matter space lying between the basal ganglia (see Fig. 13). These latter grey matter nuclei include the caudate nucleus (the 'head' of which lies anteriorly), putamen (lying laterally), and thalamus (lying posteromedially). (The caudate nucleus and putamen are collectively termed the 'striatum' because of their striped appearance; see Chapter 4). On each side of the brain, these three structures lie in close proximity to each other so that (when viewed from above, in cross-section) they appear to leave a narrow channel of white matter (the internal capsule) shaped like '>' (left) or '<' (right), through which the corticospinal tracts must flow if they are to reach the spinal cord below (see Fig. 13). Again, there is a pattern to the spatial distribution of fibres lying within this 'capsule':

i) Those fibres lying furthest forward, in the capsule's 'anterior limb', constitute the neighbouring 'frontopontine tract', a pathway connecting the frontal lobes with the pons below (see Fig. 14).

ii) Next is the corticobulbar (corticonuclear) tract, running from the cortex to the brain stem nuclei (below the pons; Table 2).

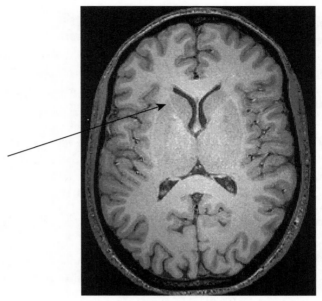

Fig. 13 A structural magnetic resonance imaging scan of a healthy human brain, in the transverse plane. The arrow indicates the position of the anterior limb of the left internal capsule. Medial to the tip of the arrow is the head of the left caudate nucleus, which appears to bulge into the left lateral ventricle. Beneath the tip of the arrow is the left putamen (which is slightly darker than the surrounding structures).

iii) At the middle, the 'genu' (or 'knee') of the capsular '<', the corticospinal tract begins to feature, at first containing those elements involved in the movements of our subject's head.

iv) Moving backwards, between the putamen (laterally) and thalamus (posteromedially), along the anterior two-thirds of the 'posterior limb' of the capsule, the corticospinal tract comprises those axons involved in the movements of our subject's neck, his (contralateral) upper limb, trunk, and lower limb, again arranged in a topographic sequence (i.e. comprising another potential 'map').

v) Throughout the internal capsule, there are also returning sensory fibres, the 'thalamocortical tracts', running in the opposite direction (conveying information from the thalamus to the cortex, 'corticofugally').

Now, the narrowness of the internal capsule is such that it serves to concentrate many critically important structures within a relatively small volume of brain tissue. Hence, a lesion of this region could wreak havoc on our subject's

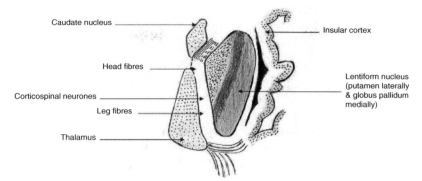

Fig. 14 Diagrammatic representation of the right internal capsule, showing the main components of the basal ganglia. Note that the posterior limb of the capsule has a somatotopic distribution of corticospinal tracts: those involved in head movement are represented at the junction of the anterior and posterior limbs, and the tracts involved in leg movement are located within the posterior limb of the internal capsule.

brain and, via his brain, his voluntary behaviours. Indeed, this is what happens when a 'stroke' (a 'cerebrovascular accident', comprising either a haemorrhage or a thrombosis [a blood clot]) affects the blood vessels in this location. Our subject (sadly, soon to become our 'patient') may suddenly lose the ability to control the movements of the opposite side of his body: he exhibits a contralateral paralysis (a 'unilateral hemiparesis'). One side of his face, arm, and leg (on the same side of his body) may be selectively or continuously affected. The extent of this clinical 'picture' is influenced by the precise location of the lesion: this determines which body parts (and functions) will be most adversely affected (Fig. 14). Hence, this one small area of brain tissue (the internal capsule) conducts vital information between our patient's motor cortex and the opposite side of his body. It is pivotal to his voluntary movement. Therefore, it should also provide a necessary conduit for my own voluntary impulses as and when I wish to move my right index finger, 'spontaneously':

> As I flex this single finger, I know that neural signals have traversed the posterior limb of my left internal capsule.

Now, how do these signals reach the 'other side' of my body? For, remember, it is the left motor cortex that 'controls' my right index finger. What happens to the signals on their way to the spinal cord? How do they make it to the 'other side'? Well, what 'happens' is that, beneath the level of the internal capsule, the corticospinal axons, carrying their motor signals, proceed through the (ventral, anterior) midbrain, and then through the pons, on towards the 'medulla oblongata', where their appearance on the ventral surface of the brain gives rise to their being described as 'pyramids' (prominent columns of white matter, running down along the medulla's ventral surface). (The 'ventral' surface is the 'front' of the medulla; Table 1; Fig. 12) Furthermore, at this level, most corticospinal axons (60–90%; estimates vary) cross to the other side of the brainstem (i.e. they are said to 'decussate'). Those fibres that cross the midline then form a pathway through the spinal cord called the (right) 'lateral corticospinal' tract, whereas those that do not cross go on to form the (left) 'anterior (or ventral) corticospinal' tract. From then on, the former pathway runs down the *lateral* aspect of the *right* side of my spinal cord, where its axons will eventually synapse with the (lower) motor neurons controlling the right side of my body. Those fibres running in the left anterior corticospinal tract will also, mostly, innervate the right side of my body (though they cross the midline 'later', once they have traversed the spinal cord and are close to the level of their target lower motor neurons; Fig. 12). Hence, my *left* motor cortex gives rise to corticomotor neuronal axons, most of which will ultimately flow within my *right* lateral corticospinal tract (a pathway that consists of ~1 million nerve fibres), until they reach the level (or segment) of my spinal cord that contains the lower motor neurons, which will in turn communicate with the voluntary musculature moving my right index finger. In fact, the relevant segment of the spinal cord is located at the junction of my cervical (neck) and thoracic (chest) spine, extending over the levels of the seventh cervical and first thoracic vertebrae (the movements of my shoulders are 'represented' a little higher up, at the level of the fifth and sixth cervical vertebrae).

The spinal cord

If we were to examine the spinal cord in transverse section (at right angles to its longitudinal axis), we would find that the bilateral, descending, lateral corticospinal tracts lie in close proximity to the so-called rubrospinal tracts (carrying descending fibres from the red nucleus of the midbrain; Table 3; Fig. 15). Both of these tracts are involved in the movement of ipsilateral voluntary musculature. However, for their signals to result in movement, the messages from their constituent 'upper motor neurons' (called so because they originate *above* the level of the spinal cord) must be conveyed to 'lower motor neurons', those motor nerves that have their cell bodies located within the ordered segments of the spinal cord. These lower motor neurons are located ventrally, in the 'anterior horn' of the spinal cord (Figs. 15 and 16), and are pivotal to distal limb control (e.g. the fine control of finger movement). We shall return to them shortly.

However, there are other tracts descending within the spinal cord that influence ongoing movements: the so-called 'extrapyramidal tracts' of the

Table 3 Identity and characteristic contributions of the descending tracts located in the human spinal cord

Tract	Contribution
Corticospinal, pyramidal	A tract originating in the primary motor, premotor, and somatosensory cortices. It is important for the execution of independent finger movements.
Rubrospinal	A tract originating in the red nucleus of the midbrain. Similar to the pyramidal tract, it projects to lower motor neurons, specifically those concerned with distal motor control.
Vestibulospinal	A tract originating within the medulla, from the vestibular nuclear complex (of the vestibulocochlear nerve). It mainly innervates extensor and axial muscles involved in the control of posture and balance.
Reticulospinal	A tract originating in the reticular formation of the pons and medulla. It exhibits both excitatory and inhibitory input to spinal cord interneurons and lower motor neurons, and serves to 'damp' down activity in the spinal cord. Dysfunction leads to increased extensor tone. This pathway is crucial for controlling the paralysis that occurs during normal dreaming (rapid eye movement [REM]) sleep (see Chapter 4).
Other descending influences*	
Locus coeruleus and raphe nuclei (noradrenergic and serotonergic innervation, respectively; see Chapter 4)	These systems send diffuse projections to the spinal cord. They are activated during the expression of emotions such as laughing or crying. They are thought to lower the firing threshold in lower motor nuclei, thereby facilitating activation by *other* descending pathways (mentioned earlier).
Lateral tegmental interneurons	These receive projections from 'limbic' regions and exert an influence on rhythmic behaviours: respiration, vomiting, swallowing, chewing, and licking.

*These influences are more diffuse and less circumscribed than those of the tracts described earlier.

Source: Adapted from Barker and Barasi (2003), and Brunia and van Boxtel (2000).

vestibulospinal, and reticulospinal pathways (Table 3). These run *anterior* to the ventral horn of the spinal cord and innervate the more ventromedially located lower motor neurons, those playing a key role in the control of the 'axial' musculature of the trunk. Hence, these motor neurons are more concerned with balance and posture than with the fine movements of the distal limbs.

It is also worth noting that, as was the case with the cerebral cortex, the spinal cord contains a great many interneurons, neurons that are confined to adjacent levels within the cord: that is, they do not enter the spinal cord from above or leave it laterally or below; instead, they communicate within adjoining

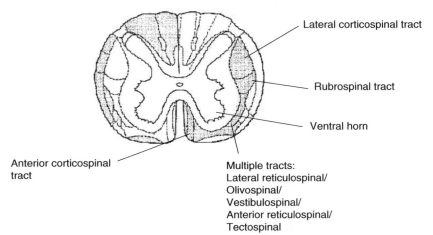

Lateral corticospinal tract

Rubrospinal tract

Ventral horn

Anterior corticospinal
tract

Multiple tracts:
Lateral reticulospinal/
Olivospinal/
Vestibulospinal/
Anterior reticulospinal/
Tectospinal

Fig. 15 Diagrammatic representation of a transverse section of the spinal cord. The important motor pathways within the cord are labelled as shown. From Wikimedia.

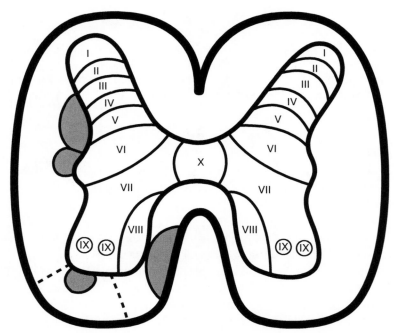

Fig. 16 Diagrammatic representation of a transverse section of the spinal cord indicating the approximate positions of Rexed's laminae within the spinal cord grey matter.

segments of the spinal cord and exert a crucial influence over automatic, rhythmic behaviours, exemplified by the locomotion constituting our gait (the way in which we walk). Such interneurons may form networks with their own intrinsic activity, so-called 'central pattern generators'. Though ascending and descending neural pathways can influence such networks, the latter may also execute autonomous functions. These are particularly relevant when we come to considering reflex reactions.

In a sense, the spinal cord exhibits an organization resembling an inversion of that seen at the level of the cerebral cortex: the cord's grey matter lies at its core (comprising 10 layers, the so-called 'Rexed's laminae'), and its white matter constitutes the surrounding mantle, a mass of vertically ascending and descending axonal pathways. However, as with the cerebral cortex above, there appears to be a pattern to the distribution of neural elements within both the grey and white matters of the spinal cord. In the white matter, this is seen in the arrangement of its tracts, its axonal pathways; in the grey matter, it is apparent in the arrangement of neuronal cell bodies.

The spinal cord's grey matter exhibits a profile rather similar in shape to that of a butterfly (Fig. 16). On each side, it contains laminae that are numbered I–X, from the dorsal (posterior) horn, behind, through to the ventral (anterior) horn, in front. The dorsal horn receives afferent, sensory, information, from the periphery, via incoming sensory neurons (their cell bodies being located in the 'dorsal root ganglia'), which synapse in its grey matter. Hence, laminae I–IV contain mainly sensory neural elements. These regions also relay such sensory information back to the parietal cortices.

Corticomotor axons (arising from both primary motor, BA 4, and premotor cortices, BA 6) terminate most often on interneurons within laminae V–VIII of the spinal cord. They mostly exert their influence over lower motor neurons via such interneurons, although they can also exhibit direct (monosynaptic) junctions with some of the former (the largest), called 'alpha' motor neurons. This is particularly the case in those regions of the spinal cord where the alpha motor neurons concerned 'control' the muscles of the upper and lower limbs (from the cervical and lumbosacral expansions of the spinal cord, respectively). Laminae V and VI are generally involved in the regulation of limb movement, and lamina VII is involved in the regulation of posture; lamina IX contains the cell bodies of lower motor neurons and related interneurons. At each segment (or level) of the spinal cord, the lower motor neurons send their axons *away* from the nervous system, via the *ventral* nerve roots; these axons then synapse with distal structures (beyond the spinal column; Fig. 16), such as the muscles of the hand.

Lower motor neurons may be categorized into two important groups:

i) As noted already, the most prominent motor neurons in the anterior horn (of the spinal cord) are the alpha motor neurons, comprising one of the largest categories of neurons described within the entire human nervous system. They innervate voluntary ('skeletal') muscle fibres, located in the periphery. Those that innervate the muscles of the arm and hand emerge from cell bodies located within the cervical cord (that section of the spinal cord traversing the subject's neck). Here, the ventral horn of the spinal cord provides another illustration of a topographic ('map'-like) distribution of neural components: those motor neurons lying more *laterally* innervate those muscles located more *distally* (e.g. those of the hand), whereas those located more medially innervate more proximal musculature (e.g. that of the shoulder). Alpha motor neurons are large cells and their metabolic activity must be sufficient to support the long axonal processes that leave the spinal cord, in order to innervate the voluntary musculature beyond. It is at the 'end plates' of so-called 'extrafusal' muscle fibres that alpha neurons terminate (Fig. 17). There they utilize acetylcholine as their neurotransmitter (in contrast to glutamate and aspartate, utilized by upper motor neurons).

Alpha motor neurons may be further subdivided. There are those with a 'tonic' pattern of activity, that 'fire' or signal at a low rate, and which exhibit a low speed of signal transmission (i.e. a lower 'conduction velocity'). These neurons innervate so-called 'type S' muscle units. In contrast, there are 'phasic' neurons that exhibit a higher conduction velocity and supply so-called 'fast twitch', 'FR' and 'FF' muscle units.

ii) The anterior horn also contains 'gamma motor neurons': these are neurons that innervate the 'intrafusal' fibres of 'muscle spindles'. The latter are sensory organs, located within the voluntary musculature, that are intimately involved in mediating the simple stretch reflexes underlying tendon jerks (those reflexes that the doctor elicits with her tendon hammer!). Gamma motor neurons also exhibit several forms: for example, those with 'static' and 'dynamic' response characteristics.

Lower motor neurons receive a variety of inputs from other neuronal groups. From above, they receive signals from corticospinal and vestibulospinal tracts (these may include direct 'monosynaptic' communications, i.e. where a corticospinal neuron 'speaks' directly to a lower motor neuron, without an intermediary interneuron). At its own level, a lower motor neuron also receives signals from incoming sensory fibres (the dorsal afferents, referred to earlier). These may originate via direct monosynaptic connections, for example, carrying proprioceptive (joint position sense) information from the same level or

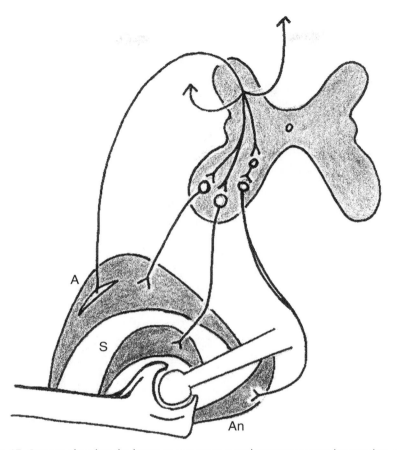

Fig. 17 Cartoon showing the lower motor neuron and sensory neuron innervation of the agonistic (A), synergistic (S), and antagonistic (An) muscles moving a peripheral joint. The agonist muscle contains stretch receptors, which send sensory information back to the spinal cord, where sensory information is further relayed to structures higher up within the human nervous system. Also at the level of the spinal cord, inhibitory interneurons serve to inhibit motor output to the antagonistic muscles, thereby allowing them to relax while the agonist and synergist contract.

a neighbouring cord segment. Alternatively, they might originate as collaterals from dorsal horn neurons and interneurons. These connections have relevance when we come to consider reflexive responses.

Spinal reflexes

A spinal reflex usually comprises a brisk automatic movement about a joint following peripheral stimulation. The knee jerk is an obvious example, but there are many reflexes that can be elicited during a neurological examination (e.g. those at the elbows, the wrists, and even the fingers). Such reflexes may be 'simple', in that the neurons responsible for their appearance make up a simple ('monosynaptic') arc: an incoming (afferent) sensory fibre (accessing the spinal cord via the dorsal root) and its direct (monosynaptic) communication with an outgoing (efferent) motor neuron (i.e. a lower motor neuron, with its cell body located in the ventral horn, the axon of which leaves the spinal cord via the ventral root, terminating on the agonist muscle, which produces the 'jerk'). Alternatively, an interneuron may act as an intermediary in such a sequence, conducting signals between the sensory and motor nerves. Hence, interneurons are implicated in 'polysynaptic' reflexes, where the motor response involves more than one level of the spinal cord (e.g. if I burn my fingertip, my whole arm is likely to retract, flexing at multiple joints.) The reflex itself is stereotypic (assuming it is unimpeded, its expression is automated). However, 'higher' centres may also supervene to exert their influence (i.e. to 'modulate' lower centres). So, for example, if a doctor taps your patellar tendon with a hammer, you can always 'try' to suppress the reflexive jerk of your knee.

Furthermore, the modulation of reflexes by higher centres alerts us to another interesting (and recurrent) pattern discernible within the organization of the central nervous system. Many of the reflexes that a newborn baby might exhibit are sequentially suppressed during subsequent development. This is not achieved consciously but appears to arise spontaneously as a consequence of 'higher' centres modulating or suppressing the reflexive behaviours of those centres located 'below' them (in the neurological hierarchy). In other words, as we develop and mature, our reflexes become harder to elicit. However, if (subsequently) our higher centres should undergo pathological change, or are subjected to physical trauma in some way (e.g. through a penetrating head injury), then their 'control' over our lower reflexes may be diminished. Hence, reflexes may reappear once more or become more pronounced (exaggerated) if our patient develops a stroke or frontal lobe disease. What was once apparent (a reflex) and then suppressed (during normal development) may later re-emerge (in the context of pathology). Hence, those reflexes that are not apparent in the healthy adult state are, by implication, 'latent': they may re-emerge if or when the motor system is damaged.

A good example of this principle is seen in the case of the plantar reflex, named after Babinski, the physician who first described it. This reflex involves the big toe of the 'affected side' of the body. Under normal conditions, when the sole of the foot is gently stroked or scraped, for instance, with the head of a patellar hammer, the big toe will be seen to turn downwards (in 'plantar flexion'); this is an example of the body's automated, flexion response to pain or discomfort. Under normal conditions, it would serve to remove the foot from further irritation. However, under certain pathological conditions, the big toe may respond by pointing upwards (in so-called 'dorsiflexion'). This characteristically accompanies pathology affecting the upper motor neurons, the pyramidal tract. An example would be a 'stroke' affecting the contralateral internal capsule (Fig. 14). The loss of input from contralateral corticospinal neurons serves to 'release' the reflex arc at the level of the spinal cord mediating the plantar reflex (i.e. at the fifth lumbar region); hence, this reflex becomes exaggerated. Thus, a fully integrated input from higher centres targeting the spinal cord serves to 'dampen' certain of its (spinal) reflexes, so that the latter are only *released* when such descending influence is interrupted by pathology.

Stretch reflexes

As a slight aside, it is also worth considering those reflexes that are not concerned with dramatic, demonstrable excursions of our limbs but with 'quietly' maintaining our posture, the balance of our bodies in space. As a species, we humans require our skeleton to remain upright, or at least stable, even while carrying out a host of complex actions over a variety of terrains. Our ancestors may have had to run after their food, while throwing spears, but we might wish to read a book while standing in a tube train, without holding onto the bars! Our posture depends very much upon our joints maintaining their positions in space, in supple (and subtle) ways, through the interplay of muscles that would otherwise be acting in opposition to each other (i.e. agonists and their respective 'antagonists').

So, if I am holding a book in my left hand, and if I turn the pages with the fingers of my right, while standing in that train, then I am maintaining the balance of my frame through the muscles and joints of my feet, legs, hips, and spine; but, I am also maintaining the position of the book in space through my use of my elbows, hands, and (predominantly, left-sided) fingers. My elbows are probably held in a flexed position, at something less than 90°, and on each side, my biceps and triceps are held in potential opposition. However, I really need them to 'work together', in cooperation: I need the triceps to relax if I flex my elbow (with the biceps) and I need the biceps to relax if I extend my elbow ('using' my triceps). Of course, I am not usually thinking about any of this. It occurs 'automatically', while I am attempting to read my book without falling over. So, it is here that we need to consider the vital contribution of so-called 'muscle spindles'.

Muscle spindles are sensory organs that are located within our voluntary musculature. Their ('intrafusal') fibres run parallel to those of the muscle itself (termed 'extrafusal'). When a spindle detects that the muscle is stretching (through its own intrafusal fibres), it sends an afferent signal, via the dorsal root to the spinal cord, to make a synaptic connection with the alpha motor neurons innervating that same muscle (the 'homonymous' muscle) and its synergists (those muscles that will contract in unison with it). The latter respond with an efferent response, stimulating the muscle to contract. However, at the same time that the agonist and its synergists are contracting, there is also an interneuron-mediated *inhibition* of those alpha motor neurons controlling the (potentially opposing) 'antagonist' muscles. The contraction of agonists is therefore timed to coincide with the relaxation of antagonists.

Hence, if the stretching of a muscle spindle had been detected in my biceps, while I was reading on the train, then the biceps would have been stimulated to contract whereas the triceps would have been inhibited (i.e. while it was 'relaxed'). So, it is that I may hold my book steady in space, automatically (though of course similar adjustments are occurring simultaneously in many other joints and muscle groups). Indeed, the impulses arising from my muscle spindles are also being simultaneously relayed beyond their spinal cord segment, further 'up' the nervous system, to the cerebellum and somatosensory and primary motor cortices via my ascending sensory pathways. Hence, a host of adjustments may be initiated (outside of my awareness).

Flexor reflexes

Finally, let us consider another reflex, which impacts upon the way my limbs arrange themselves in space. This one also has a readily apparent evolutionary 'reason' for its existence—the avoidance of pain. If my hand is suddenly the focus of a painful stimulus, for example, if I inadvertently place my right index finger on the hotplate of a grill, then the limb itself flexes. When my finger is the 'victim', it flexes, the hand retracts, flexing at the wrist, the arm withdraws, flexing at the elbow, and depending upon the severity of the pain, my shoulder (and torso) too may rotate in space. Most of what occurs is therefore a withdrawal from pain, through sequential flexions (and as noted earlier, this is also the case during the elicitation of a 'normal' plantar reflex: the big toe flexes as do the ipsilateral ankle and knee.) Such a 'flexor' reflex is mediated via spinal cord interneurons. Indeed, in order for it to be successful, it requires the coordinated contraction of limb flexors at the same time as the limb's extensors relax, cooperatively (if my triceps were to extend, inappropriately, then it would oppose the flexion of my biceps and impede my arm's retreat to safety). Additionally, at the same time as this unilateral, ipsilateral, flexion of my right arm is taking place, the interneurons of my spinal cord may be stimulating the contralateral alpha motor neurons at the same and neighbouring cord levels to contract the contralateral extensors; hence, while my right arm flexes, my left extends—the so-called 'crossed extensor reflex'.

Again, higher centres may modulate or suppress the extent of such a reflex, the magnitude of its expression. Indeed, when there is pathology 'higher up', the flexor reflexes may become exaggerated. One of the most distressing 'signs' to elicit in another human being is the widespread, bilateral flexion that emerges following a painful stimulus administered to someone who has suffered extensive brain injury. It is an awful thing to see.

Towards the periphery

Now, let us pause, to recap, to consider what we have learned so far.

In order for me to be able to move my right index finger as I please, the motor signal originating within the 'finger area' of my left motor cortex, more specifically within the pyramidal (upper motor) neurons of my left BA 4, has had to travel inferiorly, caudally, within my left corticospinal tract. Initially, it traversed the corona radiata, and then the left internal capsule; subsequently, it may have bifurcated, as the tract itself underwent bifurcation at the level of my medulla oblongata. At this point, most of my descending left-sided corticospinal tract fibres 'decussated' and came to form the lateral corticospinal tract on the right side of my spinal cord. They then descended further, to the spinal cord segments in my cervical (neck) region, where they (and the remnants of their former neighbours, which, having travelled within the left anterior corticospinal tract, 'eventually' came to cross the midline) synapsed on interneurons and lower motor neurons located in the ventral horn of my cervical spinal cord. At this level, it was the large, alpha (lower) motor neurons that took up the motor signal. Moreover, theirs was an intermediary role, for they conveyed our motor message to the 'striated', voluntary musculature of my upper limb, my right arm, where the message eventually terminated at the muscle 'end plates', where acetylcholine is deployed to transmit efferent motor signals. So, finally, muscles contract and a finger moves. Is that it? Have we now reached the end of our journey?

Well, no, we have not.

For the next stage of our quest concerns the accurate identification of those nerve routes that will convey the messages from my spinal cord to my right hand and index finger, and the identities of those muscles that will execute these final movements. There are still precise and specific tasks to be undertaken by the components of my upper limb. Hence, I need to describe how the signal completes its journey, from the spinal cord to the muscles, of the hand and the finger.

Thus, if we pick up our story at the level of my cervical spine, and those ventral nerve roots that carry efferent (motor) messages to the periphery, then we next encounter a complex web of nerve fibres making their way towards my right arm. These emerge from the spinal cord to form a structure called the 'brachial plexus', difficult to describe in words and easier to explain in images (see Fig. 18). The ventral nerve roots that emerge from the fifth cervical segment to the first thoracic segment of the spinal cord (C5–T1, respectively) interdigitate to form the medial, lateral, and posterior 'cords' of this plexus. The latter then undergo further division and coalition, and eventually, we can identify the emergence of three major neural pathways innervating the arm: the ulnar, median, and radial nerves (Fig. 18). Each of these brings its own characteristic contribution to the movement and sensation of the upper limb. Two of them, the radial and median nerves, are particularly germane to our story: the eventual movement of my right index finger. Let us now sketch out what it is that they each contribute.

The radial nerve

This nerve derives its roots from all of the origins of the brachial plexus (C5–C8 and T1), and later emerges as a continuation of the plexus' posterior cord. In the upper arm (between the shoulder and the elbow), it runs in the spiral groove of the humerus and, after passing through the so-called 'posterior extensor compartment', innervates the triceps. Hence, if I extend my right arm

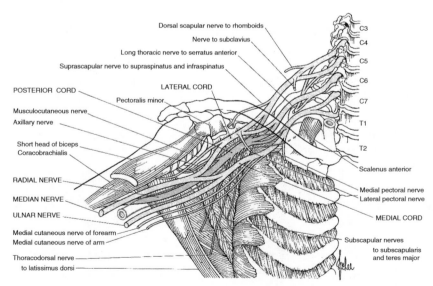

Fig. 18 Diagram showing the structures comprising the right brachial plexus. The radial and median nerves are particularly implicated in the extension and flexion of the right index finger. (Diagram reprinted with permission from Medical Research Council's 'Aids to the examination of the peripheral nervous system' Memorandum No. 45). From HMSO. (See colour plate section).

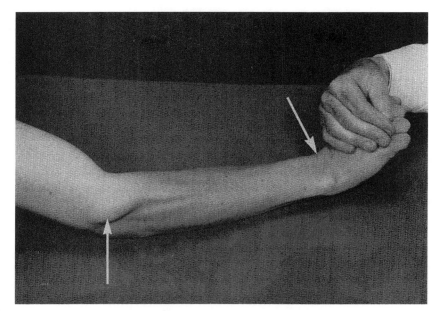

Fig. 19a A photograph demonstrating a clinical examination for the integrity of the posterior interosseous nerve (a branch of the radial nerve). The patient is extending his wrist against resistance. The muscle indicated by the arrows is the extensor carpi radialis longus. (Reprinted with permission from Medical Research Council's 'Aids to the examination of the peripheral nervous system' Memorandum No. 45). From HSMO.

(i.e. 'straighten it out'), I am contracting my right triceps, thanks largely to the contribution of my right radial nerve. Further on, as it enters the forearm, the radial nerve gives off a branch called the 'posterior interosseous nerve', which innervates the muscles of the forearm's 'extensor compartment' (Fig. 19a). Hence, the posterior interosseous nerve supplies all the 'extensor' muscles located there (the extensors being those muscles acting on the finger joints to extend, i.e. straighten, the fingers). Therefore, the right posterior interosseous nerve is responsible for the innervation of those ('extensor digitorum') muscles that act to extend the digits of my right hand (Fig. 19b). Indeed, of especial relevance to our story is the 'extensor indicis', a muscle that specifically extends the index finger (see Fig. 20). The contributory fibres of the radial nerve and (subsequently) the posterior interosseous nerve, supplying these extensor digitorum muscles, are largely derived from cervical roots C7 and C8.

The median nerve

This nerve takes its origins from the sixth to the eight cervical (C6–C8) and the first thoracic (T1) ventral nerve roots. It subsequently emerges from the terminal branches of the lateral and medial cords of the brachial plexus. Unlike the

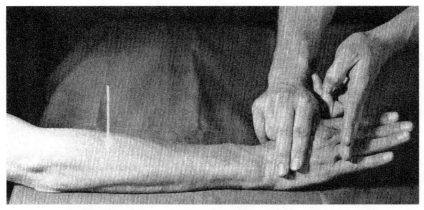

Fig. 19b Photograph showing an examination for the integrity of the posterior inter-osseous nerve. In this case, the patient is extending their fingers against resistance applied by the examiner's left hand. The muscle indicated by the arrow is the extensor digitorum. (Reprinted with permission from Medical Research Council's 'Aids to the examination of the peripheral nervous system' Memorandum No.45). From HMSO.

radial nerve, the median nerve gives off no branches within the upper arm. However, as it enters the forearm, it gives off its own subsidiary branch, called the 'anterior interosseous nerve', which supplies most of the muscles in the 'flexor compartment' of the forearm (i.e. the origins of those muscles that act to flex, bend, the fingers) (Fig. 21). The muscles innervated include the radial por-tion of the flexor digitorum profundis (which serves to flex the index and middle fingers and the hand). The median nerve then goes on to supply the flexor digitorum superficialis and two 'intrinsic muscles' within the hand (the two most radial 'lumbricals', which also act on the index finger). Hence, we can say that the median nerve 'supports' my ability to flex my right index finger (Fig. 19a and 19b), just as the radial nerve 'supports' my ability to extend that same digit. Indeed, they seem to act in functional opposition to each other.

A finger moves

So, now we can see that much of my ability to move my right index finger, in extension or flexion, as I please is dependent on the integrity of my cervical spinal cord, my right brachial plexus, the right radial and median nerves, and their branches (the posterior and anterior interosseous nerves, respectively). As I sit and move my index finger, in the manner of a Libet volunteer, I am utilizing a long pathway that we have now traced out, connecting the upper motor neurons of my motor strip (in left BA 4) with the muscles acting on one specific digit—the right index finger. Hence, we have described much of what it is that is necessary, though by no means sufficient, for me to be able to

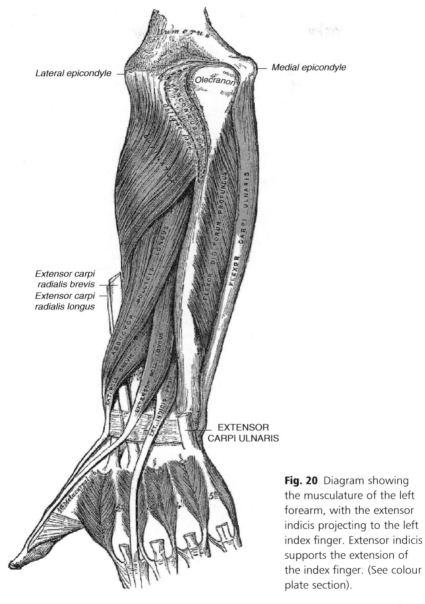

Lateral epicondyle

Medial epicondyle

Olecranon

Extensor carpi
radialis brevis

Extensor carpi
radialis longus

EXTENSOR
CARPI ULNARIS

Fig. 20 Diagram showing
the musculature of the left
forearm, with the extensor
indicis projecting to the left
index finger. Extensor indicis
supports the extension of
the index finger. (See colour
plate section).

produce what Libet requested—'spontaneous' movements of a single digit.
However, it is readily apparent that we have delineated only the bare minimum
necessary to perform such an act, the critical links in a causal chain. Nevertheless,
it is also clear that we may now begin to anticipate how that chain might break
down in a variety of circumstances, consequent upon the diseases that afflict
humankind.

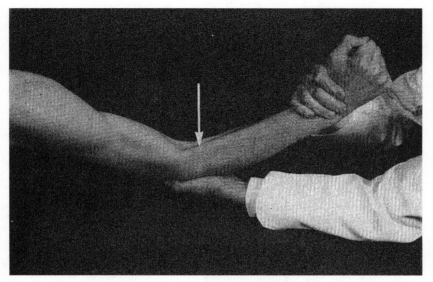

Fig. 21 Photograph showing a clinical examination for the integrity of the median nerve. The patient is flexing the forearm against resistance. The muscle indicated by the arrow is the brachioradialis. (Reprinted with permission from Medical Research Council's 'Aids to the examination of the peripheral nervous system' Memorandum No. 45). From HMSO.

A 'stroke' or tumour within the left internal capsule would interrupt the signal leaving the motor cortex. Motor neuron disease could disrupt the corticomotor neurons themselves (impacting the signal's source) and/or the lower motor neurons (impacting the signal's transmission). A spinal cord injury might also interrupt transmission, as might a demyelinating disease such as multiple sclerosis, impacting the integrity of the system's white matter; so too might the polio virus, by attacking the cord's ventral horn. Peripheral nerve lesions could also stop the signal, literally in its tracks, just before it reaches its target. Finally, in myasthenia gravis, a curious disorder of the muscle end plate, transmission of the signal might itself be interrupted, intermittently, the motor act seeming to wax and wane (fading with exertion; see Table 4).

Hence, we have described much of what is absolutely necessary for an index finger action to occur. We have described a substrate, a 'supporting structure', of neurological tissue. However, we have provided insufficient 'cause' for such an act. Why would I move my finger at all? Why should I move it 'now' and not 'then'? Why might I agree to participate in such an experiment in the first place? The motor chain tells me none of these things. It provides the road but does not justify the journey. In a sense, it is causally 'silent'; the actions (the 'reasons' for that journey) are located 'higher up'. In other words, in order to

Table 4 Examples of three neurological conditions impacting neurotransmission of motor signals and movement performance

Condition	Comments
Motor neuron diseases	A family of diseases characterized by selective loss of function in the upper and/or lower motor neurons. The lower motor profile is one of muscular wasting, fasciculation (twitching, attributable to the spontaneous and simultaneous discharge of all muscle fibres within an affected motor unit), and flaccid weakness. The upper motor profile is one of spasticity (abnormally increased muscle tone), clonus (muscle spasms), extensor plantar reflexes, and spastic weakness. Where the upper motor neuron involvement produces a 'pseudo-bulbar palsy' (see Table 2), there may be pronounced emotional lability (Donaghy, 2005).
Multiple sclerosis	Demyelination, loss of the myelin sheaths from axons, leads to failure of saltatory conduction, so that electrical nerve signals are interrupted, slowed, or misdirected to neighbouring axons ('ephaptic' transmission). If the spinal cord is affected, there is slowness and weakness of movement, differentially affecting the extensor muscles of the arms and the flexors of the legs. The pattern is one of 'upper motor neuron' involvement, so spasticity (increased muscle tone) and exaggerated reflexes occur. If the cerebellum is involved, there is incoordination of speech (dysarthria), swallowing (dysphagia), eye movements (giving rise to nystagmus), abnormal limb movement (an 'intention' tremor, on purposive movement), and loss of balance. Damage to the superior cerebellar peduncle or red nucleus precipitates a proximal 'wild flinging tremor'. Lower motor neuron signs (flaccid paralysis) may be found if there is extensive demyelination in the region of the dorsal root entry zone, of the spinal cord. Optic neuritis can give rise to blindness (Compston, 2005).
Myasthenia gravis	An autoimmune condition targeting the acetylcholine receptors on the muscle end plate (of voluntary, skeletal muscles). It is characterized by muscle weakness and 'fatigability': a weakness demonstrable through repeated or sustained muscular activity. A characteristic disease progression would be extraocular muscle involvement (manifest as diplopia and ptosis) followed by lower facial and bulbar weakness (manifest as dysphagia and dysarthria), neck involvement (with the head falling forwards, due to impaired extensor tone), and finally, limb weakness (Hilton-Jones and Palace, 2005).

Source: From the *Oxford Textbook of Medicine* (2005).

address these questions, we need to step beyond the motor cortex, at least at the level of the cerebrum, and this is what we shall attempt to do in Chapter 2. We shall be 'walking' towards the anterior brain. However, in the mean time, I would like to pause for a while, in order to refine our concept of the 'necessary', through one further question: How is it that *discrete* movements at the periphery have 'become' possible for human beings?

A finger moves, discretely

We might take it for granted, but we are actually rather unusual among mammals in that we are able to move an index finger, a single digit, independently, on its own. How is this possible and what is it that has happened, in evolutionary terms, for such precision to emerge? The answer lies in the relationships pertaining between our motor cortices and our spinal cords. To be specific, it is the relationship between the corticospinal (upper) motor neurons and the alpha (lower) motor neurons of the spinal cord that is of central importance to our inquiry, as it determines the extent to which an organism is capable of dexterous, coherent action (rather than clumsy, reflexive responding). So, to begin with, consider some observations drawn from our 'nearest relatives', the (non-human) primates.

A monkey's corticomotor neuron will fire during a movement of a given type (e.g. a precision grip) but not during a movement of a different type, *even though the same muscle groups are utilized in both sequences of movement*. This implies that

i) It is the movement performed, rather than the muscle group targeted, that is 'represented' at the level of this cortical neuron;

ii) More than one corticomotor neuron *must* synapse on each lower motor neuron (in order for the latter to be involved in the execution of more than one type of movement, via the same muscle effector); and

iii) The muscle group involved must be represented (in some way) more than once at the level of the motor cortex (as it is potentially included in representations of multiple specific movements, instantiated via multiple corticomotor neurons).

Furthermore, it is known that this complex relationship is reciprocal: that is, while more than one corticomotor neuron synapses on each lower motor neuron, it is also the case that more than one lower motor neuron receives projections from each corticomotor neuron (highlighting the importance of movement 'schemata', or patterns of action, being represented cortically rather than in individual muscle groups per se; Jeannerod, 1997, pp. 41–43). Hence, a corticomotor neuron 'talks to' multiple lower motor neurons, involved in the performance of a given movement (possibly implicating multiple muscles), while a lower motor neuron is 'listening' to multiple corticomotor neurons, each contributing to a different movement programme (yet requiring the contribution of 'its' specific muscle or motor unit, within a broader context).

So, what is it that the motor cortex is 'representing'? What does it 'code' for? Direct, unit recordings, using electrodes inserted into monkey motor cortex, have revealed that single cortical neurons may exhibit a 'preferred' direction of response during limb reaching, and that this directional 'vector' is broadly 'tuned' (Georgopoulos, 1995). Hence, a population of neurons (as few as 100–150 cells) may carry an unambiguous directional signal, the emergence of which precedes the execution of the ensuing movement by approximately 160–180 ms. This signal appears to be shared across both the upper (II and III) and lower (IV and V) laminae of the relevant motor cortex (thereby facilitating information distribution to the different projections arising from these upper and lower cortical levels; Georgopoulos, 1995). In addition, this population vector may be held 'on line' while the cue to respond is awaited, and may itself 'rotate' if the specified response direction has to be changed, the change in the response vector being accompanied by sequential recruitment of *different* cortical neuronal populations (i.e. those 'tuned' for the different, 'new' direction). Furthermore, the latter change of direction appears to be lawful: that is, the length of time it takes to happen is related to the magnitude of the change in terms of the *angle* of response required (for a review, see Georgopoulos [1995]). In other words, the greater the discrepancy between the initial and desired angles of response, the longer the time it takes to recruit more appropriate motor cortical units (in order to make the change in movement direction 'happen').

So, it looks as if the motor cortex is very much concerned with the coding of fine distinctions during the execution of emergent, discrete, voluntary behaviours. However, we also have to acknowledge that although it is pivotal to the acquisition and performance of such skilled movements, it is *not* essential for the performance of non-learnt, automated movements, such as walking and reaching, grooming and nursing. Animals can perform these movements, albeit less accurately, even if their motor cortices have been surgically removed, suggesting that subcortical regions may be sufficient to support such *automated* routines (Passingham, 1993).

Hence, the motor cortex seems to be pivotally important for the execution of *skilled* movements, movements that have had to be *learnt*, and which retain a potential for *adjustment* (or fine-tuning) according to the current, prevailing circumstances.

This brings us to our final point regarding movement precision: a lot depends upon the ratios of upper motor neurons to lower motor neurons, and of lower motor neurons to the size of 'their' respective muscle groups. In general, precise movements of a single distal structure, such as my right index finger, are reliant upon small muscle groups receiving relatively rich innervations (via lower motor neurons that are themselves richly innervated by upper motor neurons). Consider the following evidence, marshalled by Passingham (1993, pp. 22–29):

i) Monkeys cannot move their fingers independently if the pyramidal tract is completely severed. They have to use the whole hand rather than discrete digits.

ii) The rhesus monkey develops independent finger movements at age 7–8 months; this coincides with the time at which its descending corticomotor neurons form synapses with its lower motor neurons. If the pyramidal tract is cut, the monkey fails to develop independent finger movements.

iii) Mammals with paws (e.g. rats and cats) exhibit few corticomotor neurons and lack the ability to perform independent digit movements.

iv) Mammals with 'hands' that lack precision grip (e.g. the bush baby and squirrel monkey) have very limited corticomotor input to the lower motor neurons innervating their distal musculature.

v) In contrast, primates exhibiting precision movements (e.g. the macaque monkey, the baboon, and the chimpanzee) have pronounced corticomotor projections to the ventral horn of the spinal cord.

vi) One carnivore, the racoon, has a very capable hand, but its foot is no more specialized than those of other carnivores. Why might this be? Neuroanatomically, the racoon exhibits a rich supply of corticomotor innervation to the level of its 'hand' representation in the cervical spinal cord but not to its 'foot' region, lower down.

Hence, the ability of an animal to move a digit or finger, individually, with a high degree of precision appears to be critically dependent upon the richness of its upper motor neuron innervation synapsing on the relevant lower motor neurons in the ventral horn of its cervical spinal cord. The richer this supply, the greater its potential fractionation across muscle groupings, and the more precise the movements that may be generated using the animal's hand.

Hence, the motor cortices provide a

'[M]echanism for the execution of fine movements which are selected in voluntary action. The ability to perform discrete movements depends on the direct connections from motor cortex to the motor neurons in the spinal cord.'

(Passingham, 1993, p. 37).

Freedom and constraint

We saw (in the Prologue) that even such a simple act as moving an index finger was capable of stirring up controversy when the finger concerned was moving during the course of an experiment performed by Benjamin Libet. In this chapter, we have demonstrated that this deceptively simple act rests upon a concatenation of linked neural and muscular events, and that the precision with which it might even be attempted (one finger moving, independently of its neighbours), let alone achieved, is a consequence of evolution and anatomy. If I were to lack corticomotor innervation of my spinal cord's ventral horn, then I would not be able to move my right index finger with such discrimination, whether I wished to or not. Hence, we have described a motor system that is *necessary* for the performance of such an act, a system that facilitates action while setting limits on its possible excursions. For, although all the links of the causal chain are necessary for my right index finger to be able to move on its own, had that chain been 'assembled' differently (in the course of evolution), I might never have experienced independent digital movement in the first place. Stated simply, anatomy provides the *means* to an end, yet it sets certain absolute physical constraints upon that end: I can move a single finger independently, whereas a squirrel monkey cannot!

In Tables 5 and 6, we set out some of the other attributes that distinguish modern humans from their primate relatives, both 'current' and extinct. There is, necessarily, a speculative aspect to some of the functional distinctions

Table 5 Objective attributes distinguishing humans from *other apes*

Selected traits
Body shape and thorax
Cranial properties (brain case and face)
Relative brain size (but see Table 6)
Relative limb length
Longer ontogeny (development) and lifespan
Small canine teeth
Skull balanced upright on vertical column
Reduced hair cover
Elongated thumb and shortened fingers
Dimensions of the pelvis
Presence of a chin
S-shaped spine
Language
Advanced tool making
Brain topology

Source: Adapted from Carroll (2003).

Table 6 Possible impacts of evolutionary adaptations on the *modern* human response repertoire

Adaptation	Possible impact on repertoire
Increased brain volume	It facilitates greater cognitive complexity, intelligence (and, ultimately, language). However, the total volume may *not* be greater than all other primates, if body size is taken into account; instead, what probably remains 'larger' (having controlled for body size) is the volume of the brain devoted to 'higher' centres, such as the prefrontal cortex (PFC; Preuss, 1995).
Increased skull size	This accommodates increased brain volume. However, the timing of birth relative to the trajectory of skull development also had to adapt in order to allow satisfactory childbirth (i.e. human infants are born relatively 'early', with respect to their brain size, 'in order to' be able to pass through the maternal pelvis). Although facilitating a safer delivery, this development precipitates a longer period of post-natal development and dependency (in other words, vulnerability).
Jaws and teeth	These change in shape to facilitate changes in diet: the move from vegetarianism to meat eating (hence, a protein-rich diet).
Foramen magnum	It is the opening at the base of skull through which the brainstem merges with the spinal cord. This has 'moved' centrally within the skull, relative to non-human primates, facilitating an upright (vertical) posture.
Pelvis	It changes in shape to facilitate upright posture and gait.
Semicircular canals	Located in the inner ear, these are larger in humans than in other primates. They are involved in the control of balance and hence facilitate upright, bipedal locomotion.
Venous drainage of the skull	Changes in circulation around the brain and skull to enhance local temperature control. These 'allowed' early humans to adopt a more athletic lifestyle (compared with relatively sedentary non-human primates), such as running over long distances.
Thumb	The 'opposable' thumb facilitates fine motor skills, including the 'precision grip' (e.g. that seen when picking up a small stone or seed).
Hands	The shape of the hands facilitates an extraordinary range of possible procedures, including both precision and 'power' grips (the latter involving the palm, e.g. when holding a spear).
Shoulders	Adaptations in the shoulder girdle facilitated an increased range of arm and hand activities (relative to non-human primates). A 'stable' shoulder allows powerful use of the arms (in attack) and also the forceful throwing of objects, such as stones and spears.
Corticomotor neuronal innervation	The ratio of upper motor neurons to lower motor neurons (at their adjacent synapses) affects the quality of motor discrimination possible during peripheral (distal) action: for example, the pronounced (corticospinal) input to the lower motor neurons innervating the upper limb musculature facilitates the dexterous movements executed using the fingers.

Table 6 (continued) Possible impacts of evolutionary adaptations on the *modern* human response repertoire

Adaptation	Possible impact on repertoire
Handedness	The modern predominance of right-handedness (~90% of the population) is also apparent in early human artefacts, such as the early stone shavings that would have been used as tools for scraping hides. Consistent patterns of hand preference have implications for synchronized group activities, and the teaching and acquisition of motor skills. The emergence of cerebral 'dominance' (of the left hemisphere) is implicated in the development of language.
Brain asymmetries	'Language areas' are larger in the left hemisphere of the human brain (among those who are right-handed). Interestingly, there are similar asymmetries among the brains of chimpanzees, suggesting that such areas 'in humans might [comprise] elaborations of a pre-exisiting communication centre in a common ancestor of apes and humans' (Carroll, 2003, p. 852).
Larynx	Relative to other mammals, the human larynx is positioned 'low' in the throat, thus facilitating the formation of a 'sound chamber' in the pharynx, with the reverberation of the vocal cords. This (together with many other attributes) allows the production of a wide range of sounds, and hence, the possibility of speech. However, it comes at a price: unlike other primates, we cannot drink and breathe at the same time—'We exhibit the dubious liability for choking' (Leakey, 1995, p. 130).
Body size	Early humans were 'no longer' sexually dimorphic: that is, in contrast to certain other primates, males were not *markedly* larger than females. This suggests that (alpha) males did not compete for sole control of all the females in a group, and that males might have cooperated (e.g. during hunting). Greater cooperation also has implications for the (subsequent) development of 'culture'.

Source: From Carroll (2003), Leakey (1995), McManus (2002), Preuss (1995), and Wilson (1998).

identified and we are obviously on firmer ground with respect to structural, anatomical, differences (i.e. we cannot 'know' the behaviour of a species that no longer lives, though we can derive some inferences from those bones that survive within the archaeological record.) As far as one can glean from the current literature, the proposed mechanisms by which such differences came about seem to constitute multiple (polygenic) changes of gene regulation (rather than the emergence of 'new' genes per se; e.g. Carroll, 2003; Pollard et al., 2006). We may be 5–7 million years away from our last common ancestor with the chimpanzee (*Pan troglodytes*), but our own species (the modern human, *Homo sapiens*) has been around for 'only' approximately 200 000 years—indeed, only the lattermost 3% of that period during which the *Homo* species have existed here (Carroll, 2003). Our last 'hominin' relatives, the

Neanderthals (*Homo neanderthalensis*), probably became extinct about 30 000 years ago, despite having larger brains than us (Carroll, 2003). A large brain seems to be no guarantor of perpetuity.

Nevertheless, we may still sense that there is something 'special' that happens when a human subject makes a movement that is unprovoked and seemingly 'free'. When I am *not* compelled to do something, when I am 'free' ('to do what I like'), something emerges, and even though the limits of that 'something' may have been constrained (already) by my inherited anatomy (e.g. the ratio of 'my' corticomotor neurons to 'my' alpha motor neurons, conducting 'my' motor signals towards 'my' index digit), I nevertheless know that had I not acted this movement would not have existed. The world becomes different, it exists in a different state, following an act (or, indeed, its forbearance): if I do not start the car, the journey does not begin; if I do not write the letter, the recipient will never read it; if I do not use the phone, the other person does not hear my voice. An action creates a new event in the world. Michelangelo's hands created images that had not existed previously; Charlie Parker's fingers improvised new melodies. Before these movements were made, there were 'gaps', potential spaces for action.

Chapter 2

Assembling a 'will'

Suddenly, pacing by the water, he was overcome with astonishment. He found himself understanding the weariness of this life, where every path was an improvisation and a considerable part of one's waking life was spent watching one's feet.[5]

If left to themselves, human affairs can only follow the law of mortality, which is the most certain and the only reliable law of a life spent between birth and death. It is the faculty of action that interferes with this law ...[6]

In the first chapter, we described what it was that was anatomically 'absolutely' necessary for me to be able to move my right index finger, independently, discretely. We did not describe 'every' functional, anatomical condition that must be satisfied in order for such a performance to succeed, but we did identify a bare minimum: a chain of neurological connections and events that would have to be in place for me to be able to move my finger at all. We saw that, at the very least, an upper motor neuron, emerging from my left primary motor cortex (Brodmann area, BA, 4) would have to have projected inferiorly, caudally, in order to make contact with lower motor neurons residing in the ventral horn on the right side of my spinal cord (at the level of my cervical spine). We then described how such lower motor neurons were responsible for conveying ongoing motor impulses to the distal musculature of my right forearm, whence, the latter would eventually act upon the joints of my right index finger, to flex or extend that single digit. Hence, as a bare minimum, such a chain of neurological processes would have had to be intact for me to have been able to act in such a way. Had the links been disrupted, for instance by a neurological disease (Table 4), then I would not have been able to make my finger move.

5 Golding W. *Lord of the Flies*. London: Faber & Faber, 1958 (first published 1954), 81.

6 Hannah Arendt, cited in Altenbernd Johnson P. *On Arendt*. Belmont, California: Wadsworth/Thomson Learning, 2001, 1.

However, the chain that we have just delineated constitutes only the very basic 'medium' via which the 'message' to move must be conveyed (yes, we have just purloined the terminology of Marshall McLuhan). By itself, it does not tell us 'why' the message appears when it does; nor does it tell us what the message 'is meant' to achieve. We happen to know (because I told you) that I was imagining making my finger move for purely artificial purposes: as interspersed action episodes during the course of a simple behavioural experiment conducted by Benjamin Libet (see Prologue). We happen to know that I was 'not' thinking of pressing a piano key, an exit code or an alarm button. However, from the point of view of the chain itself (if upper and lower motor neurons may be briefly conjectured to experience such a 'point of view') we may suspect that it hardly matters 'why' the message appeared. A signal is conveyed, a movement executed: the chain itself appears 'blind' to its purpose. The latter is certainly a bold statement, but what do I mean exactly?

Well, as we discussed in Chapter 1, had an electrode been implanted in my left motor cortex, and stimulated with sufficient energy, then it too might have elicited finger movements on the right side of my body. There was no 'need' for an intention, on my part, in order for this to happen. An electrode, controlled by someone else, an experimenter 'in a white coat' perhaps, might have been quite sufficient. Furthermore, we know that such movements need not have resembled merely a muscle twitch; they might have exhibited an:

> [A]spect of purpose or volition ... of the same nature as those which the animal makes in its ordinary intelligent action'
>
> Ferrier, 1876; cited in Jeannerod, 1997.

So, although we have delineated the neural chain that ultimately executes my potential action, we have said very little about how, when or why such an action emerges, in the 'first place'. It is the purpose of this chapter to try to understand what it is, what structures and processes within the human brain are involved, that determine 'how' and 'when' the motor system acts and 'why' it does so. We have considered some of what it is that constitutes the 'medium'; now we wish to find out what it is that assembles the 'message'. To do this, we must go beyond and 'above' the primary motor cortex (MC). Hence, although in Chapter 1 we located MC (BA 4) at the head of a chain—the apex of one form of neurological hierarchy—here, we need to recognize a different neurological hierarchy, one in which, this time, the motor cortex is rather more 'inferiorly' located. In other words, in this chapter, we need to consider the 'anterior' frontal lobes.

Table 7 Examples of the terms used by cognitive neuroscientists to describe 'higher' control centres in the brain.

Author(s)	Putative function	Identified location
Baddeley and Della Sala (1996)	'Central executive'	Frontal lobe/PFC
Devinsky et al. (1995)	'Emotional will power'	ACC
Dolan et al. (1993)	'Alogia' (the absence of spontaneous speech, a dysfunction)	Left DLPFC (BA 9)
Frith (1987); Frith et al. (1991a, 1991b)	'Internal generation', 'willed action'	DLPFC (and ACC)
Fuster (1980)	'The proper temporal organization of motor action'	PFC
Goldman-Rakic (1987), Goldman-Rakic et al. (1992)	'Inhibitory control'	PFC
Goldman-Rakic (1996)	'Domain-specific central executive'	DLPFC (for spatial information), orbitofrontal cortex (for object-related information), and left BA 45 (for verbal information)
Ingvar (1994)	'Wilful mobilization of inner representations of future events', 'action programmes'	PFC
Jahanshahi et al. (1998)	The 'controller' of a random response generation network	Left DLPFC (BA 9)
Jeannerod (1997)	The 'prior intentions to act'	DLPFC
Luria (1966)	'Ideational apraxia', the loss of 'goal' (a dysfunction)	PFC
Passingham (1995)	'Response generation'	DLPFC (BA 9?)
Passingham (1996)	'Attention to action'	DLPFC and ACC
Petrides (1996)	'Monitoring' of action, 'self-ordering' of tasks	DLPFC
Shallice et al. (1989); Shallice and Burgess (1996)	'Supervisory attentional system' (SAS), 'will', 'monitoring'	Frontal lobe/PFC

The question mark denotes the speculative nature of Passingham's remarks regarding the role of BA 9 in response generation.

ACC, anterior cingulate cortex; BA, Brodmann area; DLPFC, dorsolateral prefrontal cortex; PFC, prefrontal cortex.

A note, concerning the 'Will'

However, before returning to a detailed description of our human actor's neuroanatomy, I should like to situate this inquiry within a broader context, one that we shall return to on and off throughout the remainder of this book. For, as will become clear, when we ascend the neurological hierarchies discernible across the frontal lobes of the primate brain we seem to encounter components of what a philosopher or theologian (or indeed, certain cognitive neuroscientists; see Table 7) might conceive of as components of a 'Will'. If we start to talk about 'choices', intentions and motivations—the 'reasons' why human agents 'do' the things that they do—then we inevitably begin to probe the foundations of some very important behaviours: moral conduct, immoral conduct, that which is harmful to others, etc. Do we do these things because we are 'free' to do them or because we are 'determined' (i.e. predestined) to do so? These are complex questions; indeed, they have occupied human minds for centuries. So, without wishing to obscure the neuroanatomical data that we are about to rehearse, I do need to point out what it is that we 'should' be looking for among the neurological mechanisms that we shall next encounter—mechanisms which shed light upon complex human behaviours, behaviours that require more than 'just' the simple flexion of a finger. If we believe that there is such a thing as a 'Will', then what should 'it' look like?

Is any behaviour ever 'Willed'?

Well, there seems little doubt that complex behaviours may 'appear' 'intended', 'purposeful' or 'Willed'. Do we not often have the impression that others (and ourselves) are acting 'on purpose'? Yes, indeed we do, but what do we mean by 'purpose'? Well, according to one dictionary, purpose is 'the idea or aim kept before the mind as the end of effort ... an end desired' (Chambers, 1997). It seems to be what we are aiming at, our 'goal'. Indeed, often we may have to aim, or pursue, such a goal over quite extended periods of time (think of Michelangelo, painting the Sistine Chapel, year upon year, squinting upwards, through the paint and the dust). Our 'purpose' is something that we may well find ourselves 'living with', throughout protracted epochs of conscious awareness (learning the piano, training to be a doctor, raising a family, etc.). We might even 'live and breathe' it. Hence, if we do, and if we are in 'agreement' with our aims and our goals, then are we not 'responsible' for them? Well, yes, in 'folk psychological' terms, indeed 'we are': in everyday life we do treat people as if they are responsible for what it is that they have wished to bring about. Michelangelo is credited with painting the ceiling (and one wall) of the Sistine Chapel: 'he' did it.

However, in a world 'after-Libet' is this 'really' an exhaustive attribution? Yes, the body of Michelangelo was the one that 'exhibited arm movement' and conveyed paint towards the ceiling (and a wall) of the Sistine Chapel. Yes, we can surely identify the organism concerned. Yes, we know 'which one' was there at the time of the painting behaviour. Nevertheless, we often seem to want to know something more. We want to know 'where' the ideas came from, where the inspiration was found, we may even wish to know what it was that 'kept Michelangelo going'. Would it matter if he had come from a long line of painters, with enhanced visuo-spatial acuity, would it matter if he had studied Giotto, would it matter if he had experienced a very subtle form of colour-blindness? I am inventing these questions, but they do serve to localize a problem—a problem that is exemplified by our thinking 'after-Libet'. For, what is it that generates our conscious awareness? What is it that 'chooses' the goals or purposes that enter our minds and then preoccupy us so, while they are 'there'? It seems to me that we are inevitably returned to our 'Libet-problem'. How can we be responsible for 'our' thoughts and actions if we only become aware of them 'after' they have been generated? How may we avoid slipping into some sort of very strange circumlocution concerning 'thoughts that are thought before we think them'? How may we remain coherent? How can we 'understand' Michelangelo's 'behaviour'?

Well, let us first cleave to what we might regard as common sense: Michelangelo painted the Sistine Chapel. Let us defer judgement on the Libet-problem until we have travelled a little further along, through the text. Instead, let us target what a 'reasonable person' might regard as purpose and responsibility and then see whether they 'make sense'. Consider the following.

A man cheats on his wife though he tells her that he loves her. He maintains complex sequences of behaviour over months, sometimes even years, at a time. He tells conflicting stories to different adult interlocutors, yet he manages to keep two narratives in play. On some occasions he is a doting father, a loyal spouse, on others he is a philanderer, furtively deployed among serial hotel bedrooms. Surely he must 'know' what he is doing. He has had to conjure so many items of information, so many modes of behaviour, just to maintain his subterfuge; he must be aware of his behaviours, must he not? Well, in 'ordinary life' one suspects that our adulterer would have to admit duplicity; he would have to accept 'responsibility'. Yes, his actions were 'intended'; yes he enjoyed what he did (at the time). However, among the loftier realms of humanity, one sometimes encounters qualifications, justifications and excuses for very similar behaviours. A film star might book himself into a celebrity clinic and claim to have been a victim of 'sex addiction' while he engaged in similar pursuits, a pop star might go back into 'rehab' (it was the alcohol and cocaine that 'made' him behave in this way; note: the implication is that he too is a 'victim'), a politician may claim that what he did was 'stupid', an 'error' (note: it was not 'wrong', it was a 'mistake'; the moral has been substituted by the cognitive). So, across many settings the casual observer may witness very capable people claiming to have 'not' been responsible for the things that they did or at least not fully 'cognizant' of them (at the time); even when their actions had clearly required a considerable amount of deliberation, extended periods of behavioural control and where the consequences for these individuals had been rather enjoyable (at the time). Nevertheless, control and volition, intent and responsibility, are mysteriously denied. Clearly, there are times when people go to great lengths to deny their own freedom, their own volition. (Note also: the subtle elision between moral failure and intellectual error. In Britain, at the moment, it is unusual to hear of a politician (or, indeed, any 'personality') admitting that they did something 'wrong', there is instead an identification of error: 'it was a stupid mistake'. The 'moral' becomes 'cognitive'). Do we take such accounts at face value? Does anyone ever do anything that they realize is 'bad'? (Well, sadly, yes they do and we shall meet them in Chapter 9).

Someone else feigns an illness to avoid going to work. He winces with pain when the doctor touches him. He limps when he knows that he is being observed. He cannot go to work but he can go for a run. He receives invalidity benefits though he plays soccer at the weekends. He must know what he is doing; he must 'intend' to do it, must he not?

And what about the Machiavellian manager? This person spreads a rumour that he knows to be untrue. He speaks quietly, modulates his tone. He tells some people some details and other people others. Is he in 'control' of his actions; is he 'responsible' for his words? Are these behaviours 'willed'?

Admittedly, it can be difficult to find a definition of the 'Will' (and 'willing') that might be agreeable to everyone. Indeed, the *Oxford English Dictionary* offers several definitions, in the context of voluntary behaviour:

> The action of willing or choosing to do something; the movement or attitude of the mind which is directed with conscious intention to (and, normally, issues immediately in) some action, physical or mental; volition.
>
> The power or capacity of willing; that faculty or function which is directed to conscious and intentional action; power of choice in regard to action.

These definitions echo the philosopher John Locke (as cited by Berrios & Gili, 1995):

> [T]his power that the mind has to order the consideration of any idea, or the forbearing to consider it; or to prefer the motion of any part of the body to its rest, and vice versa, in any particular instance, is that which we call the will.

He goes on: 'The actual exercise of that power, by directing any particular action, or its forbearance, is that which we call volition or willing.'

So, to John Locke, the Will comprises a 'capacity' to choose and volition (willing) is its enactment, its execution. The cheating husband, the malingering employee and the devious manager exercise their Wills; they make choices. They 'are' responsible for what they have done, at least in the everyday, 'commonsense' terms that 'normal' humans seem to understand, while deploying the 'folk psychology' of beliefs, desires and actions.

Philosophical differences

However, it is also clear that several different 'Wills' are discernible among the ways in which other philosophers use this word. Some authors focus on the 'choice', the decision that is made, others on the actor's determination; their sticking to that decision over time (e.g. when exhibiting 'will power'), in contrast to those who exhibit 'akrasia' (weakness of the will), 'changing their mind' in the face of 'temptation'. Other authors seem to mean the voluntary process itself (manifests 'the Will'), the performance of actions. Here are just a few statements taken from a recent monograph by Dilman (1999):

> Willing is the action itself trying, attempting, making an effort
>
> (Ludwig Wittgenstein; p. 123).

> I will to write and the act follows, I will to sneeze and it does not
>
> (William James; p. 119).

> We learn the influence of our will from experience alone; and experience alone teaches us how one event constantly follows another
>
> (David Hume; p. 119).

Dilman himself is clearly interested in a Will that is cognitively complex and 'supervisory' (in a sense that we shall rehearse, later, in Chapter 4):

> I am saying that our will, as it finds expression in our intentions, choices and decisions, belongs to us, flesh and blood beings, and it is embedded in situations of human life in which we act. We enter these situations as beings with a specific history in the course of which we have learned a great many things and have become the particular individual who *judges, deliberates, takes decisions, acts*. We bring much of this to bear on the situation in our assessments and considerations before acting. It is as such that *we determine our actions in accordance with considerations* and, therefore, not arbitrarily: our actions are not gratuitous acts.
>
> (263; the italics have been added).

Now, for our present purposes, I am going to retain Dilman's description of the 'Will'. As such, I am retaining a description that is necessarily rather loose and open and I do this for a specific reason. I propose that, in the course of this chapter, we shall encounter many different attributes (of the frontal brain) that we might understand as contributing to such a complex (hypothetical) construct as the 'Will'. Hence, I think that it maybe helpful to keep an open mind at this stage concerning its attributes: a hypothetical Will might have many components, not least those concerned with choice and endurance (below).

However, I should also alert the reader to an interesting distinction that will become increasingly apparent over the course of this chapter: that of the 'precision' of an act (i.e. the 'success' with which it is enacted) and its 'quality' (i.e. whether it accords with the pre-existing, 'moral norms' of a given individual, an actor). This distinction may be regarded as having a neurological underpinning, manifesting the consequences of a kind of 'gradient' instantiated across the 'higher' centres of the brain, from lateral to medial, from dorsal to ventral. Hence, we shall see that dorsolateral brain systems are often implicated in actions that 'go wrong', i.e. movements that are performed 'badly', while ventromedial systems are often implicated when an action is inherently 'wrong', i.e. when it carries some harmful or immoral valence. I shall defend these predictions towards the close of this chapter.

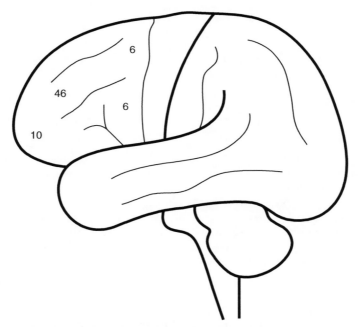

Fig. 22 Cartoon showing the lateral aspect of the human cerebral cortex. The numerals indicate Brodmann areas 6, 46, and 10.

Premotor cortex (Brodmann Area 6)

Immediately anterior to the primary motor cortices (BA 4) are the PMCs (BA 6; see Figure 22). If the former can be regarded as relatively low-level 'output' regions within the cortical motor system, then the latter may be thought of as relatively 'higher up': engaged in the programming of motor activity. Furthermore, when I use the word 'programming', I am really using a form of shorthand, currently associated with computer science, indicating that the premotor regions have a role in determining the 'script', the 'pattern' of motor events, that the motor cortices (and other motor regions) may be subsequently called upon to execute. The eminent French motor physiologist Marc Jeannerod (2006), and his contemporaries Brunia and Van Boxtel (2000), ascribe the use of such terminology to the work of Steven Keele (writing in 1968), a motor programme being, in his view:

> [A] set of muscle commands that are structured before a movement sequence begins, and that allows the entire sequence to be carried out
>
> (Keele, cited by both Jeannerod, 2006, p. 10, and Brunia & Van Boxtel, 2000, p. 510).

Hence, in order to compose such a script, premotor cortical regions should require at least two fundamental forms of data:

1. A *goal* (i.e., what it is that the script is 'meant to achieve'), and

2. A *repertoire* or 'tool-box' (a collection of motor sequences, previously acquired and honed (i.e. learned), that may be deployed, or delegated to other regions, to achieve the specified goal).

As we shall see (below), there are good grounds for believing that prefrontal regions (anterior to PMC) play pivotal roles in determining such goals ('1', above), while PMCs themselves can be shown to be particularly involved in motor learning and selection ('2', above). (However, although it may be tempting – and easy when writing – to lapse into a narrative that describes the components of the motor system as if 'they' were 'determining goals' or 'writing scripts', we must continually endeavour to remind ourselves that we are describing biological systems and events: physiological processes. While it is again, of course, tempting to deploy teleological (and anthropomorphic) terms when describing brain regions, we should not say (or imagine) that the PMC has a 'plan'. The PMC is a component within a larger system; and that system has other components that (somehow) help to generate plans; but it is the system as a whole that exhibits any 'purpose' that we may identify and attribute. In humans, it is common to attribute purpose to a person, as in: 'the philosopher went to the refrigerator to take out a bottle of beer'; we do not attribute a

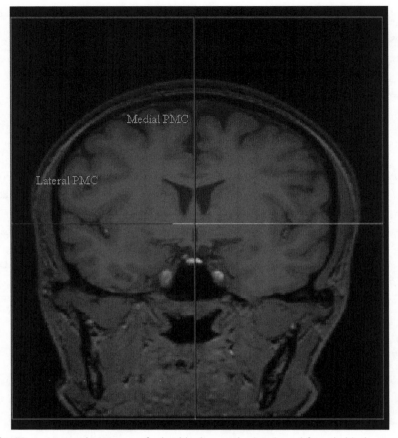

Fig. 23 A structural MRI scan of a healthy human brain, viewed from behind in the coronal plane, showing the medial and lateral premotor cortices of the left hemisphere. (See colour plate section).

purpose to his BA 6! Nevertheless, it can be difficult to avoid such lapses when describing 'his' brain.)

While PMCs, in general, can be shown to share an ability to learn and construct new motor routines (below), they also exhibit regional sub-specializations, the most pertinent of which is apparent over the lateral-to-medial convexity (in the coronal plane; see Figure 23).

Those premotor regions located 'laterally' are most implicated in responses (reactions) to prompts or cues discernable within the current external environment. For example, a monkey may have been taught that, upon hearing a bell, he should press one button rather than another in order to receive a reward. So, when he hears the bell, he pushes the correct button. He receives his reward (often a peanut). The bell constitutes the cue and the monkey responds, explicitly. He has been 'conditioned'. This response can be shown (below) to rely upon the integrity of the monkey's lateral PMC. Lesions in this region disrupt this form of learning and responding. In other words, lateral PMC lesions seem to interfere with the monkey's ability to use the 'external environment' as a guide to his ongoing behaviour. In contrast, the 'medial' PMC seems to be especially important in the performance of actions that occur in the 'absence' of such an explicit, external cue: so-called 'internally initiated' actions. Hence, the medial PMC is implicated in those situations where a monkey has been taught that spontaneous acts might elicit a reward. As a result, in this latter scenario, there is no explicit cue or prompt emerging from the environment. Instead, at some unspecified moment, the monkey uses his hand to press a lever and, as a consequence, a peanut appears. Note: there was no external cue. So, what made the monkey do it? Perhaps he was hungry. In other words, we might infer that there was indeed a cue, but one that was actually 'internal' (i.e. located within the monkey).

The Oxford physiologist Dick Passingham (1993) has provided an elegant and extensive review of the consequences of localized lesions of the lateral and medial PMC in non-human primates. Most prominent, following a lateral lesion, is an inability to learn new contingencies, a failure to respond to external stimuli. In contrast, following medial lesions, a monkey is unable to initiate spontaneous behaviours such as the one just described (i.e. he will not initiate the spontaneous lever press that would have brought him the peanut).

This distinction – between 'externally cued' and 'internally initiated' acts – is crucial when we come to consider what could be 'going on' in Benjamin Libet's experiments: the notion that a human actor may have acted from purely 'internally determined' conditions. Indeed, Libet's experiment (as described in the Prologue) looks very much like the ideal procedure for eliciting activity within the medial PMC: his subjects were sitting in silence, there were no cues to action, and they moved spontaneously when they experienced an 'urge' to do so. Hence, when Mike Hunter and I repeated Libet's experiment – albeit within the confines of a magnetic resonance imaging (MRI) scanner, using a functional neuroimaging technique to examine regional brain activity – we were unsurprised to find significant activation in the medial PMC and the primary motor cortex (see Figure 24). So, there is clearly a connection between medial PMC activity and the onset of 'internally initiated' action. (Indeed, if, in the course of neurosurgery, the medial PMC is directly stimulated with an electrode, then human subjects experience a similar subjective 'urge' to move (see Fried et al. 1991; Fried, 1996)).

Left   Left

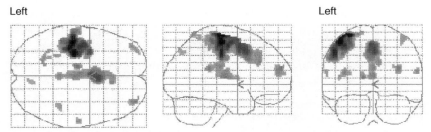

Fig. 24a Statistical parametric maps showing areas of increased activation in the instant during which normal healthy males moved their right index fingers 'spontaneously'. There is prominent activation of the left motor cortex and also medial premotor regions. Activation at the frontal poles is located in Brodmann area 10 (bilaterally). These data are reprinted from *Neuroimage, 20: Hunter* et al. *Approaching an ecologically valid functional anatomy of spontaneous 'willed' action. 1264–9.* © 2003. With permission from Elsevier Ltd.

However, it is also important to heed Passingham's reminder that the absence of a current (explicit) external stimulus or cue does not necessarily imply that internally initiated actions arise within a causal vacuum, in isolation from external influences:

> We should not suppose that there is no context for self-initiated movements. The difference is only that there is no *external* context[,]… no event in the outside world.

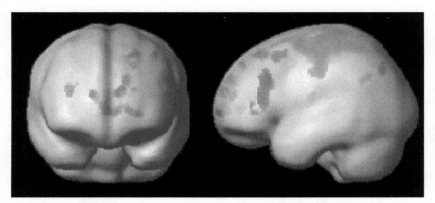

Fig. 24b Statistical parametric maps represented on a smooth brain template. The areas in red show activity during the second when normal healthy males moved their right index finger 'spontaneously'. The areas in blue demonstrate areas that have previously been activated and are relatively 'deactivated' at the moment of spontaneous action. There is prominent deactivation in the left dorsolateral prefrontal cortex (seen in the lateral view on the right). These data reprinted from *Neuroimage, 23: Hunter* et al. *Spatial and temporal dissociation in prefrontal cortex during action execution.* © 2004, with permission from Elsevier Ltd. (See colour plate section).

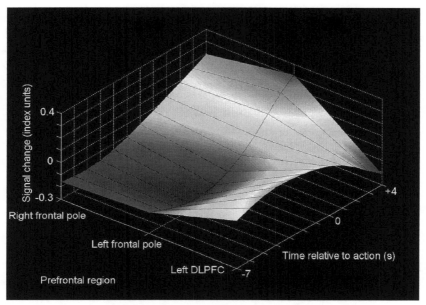

Fig. 24c Cartoon showing a graphic representation of the changes in focal activity in prefrontal regions immediately prior to a spontaneous act (in healthy human males). Seven seconds before the act (at minus seven) there is increasing activity within the left dorsolateral prefrontal cortex (DLPFC). This reaches a peak and then declines over the course of the action. In contrast, focal activity is decreased at the frontal poles prior to the action but gradually increases towards the point of activity itself. These data reprinted from *Neuroimage, 23: Hunter et al. Spatial and temporal dissociation in prefrontal cortex during action execution.© 2004,* with permission from Elsevier Ltd. (See colour plate section).

> Many of the movements that we make are appropriate in the context of our previous behaviour.
>
> (Passingham, 1993, 69, original italics)

Hence, it makes sense for the monkey engaged in the experiment (above) to pull the lever, spontaneously, because he 'knows' (at some level) from past experience that a peanut may appear.

As already mentioned, BA 6 lies immediately anterior to the primary motor cortex (BA 4) and, in common with its neighbour, is cytoarchitecturally 'agranular' (i.e. it lacks numerous granular cells in laminae II and IV, the outer and inner granular layers of the cortex, respectively; Chapter 1, Figure 8). It also possesses far fewer Betz cells (in lamina V) than BA 4 and consequently, although electrical stimulation of BA 6 may elicit some peripheral movements;

these emerge far less readily than they would have from stimulation of BA 4 (primary motor cortex).

Medial and lateral BA 6 each send reciprocal projections back to motor cortex, as do further 'premotor' regions located in the lower cingulate sulcus (Passingham, 1993; 1997). (The latter region lies lower down on the medial surface of the hemisphere). Hence, there is a physical conduit via which the PMC may send 'messages' – motor signals – to the primary motor cortex.

The medial PMC also incorporates the supplementary motor area (SMA), situated high up on its dorsomedial surface. The SMA has been repeatedly implicated in human brain-imaging studies of 'internally initiated' activity (below). Indeed, it is one probable source of those electrical signals (the Bereitschaftspotentials) detected by Libet and his colleagues in their studies of spontaneous movement (described in the Prologue). It also constitutes the specific site within the medial PMC where stimulation elicits the subjective 'urge' to move (Fried et al. 1991).

Now, the PMCs may influence movement execution via several possible routes: they have direct projections to BA 4 (above) and subcortical projections to the corticospinal (pyramidal) tract (Chapter 1). They also contribute to re-entry circuits conveying information between cerebral motor regions, the basal ganglia, and the thalamus before returning to the SMA (thereby 'closing a circuit'; Figure 25). We shall address the properties of such systems in Chapter 4, but for the time being it is clear that the PMC 'programming' centres have multiple routes via which they may exert influence upon the 'output' regions of the motor cortex and corticospinal tracts. Furthermore, they also project to other, distinct, subcortical regions, including the pontine nuclei, superior colliculi, and reticular formation (these regions being implicated in facial movement, eye movement, and arousal, among many other important processes). Conversely, the PMCs receive regionally specific projections from the parietal cortex, with these also exhibiting a characteristic pattern:

1. Medial BA 6 has reciprocal connections with medial parietal lobe (BA 5);

2. Dorsolateral BA 6 has reciprocal connections with dorsal parietal lobe (also BA 5);

3. The ventrolateral region of BA 6 (lying on the outer, inferior convexity of the hemisphere) has reciprocal connections with the inferior parietal lobule (an area labelled 7b in non-human primates and BA 40 in humans).

Hence, PMCs receive incoming sensory data from parietal cortices; and such information is thought to comprise visual, proprioceptive (joint-position sense) and spatial co-ordinate information arising from those bodily structures engaged in movement. From a teleological perspective, it is apparent that integration of sensory and motor data 'should' be required for such a brain

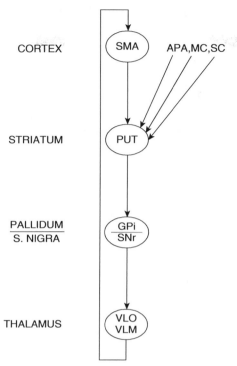

Fig. 25 Diagram showing the structure of the motor (supplementary motor area, SMA) loop in the primate cortex. The loop is semi closed in that it receives multiple projections from the cerebral cortex, targeting the putamen, relaying onto the pallidum and substantia nigra, followed by the thalamus, before a final projection closes the loop (targeting the SMA). The other cortical areas implicated are the arcuate premotor, motor and somatosensory cortices. *This image is taken from Alexander* et al. *1988. (created by an employee or agency of the U.S Government and is thus in the public domain).*

region to be engaged in efficient motor programming; for, in order to 'script' anticipated movements, the PMC 'needs to know' where the animal's limbs are in space, 'right now'.

Therefore, if we wish to consider what can happen when such (incoming) parietal communication breaks down, when a lesion of the parietal lobe or its communicating tracts interrupts volition, then a clear example is provided by the syndrome of 'ideomotor dyspraxia', a neurological condition in which humans exhibit an inability to carry out specified motor acts. Although an affected patient appears to be neurologically 'intact' grossly, with normal sensation, muscle power, and vision, they cannot 'copy' gestures. A doctor may say 'please do this', demonstrating a series of simple hand movements, but the patient cannot imitate them. Even though she comprehends the instruction, can see what the doctor is doing, and can potentially move her limbs with normal power, she cannot copy the act. The problem lies within action 'programming' – the translation of an idea into an act (hence, the label 'ideomotor' dyspraxia) – the patient 'knows' what the examiner wants her to do but she cannot 'make' her body do it; she cannot 'translate' her observations into actions. In his extensive monograph on 'handedness', Chris McManus quotes just such a case of dyspraxia, as described by one of the fathers of clinical neurology, Kinnier Wilson:

> [She, the patient] was asked to lift her right arm, but after crossing it over her body, putting her hand in her left axilla [armpit], and making various energetic but hopeless efforts, she said plaintively, 'Je comprends bien ce que vous voulez, mais je ne parviens pas a le faire' [I understand well what you want me to do, but I can't manage to do it], and there lies the whole situation in a nutshell.
>
> (Kinnier Wilson, 1908, cited by McManus, 2002, 177)

Dyspraxic patients may also experience difficulties in posting a letter or picking up a cup of tea; they may not be able to 'automatically' adapt the shape of their hand to the contours of their target (the letter box or the cup's handle, respectively). This condition serves to highlight what we normally take for granted, so long as our parietal and PMCs are intact and able to 'talk to each other', efficiently. Deprived of such communication, an 'idea' cannot be translated into an appropriate 'act'. Hence, although the lesion may reside in the parietal cortex, its influence impacts the 'ability' of the PMC to programme skilled movements. Extensive accounts of such phenomena, consequent upon parietal lobe pathology, are provided in the works of Marc Jeannerod (1997, 2006).

Now, if we leave parietal lobe pathology for the time being and return to the innervation of the PMC itself, then we find that the latter receives further projections from the anterior division of the ventrolateral nucleus of the thalamus, and the centromedian, parafascicular, and centrolateral compartments of the thalamic intralaminar nuclei. Note that two of these areas (the centromedian and parafascicular compartments) have also featured among the innervations of the primary motor cortex (Chapter 1). We shall further elaborate on the thalamus and its contribution to frontal circuitry in later sections of this book (especially in Chapter 4); however, for the time being, it is worth noting that interruptions to thalamic output (perhaps as a consequence of a thalamic 'stroke') provide another possible means by which PMC function can be disturbed as a consequence of a distant, though connected, lesion (as was the case with parietal lesions, above; a phenomenon referred to as 'diaschesis').

What is it that the cells in the PMC actually 'do' in the context of a movement? Well, as we saw in Chapter 1, it is possible to demonstrate that activity within a motor cortex Betz cell, or a population of such cells, can be studied directly via electrode ('unit') recordings, whereupon motor cell activity can be clearly shown to 'precede' that seen at the periphery (as manifest in the form of electromyography (EMG) signals or overt muscular contractions). In this way, we could justify the statement that corticomotor neurons 'initiated' movement. But what it is that the PMC adds? Actually, unit recordings from PMC cells reveal that the latter demonstrate a wide range of activity profiles, apparently related to different aspects of movement and its timing. Hence, there are PMC cells that exhibit a firing pattern related to the onset of movement – cells that fire when a movement is withheld, others that exhibit directional response profiles, and others still that remain active while a subject (in this case a monkey) holds a response 'on line' (i.e. while he waits for an external cue to move; Passingham, 1993). Therefore, at least on the basis of non-human primate work, the PMC seems pivotal to that aspect of voluntary action that interests us here: the ability of an agent to choose 'when' to act in time. It seems that PMC may 'tell' the motor cortex 'when' to go.

Furthermore, in humans studied using positron emission tomography (PET; and other functional neuroimaging techniques), the activation of the PMC can be shown to be increased under those conditions where a subject has to 'choose' their response, compared with conditions during which a stereotypic sequence will suffice (e.g. Deiber et al. 1991; Passingham, 1993; Spence et al. 1997). In other words, there is greater PMC activity when a human subject chooses the direction in which to move a joystick than there is when they simply follow a pre-specified pattern (e.g. 'keep moving clockwise'). This provides tangible evidence for the role of PMC in choosing the 'identity' (or content) of acts (as well as their 'timing'), albeit under highly constrained experimental conditions.

Additionally, there seems to be a relationship between the temporal 'progress' of an emergent act and the region of PMC that is most activated. While a movement is being prepared, more anterior elements of the PMC appear active, whereas during the ensuing execution (performance) phase greater activity is observed in the posterior PMC (e.g. Stephan et al. 1995). This prompts the suggestion that there is an antero-posterior gradient, progressing from 'programming to execution', within the PMC itself (Passingham, 1997). Indeed, the SMA (medial PMC) can be further divided into two functionally and neuroanatomically distinct regions: an anterior, 'pre-SMA', lying anterior to a line running vertically (upwards) through the anterior commissure of the brain and a posterior portion, SMA 'proper', lying posterior to that same line (Luppino et al. 1993; Rizzolatti et al. 1996; and see Cunnington et al. 2005, for a review of this literature; Figure 26). Pre-SMA exhibits greater activation during motor planning, internally-initiated acts and motor imagery

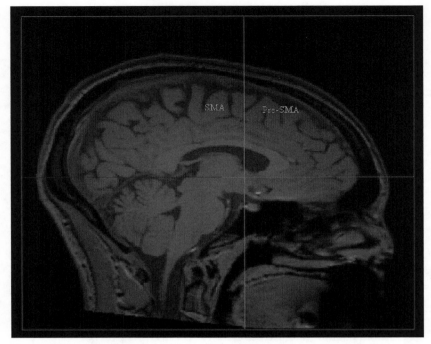

Fig. 26 Structural MRI scan of a healthy human brain showing the approximate position of the supplementary motor area on the medial surface of the frontal lobe (viewed in the sagittal plane). The ascending (green) line shows the plane passing through the anterior commissure. The SMA 'proper' lies behind this line while the so-called pre-SMA lies anterior to it. The pre-SMA exhibits executive properties while the SMA proper is a motor output region, connected to the primary motor cortices. (See colour plate section).

('imagined movements'; and see Chapter 3). SMA proper has a response profile more akin to that of primary motor cortex, with which it is intimately connected. These regions (of SMA) also receive different 'thalamic' innervations: those to pre-SMA arise in dorsomedial and anterior ventral thalamic nuclei (note: dorsomedial afferents also characteristically target the 'higher', prefrontal regions of the brain), whereas the SMA proper receives afferents from the ventrolateral posterior nucleus (of the thalamus; Brunia & Van Boxtel, 2000). Hence, there seem to be good grounds for positing a functional antero-posterior gradient within the SMA (BA 6), from movement planning (in the anterior section) to movement execution (in the posterior section).

Returning to another dichotomy that is drawn between the lateral and medial PMCs (above), it is clear that, in both human and non-human primate literatures, Goldberg (1985) and Passingham (1993) have emphasized regional functional specializations. As already noted, the lateral PMC is most active when external cues are used to guide behaviour. Medial PMC is most active when no cues are available, i.e. when the behaviour has been learned well enough for its execution not to depend upon such (external) prompts (Passingham, 1993; 1997). Monkeys with lesions of the lateral PMC exhibit deficits in motor learning and in recalling the correct response to an environmental stimulus. Monkeys with lesions of the medial PMC exhibit deficits when they have no cues to guide them; they are severely impaired at producing 'self-paced' ('internally initiated') movements.

Similar accounts emerge from the field of human pathologies: we have already seen that lateral parietal-PMC dysfunction may render a patient 'dyspraxic', i.e. unable to copy actions demonstrated to her by her doctor (a human exemplar of a stimulus located in the external environment!); however, in Parkinson's disease we witness a contrasting state of affairs: patients who are unable to initiate 'spontaneous' behaviours (implicating their medial PMC and SMA; e.g. Jenkins et al. 1992). Indeed, people with Parkinson's disease may actually fall back on their 'lateral' systems to enhance their remaining motor activity, e.g. by increasing the visual cues to movement within their external environment (Morris et al. 1996) or in response to sudden visual imperatives (e.g. the 'paradoxical kinesis' observed when an otherwise severely impaired parkinsonian patient is suddenly able to catch a ball that is thrown to them; and see Brown & Marsden, 1998).

That lateral PMC should be particularly concerned with 'learning' movements is also compatible with the specific properties of some of its cells, the so-called 'mirror' neurons. In experiments conducted on non-human primates, these cells have been shown to exhibit activation during the observation of a specific movement, whether the monkey herself, another monkey, or even a human actor performs the movement concerned. Hence, it is the 'act' (the movement) that seems to be represented at the level of the mirror neuron, not the 'agent' (the one who performs that act). It might be argued (again, rather teleologically) that such mirror neurons would be of particular utility during the acquisition (learning) of new skills, new motor behaviours, when the organism must differentiate the (target) act performed from the actor responsible. Such cells offer the possibility of vicarious learning, through imitation (below).

Indeed, if we extrapolate once more to humans, and conjecture that we too possess mirror neurons (and there are grounds for defending this proposition: Gallese et al. 1996; below), then their existence tells us something else that is rather interesting about the brain: when 'we' see someone else performing an action, that action elicits a neural response within us (though 'we' may be subjectively unaware of this and may not necessarily move, explicitly); this (implicit) response relates to a potential act (one that we 'may' perform, in future). (One is reminded, here, of the emotional investment that human observers often have in all sorts of motor performances carried out by others, e.g. the penalty kick undertaken in the course of a soccer match or the closely followed monologue spoken during a film. We are sometimes vicariously involved in others' performances.) However, there are also echoes of this facility in certain human pathological states: if we 'automatically' respond to others' actions (albeit neurologically, implicitly, and unconsciously) then there may be instances when our responses are 'unmasked' – when they may emerge – inappropriately. We see this in schizophrenia, among patients who exhibit the symptoms of so-called 'echopraxia' and 'echolalia': they repeat (i.e. 'echo') the gestures and speech of people around them in their environment; they seem to be unable to 'prevent themselves' from imitating others' behaviours.

Consideration of such phenomena also reveals how important visual information is during the acquisition of motor behaviours, and our anticipation of their deployment in the environment around us. As we noted (above), there is a specific relationship between regions of the PMC and parietal cortex, with the lateral PMC receiving projections from lateral parietal regions, and Jeannerod has stressed how these inputs include 'visual' information about objects in the environment. Neurons in (primate) lateral PMC show specific patterns of response to such incoming information:

1. While most respond to 'object-related *characteristics*' (i.e. those features of the object, such as its shape and size, that influence how it might be held, if handled),

2. Some (the mirror neurons; above) respond to 'object-related *events*' (i.e. those actions that might be performed using such an object, in other words, the uses to which it might be put; Jeannerod, 1997).

In the first case, 'grasping' neurons respond to the physical properties of the object and have a role in programming the particular phases of any subsequent physical response executed by motor cortex towards that object. In the second case, the mirror neurons exhibit a response that correlates with the overall 'action' being undertaken with that object (e.g. taking a peanut from a tray; Gallese et al. 1996; Jeannerod, 1997; above). The recognition of a 'purpose' seems to be implicit to the activation of mirror neurons:

> [T]he important point is that, in order to fire a mirror neuron, the observable hand movement has to be the same as that which would activate that neuron if the monkey performed it. For example, many mirror neurons fire when the monkey grasps a piece of food and also when the experimenter or the other monkey does so. They do not fire . . . when the experimenter makes a grasping movement without food, or when the food is grasped with a tool. . . .

(Jeannerod, 1997, pp. 49–50).

Note how there seems to be yet another form of hierarchy emerging here. Mirror neurons code behaviours that are rather more complex than those coded-for by simple 'grasping' neurons. There is the suggestion that the former code for a coherent act (evincing a 'goal'), as opposed to a component movement (a contingent muscular adjustment, a step towards that goal). This distinction is subtle, but important: it begins to take us towards an account of actions, with 'purposes'. Hence, and to reiterate, mirror neurons encode 'object-oriented actions', independent of the agent performing those actions. Therefore, action ('the act') and agency ('the actor') appear to be at least potentially dissociable within the primate brain; they can be represented separately. This is a very important point; not least, because it opens up a host of evolutionary possibilities. The greatest of these is language.

Moving forward

Now, this moment of realization has provided us with a suitable cue to cease our exploration of PMC and to turn, instead, to the next frontal lobe region that we encounter in our journey across the anterior brain. This next region is one that is crucially implicated in human language generation. I am referring to BAs 44 and 45, also known as Broca's area (though only applied to these regions when they are located within the 'left' hemisphere of the brain), which some investigators believe to have been an evolutionary elaboration of BA 6 (PMC, above). Hence, an area pivotally involved in the programming of hand movements may have 'given rise' to an area crucially involved in speech. Is there any logic to this?

Well, if a brain can distinguish actions from actors, then it has already demonstrated the potential to recognize gestures, signs, and symbols.

> *Gesture:* an action, especially of the hands, which expresses an emotion or is intended to show inclination or disposition; the use of such movements; an action dictated by courtesy or diplomacy …
>
> *Sign:* a gesture expressing a meaning; a signal; a mark with a meaning …
>
> *Symbol:* an emblem; that which by custom or convention represents something else …
>
> (All definitions taken from Chambers, 1997.)

We use these visible signals to transmit information, and that information is potentially independent of its source, its 'transmitter'. What do I mean by this? Well, obviously, there is a transmitter involved: there is the agent, the one who makes the gesture or sign. However, that gesture or sign has an existence independent of that agent: it has a 'meaning'. It is as if the agent has temporarily 'borrowed' the gesture, in order to make their point. Indeed, what gives the gesture its very utility is precisely that it 'can' be shared with others, that they may recognize it. Hence, to return to the metaphor of the message and the medium, the existence of symbolic communication means that messages may be transmitted and exchanged between numerous messengers (media). In other words, there is a basis for language.

So, when a speaker says a word aloud that word is generated in the course of an action (a speech act), but the word spoken also exists communally, independent of its speaker. Indeed, I may use many words without having any conscious recollection of how I first learned them, acquired them, or who it was that first used them in my external environment. Furthermore, this would seem especially likely given the sheer number of words that I am probably holding in my 'word store' – my 'lexicon'; Hagoort (2007) notes that a native English speaker retains approximately 60 000 words. Nevertheless, sometimes, if the word is 'strange enough', then I might recall when or where I first came across it, e.g. 'instantiation' (a word beloved of neuroimaging scientists, but often queried by anonymous reviewers. Our relationship began in the Hammersmith Hospital!).

Now, at least at a theoretical level, the existence of mirror neurons in PMC provides a basis upon which language 'might' have evolved: through neural

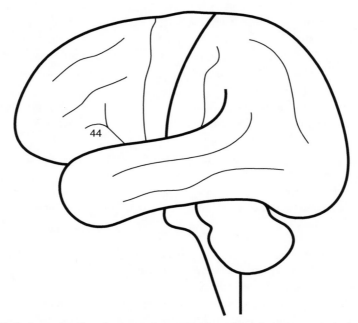

Fig. 27 Cartoon showing the approximate position of Brodmann area 44 in the human brain.

systems that were capable of distinguishing a message from its medium (above).

Broca's area (left Brodmann Areas 44/45)

In most right-handed people, the so-called 'speech centres' are located in the left cerebral hemisphere (see Figure 27; and Indefrey & Levelt, 2000). Indeed, this can be demonstrated nowadays, in healthy living subjects, through the application of modern brain-imaging techniques – i.e. we may 'scan' people while they generate words – and the methods that we use provide us with proxy markers of regional synaptic activity (e.g. Spence et al. 2000; Figure 28). However, the relationship between the left hemisphere and language performance acquired clinical salience when physicians noticed that, if a right-handed person suffered a 'stroke' affecting the right side of their body (thereby implicating the left side of their brain), they often had difficulties with their speech production as well. Hence, speech seemed also to implicate the left hemisphere. The French neurologist Paul Broca is credited with one of the major discoveries in this field, published in 1861, and a number of his close contemporaries made similarly pivotal contributions (their 'early' hypotheses and controversies are eloquently re-examined by MacMillan, 2000, pp. 189–204).

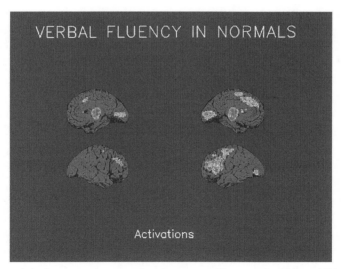

Fig. 28 Statistical parametric maps showing areas of increased activity exhibited by healthy human subjects during the generation of words. There is increased activation in the left dorsolateral prefrontal cortex, the left supplementary motor area, and also the left thalamus. These data were originally reported in Spence et al. British Journal of Psychiatry, 2000, 176, 52–60.

(Nevertheless, one cannot help but wonder whether a similar relation between speech and movement was 'noticed' very much earlier indeed, in 'Biblical times': 'If I forget you, O Jerusalem, let my right hand wither! Let my tongue cleave to the roof of my mouth ...' (*Psalms* 137: 5–6)).

Brain lesions may affect speech and language in several different ways, not all of them solely indicative of left-sided pathology:

1. It might be that a person's speech becomes slurred and physically impeded by paralyses affecting the muscles of their mouth, tongue, and larynx. In this case, the impairment may be attributable to the impact of a stroke (or strokes) upon the descending corticospinal and corticobulbar pathways (remember that the latter innervate the cranial nerve nuclei, and that these in turn innervate the muscles of speech, facial expression, mastication, and swallowing; see Table 2, Chapter 1). So, in this case, speech itself is normal in 'form', i.e. it would probably make sense if it were to be written down *verbatim*; it is its performance, the enunciation of the words, that is impaired. Such impairment is termed 'dysarthria'. It may be caused by a stroke on either side of the brain and also by diseases of the brainstem and cerebellum, i.e. it is not solely a 'left-brain' phenomenon. Note also that while it describes a defect of speech, it simultaneously denotes a preservation of language (the use of symbols in communication).

2. Alternatively, it might be that the 'form' of a person's speech, their 'language', is disturbed. In one case, words may be hard to produce, speech faltering, and the observer can see that the patient 'knows' what they want to say though they cannot seem to say it. They appear frustrated. They have difficulty finding the appropriate words. This is termed an 'expressive' or 'non-fluent dysphasia'. It implicates Broca's area (so-called, but see below), the left-sided BAs 44 and 45, their neighbouring cortical regions (including the anterior insular cortex), and underlying white matter tracts. It is this phenomenon that Paul Broca is credited with being the first to describe (or at least to publicize) in 1861, hence, the condition is also known as Broca's dysphasia (or 'aphasia', when speech is entirely absent). Notice that the lesion implicates the 'left' frontal lobe specifically and also that the patient's problem is with finding words; he seems to 'know' the concept that he wishes to convey (indeed, he is frustrated at being unable to express it); the problem is that he cannot find the appropriate word (symbol).

3. Now, there is another form of frontal dysphasia, which I think is particularly interesting, because it actually serves to show us what Broca's area can do 'by itself' and what it 'requires' other frontal regions to 'help with' (this is, admittedly, a rather gross simplification since all frontal regions are

likely to 'benefit' from their connections with, and contributions derived from, multiple other brain regions, but the example is informative nevertheless). In this 'dynamic' or 'trans-cortical motor' aphasia, a patient suffers a lesion, usually in their left anterior frontal lobe, as a consequence of which they cannot speak 'spontaneously'. However, and this is crucial, they may still be able to 'repeat' the words that are spoken to them by others. Hence, the patient seems to understand language, he detects what others are saying, and he can articulate and repeat their words (i.e. he is not dysarthric and he does not exhibit Broca's dysphasia). His 'problem' seems to be that he cannot initiate 'new' speech, new discourse. There is no originality. The lesion, in such cases, tends to be anterior to Broca's area: in other words, left BA 44 and 45 appear preserved, hence, the patient can speak to repeat words, but he does not create new sentences or new statements. This suggests that even within the left frontal cortex there is a neurological, functional anatomical hierarchy: Broca's area is located relatively inferiorly (or 'downstream') in this system compared with areas anterior to it. Broca's area may be 'necessary' for formally correct speech, but it is not 'sufficient'. Original discourse, having 'something to say' seems to 'require' the contribution of prefrontal regions, areas 'anterior' to Broca's area (Lichteim, 1885; Freedman et al. 1984; Warren et al. 2003; Figure 29).

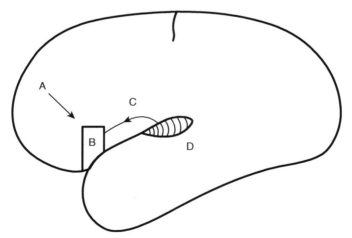

Fig. 29 Cartoon showing the brain areas where lesions produce different forms of dysphasia. A lesion in area A deprives the subject of spontaneous speech. However, they may still repeat words spoken by others. Lesions in area B give rise to Broca's dysphasia, characterized by sparse agrammatical utterences. A lesion in area C (affecting the arcuate fasiculus) affects the subject's ability to repeat words spoken to them. Lesions in area D produce Wernicke's dysphasia, characterized by fluent incoherent speech.

4. Now, consider another condition. In this case, a patient's form of speech might be disturbed thus: he produces a flowing stream of words, an excess of speech in fact, but it does not make sense. Sadly, here, the patient also fails to 'notice' that his speech is incomprehensible. This is called a 'receptive dysphasia', 'receptive' because the patient does not recognize the meaning of 'incoming' words (including his own). He cannot detect that his own speech is confused and disordered. Classically, such a dysphasia implicates a region of the left temporal lobes, traditionally known as 'Wernicke's area', in recognition of Carl Wernicke's (1848–1905) role in the elucidation of this condition: 'Wernicke's dysphasia'. Classically, Wernicke's area comprises the posterior superior and middle gyri of the left temporal lobe (Indefrey & Levelt, 2000). However, the precise regions of the left temporal lobe that are maximally implicated have also been variously described as extending across BAs 41 and 42, and even reaching the left parietal cortex (BA 39 & 40; Standring et al. 2005, p. 400). Hence, there may well be some variation in the regions implicated across individual (pathological) cases. Nevertheless, the existence of such a syndrome tells us something very interesting: that there are specific regions of the cerebral cortex which are pivotal to the interpretation of speech, and that such 'interpretation' seems to encompass 'thought' as well. For, the patient with Wernicke's dysphasia is not only incapable of understanding others' speech; he does not seem to realize that 'his own speech' is disordered; it is as if s/he is 'cut off'– 'disconnected' from the meanings of his own words. This is a deeply curious state of affairs. How can he 'not' know what he is saying? Indeed, it may be even more curious, for, it is not 'just' that such a man does not understand his own words, it is that he does not seem to 'know' that he 'does not know'; he carries on speaking, regardless. (It is as if a visitor to a foreign land continued to speak a language different from that spoken by everyone else and, moreover, that he did not spot the discrepancy because he (unknowingly) understood NEITHER language). Therefore, processes occurring in the region of Wernicke's area, or 'upstream' of it, appear to be implicated not solely in the interpretation of speech but also in our access to our own 'awareness' of its meaning. This entity has been called 'self-monitoring' – a deceptively simple term – aiming as it does to capture deeper considerations of 'higher' 'self-awareness', 'meta-cognition', our awareness of our own awareness.

5. Finally, consider another example. This one relates to the white matter pathways connecting Wernicke's and Broca's areas. We saw (above) that a lesion anterior to Broca's area deprived a person of spontaneous speech though it did not rob him of the ability to repeat others' words. He could

still hear, understand, and repeat what another person said to him. How was this possible? One answer is that an anatomical pathway connects Wernicke's area with Broca's area (it is called the 'arcuate fasciculus') and that it allows incoming auditory data (words) to be decoded and transmitted to Broca's area for their recapitulation as speech acts. (This link can be thought of, psychologically, as comprising the 'articulatory' or 'phonological' loop (Paulesu et al. 1993)). So, while a patient can repeat words accurately we know that each element in this chain is functioning adequately: Wernicke's → arcuate fasciculus → Broca's area. However, what happens if the 'loop' is interrupted, if there is a lesion of the arcuate fasciculus? What happens is that the patient loses the ability to repeat words. He can still speak spontaneously (probably using repetitive, stock phrases, if Broca's area and anterior frontal regions are intact), but he cannot repeat what others say to him.

So, there are multiple ways in which speech may be affected by cerebral disease, and what these varying pathologies serve to reveal is the seemingly specific contribution of Broca's area. Taken at face value (and there are caveats, set out below), Broca's area seems to function as an 'output' region for speech generation – one that is necessary for the production of contextually appropriate words, though it appears to be insufficient for sentence composition *per se* (consider 'dynamic aphasia', above): if one 'loses' areas 'anterior' to BA 44 and 45 (in the 'dominant' hemisphere), then one may lose novel or spontaneous speech. Furthermore, Broca's area seems to be 'released' to 'supply' contextually 'inappropriate' words if Wernicke's area is damaged (consider 'Wernicke's dysphasia', above). Hence, while Broca's area may be necessary for appropriate speech production, it is certainly not sufficient.

Therefore, it becomes possible to understand why Broca's area resembles a premotor region in some investigators' accounts (e.g. Gallese et al. 1996). It is implicated in the 'programming' of speech acts, the selection of words but – in prosaic terms – it does not seem to initiate 'speech goals' (as revealed by dynamic aphasia, above). Indeed, as we noted with respect to BA 6 (above), a premotor region requires two fundamental forms of data:

1. A 'goal' to be reached and

2. A repertoire (or 'tool-box') of practiced responses.

Therefore, we can see that although Broca's area is implicated in deploying such a repertoire of responses ('2', above, i.e. words), it requires still 'higher centres' to formulate speech goals ('1', above, i.e. to 'decide' what we 'want' to say). If we are interested in Dilman's (1999) notion of a 'Will', then the Will behind our spontaneous, freely chosen speech seems to reside at some location 'higher up' within this neurological hierarchy (i.e. it lies 'above' Broca's area).

However, there are important caveats that I should mention. For, it is possible to provide an overly 'neat' account of the contribution of Broca's area to language, and this would misrepresent the empirical data. As we shall see (below), it is likely that Broca's area is *not* the sole repository of those functions that we have just outlined. For instance, it now seems likely that cases of 'Broca's dysphasia' commonly implicate brain regions 'surrounding' left BAs 44 and 45 (indeed, such was the case with Broca's first reported patient, 'Tan'; see MacMillan, 2000, pp. 190–1). So, when we use the term 'Broca's dysphasia' as a descriptor, we may be using it 'accurately' if we do so to describe a certain form of 'language pathology' (i.e. a non-fluent, expressive dysphasia), but we are at risk of using it 'inaccurately' if we automatically assume that this specifies a specific 'focal neuropathology': for the latter is not necessarily located in, or confined to, left BAs 44 and 45; it 'might' involve the underlying white matter, it 'might' involve the left anterior insular cortex. Indeed, more recent brain-imaging findings have suggested that the simple articulation of words (their 'syllabification') may be supported by the left anterior insula and lateral PMC, i.e. it might not 'need' to recruit 'Broca's area' at all (see Wise et al. 1999).

Hence, when we speak anatomically, it is preferable to talk about left BA 44/45 rather than 'Broca's area'. Nevertheless, this is a difficult rule to adhere to because so much of the relevant literature still employs the latter nomenclature.

In terms of its cytoarchitecture, BA 44 comprises a 'dysgranular' cortex with a poorly developed lamina IV (the inner granular layer; Chapter 1) and large pyramidal cells in its lamina III (the outer pyramidal layer). (There is thought to be a homologue (equivalent) of this area in the monkey PMC (see Passingham, 1993; Pandya & Yeterian, 1996; Rizzolatti & Arbib, 1998)). The region receives diverse inputs from prefrontal, cingulate, and lateral PMC regions, somatosensory association cortex (including inferior parietal lobule; human BA 40), and the angular gyrus (parietal cortex; BA 39). It receives minimal visual input from the inferotemporal cortex. However, BA 44 also receives important projections from the superior temporal gyrus (via the 'arcuate fasciculus'; above; the medium via which a person is capable of repeating the words spoken to them by another). Finally, it receives subcortical projections from the thalamus.

The BA 44 itself projects to the primary motor cortex and its electrical stimulation (in non-human primates) elicits face, lip, mouth, and laryngeal movements.

In terms of function, it is possible to propose a distinction between the contributions of the lateral and medial PMCs, as these apply in the context of language generation if we contrast BA 44 (laterally) with SMA (BA 6, medially). The former may be particularly involved in stimulus-dependent speech (e.g. 'naming' objects) while the latter (in common with more anterior prefrontal regions) is especially implicated in 'spontaneous' speech (though this may be something of an over-simplification). Passingham's (1993) view is that language acquisition is the acquisition of 'learned responses', so that lateral speech areas (such as (left) BA 44) subserve conditional learning. (This is in keeping with the view that the 'phonological loop' (the psychological concomitant of the anatomical 'articulatory loop', of which Broca's is the articulatory, rehearsal output region) is involved in language acquisition during the course of human development (i.e. it facilitates the practicing of words and speech; see Baddeley, 1998) and, of course, we may practice words 'in our head', without having to speak them aloud.) Furthermore, 'naming' is disturbed by lesions affecting BA 44, or by its electrical stimulation (though it is also disturbed by stimulation of Wernicke's area and certain thalamic foci; Passingham, 1993). Conversely, spontaneous speech is particularly disrupted by medial lesions, affecting the SMA, medial PMC, and cingulate gyrus. However, patients with medial lesions may still be able to answer questions (Jonas, 1987), prompting Passingham to conclude that:

[W]hen the patient answers questions it is Broca's area speaking.

(Passingham, 1993, p. 254)

This sets up an interesting comparison with the implications of Wise et al.'s (1999) PET study: that when a subject is merely 'repeating' words, it may be their left anterior insula that is speaking!

As alluded to above, Broca's dysphasia is characterized (phenomenologically) by 'agrammatism': patients produce very short phrases, omit connecting words, auxiliaries, and inflexions (Benson & Geschwind, 1985). Impairment and prognosis are worse if the lesion extends anteriorly, beyond the borders of area 44/45 (in the left hemisphere). This is in keeping with functional neuroimaging studies which suggest that, although Broca's area is activated during covert articulation (silent speech; Paulesu et al. 1993), the 'internal generation' of words that are not entirely specified by the experimental protocol involves activation of area 45 and other, more dorsal, prefrontal regions (Frith et al. 1991a; Spence et al. 2000; and see Rajkowska & Goldman-Rakic, 1995).

In other functional neuroimaging studies, 'Broca's area' has been activated by 'inner word generation' (i.e. speaking silently in 'one's mind'; Paulesu et al. 1993; McGuire et al. 1996). Indeed, its activation is augmented by that of the SMA when the 'inner word' to be generated is imagined as being spoken in another's voice (a process termed 'auditory imagery'; McGuire et al. 1996). However, in keeping with the view that Broca's area is an area of PMC, it has also been shown to be activated during purely motor tasks, which are thought to be non-verbal: 'inner sign generation' (among the hearing-impaired; McGuire et al. 1997) and the preparation of limb movements (Krams et al. 1996). A meta-analysis of 10 experiments found that Broca's area supported 'not only the programming of oral/speech movements but also the programming of limb movements' (Fox et al. 1998).

Hence, BA 44 is involved in the programming of responses across motor modalities, in both demonstrably overt and subjectively covert ('silent') protocols. The more demanding tasks (requiring 'internal generation' of responses) seem to recruit other brain regions, e.g. SMA, anterior cingulate, and prefrontal cortex (PFC). These latter regions are also activated during some 'inner speech' tasks (Passingham, 1993; Roland, 1993) including that of imagining the sound of another's voice (McGuire et al. 1996; above). Hence, these regions would appear to be implicated in 'inner speech acts' (the spontaneous 'voice' that we may 'hear' in our 'minds'). (Indeed, for those who subscribe to the existence of a 'conscience', they might well ask: is this 'where' it is? Is one's 'inner voice' instantiated in a pattern of activation reverberating throughout such 'inner speech' areas? Certainly, these regions seem to be implicated in a study of what we might call 'inner prayer' (see Figure 30)).

Frontal eye fields (Brodmann Area 8)

Most of this book is concerned primarily with the control of limb and mouth movements, and their contribution to the performance of complex 'higher' behaviours, in the context of voluntary action. I shall not say very much about the control of eye movements, not because these are unimportant (obviously they are important, for all of us) but because those other literatures contain many of the data that most concern us here. Nevertheless, in order to attempt a balanced account of the frontal lobes' contributions to behaviour, it is essential that I now say at least a little about those frontal regions that are implicated in the control of 'voluntary' eye movements. These regions comprise bilateral BA 8, lying just anterior to the PMCs (BA 6, above).

Whereas the primary motor cortex (BA 4) governs the movement of the limbs and face, the frontal eye fields (BA 8) govern eye movement. Indeed, although they lie just anterior to BA 6, these fields exhibit a radically different pattern of afferent and efferent projections. They receive inputs from all the visual regions of the cortex 'above' (i.e. 'upstream of') the primary visual cortices (located to the posterior of the cortex, in the occipital lobes) and additional widespread inputs arising from inferior and superior temporal regions. Also, the parietal input to the frontal eye fields (in BA 8) is distinct from that projecting to the PMC (BA 6). Whereas the latter receives crucial proprioceptive

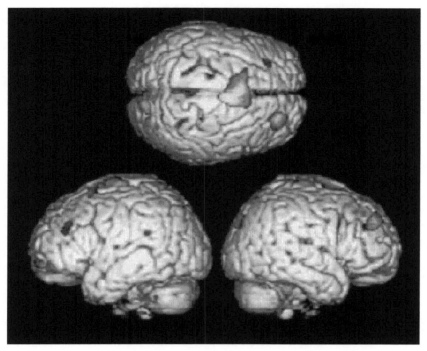

Fig. 30 Data showing those areas of the brain where there is greater activity during 'inner prayer'. Most prominent is the bilateral activation of the supplementary motor area (Brodmann area 6). Taken from *Azari* et al, *'Short Communication. Neural Correlates of religious experience'*, *European Journal of Neuroscience* with permission of Blackwell Publishing. (See colour plate section).

(joint-position sense) information, BA 8 receives rich data from the 'external senses' (e.g. visual and auditory modalities; Passingham, 1993). BA 8 has strong reciprocal connections with the lateral intraparietal area (in the intraparietal sulcus), and both of these (interconnected) areas also project subcortically to the superior colliculi (brainstem nuclei implicated in visual processing and the integration of ocular and bodily movement); hence, they are strongly implicated in the control of 'saccadic' eye movements (those sweeping movements that we make when surveying our visual environments). In contrast, connections with the medial superior temporal area and the fundus of the superior temporal sulcus are implicated in the performance of 'pursuit' eye movements (those responses we engage in when we follow the path of a specific stimulus in our visual field; Milner & Goodale, 1993). Hence, the control of saccadic and pursuit eye movements implicate distinct neural circuits originating within BA 8 (Brunia & Van Boxtel, 2000). The latter also projects to other subcortical regions known to be implicated in the control of eye movements, including the reticular formation and parts of the parvocellular red nucleus (Passingham, 1993).

Passingham (1993) has proposed that there maybe another lateral/medial distinction to be discerned among the functions of the frontal eye fields (akin to that seen within premotor cortex, BA 6, above). Hence, the lateral regions may be more specialized for 'select[ing] things in the outside world' to attend to; and both monkeys and humans with lesions in the lateral BA 8 are poor at voluntarily directing their gaze on the basis of a 'learned' context. The medial region may be more concerned with movements that are not determined by visual targets (Passingham, 1993). (The precise functional localizations of frontal eye field components have been extensively reviewed and critiqued by Paus (1996)). We shall say no more about them here.

Dorsolateral prefrontal cortex (Brodmann Areas 9 and 46)

Now, we move on to consider a region of the PFC that we shall encounter repeatedly throughout the course of this book: the dorsolateral prefrontal cortex (DLPFC), comprising BAs 9 and 46. This region extends over the lateral convexities of both frontal lobes and is an area of 'multi-modal association' cortex, reaching its apogee, its most marked elaboration, in humans.

At present, when we use the term 'multi-modal association' cortex, we mean at least two things:

1. That the DLPFC is capable of processing information from across a wide variety of different neural sources, carrying different modes of information (e.g. visual and tactile data streams), and

2. That it can process such streams of information to create new, 'higher' level, representations (e.g. in the generation of 'novelty'). Hence, it is an area where information may be represented in relatively 'abstract' patterns of data.

In monkeys, area 46 surrounds a structure called the principal sulcus and lies inferior to area 9 (see Figure 31). Both areas are heavily interconnected and share many common afferents and efferents.

Whereas the orbitofrontal (ventral) PFC (see Figure 32; below) receives most of its afferents from the temporal lobe (which can be characterized as being concerned with the 'identity' of objects in the external environment; giving rise to a 'what is it?' information pathway; Ungerleider & Mishkin, 1982; Milner & Goodale, 1993), DLPFC receives its major inputs from the parietal lobe (a locus that may be characterized as being especially concerned with 'spatial' information; giving rise to a 'where is it?' pathway; Figure 32). In the

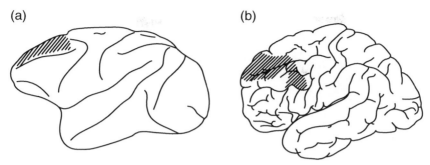

Fig. 31 Cartoons showing the approximate position of the dorsolateral prefrontal cortex (a) in a monkey brain and (b) the brain of a human. Figure 6.2 (p.125) from *"The Frontal Lobes and Voluntary Action" by Passingham, (1993)* with permission of Oxford University Press.

monkey brain, such parietal inputs arise from area 7, an area that also incorporates the monkey homologue of BA 40 (the inferior parietal lobule) found in humans. Parietal inputs carry information about the animal itself (its proprioceptive state, its position in space), the direction of its gaze (originating in the posterior parietal cortex), and the spatial position of objects in the 'outside' world (the latter being coded in 'egocentric' spatial coordinates: their location identified relative to the position of the animal's body). Hence, it follows that the DLPFC is ideally suited for sampling information pertinent to spatial forms of memory (below). (I should re-emphasize: parietal space is coded relative to the body, it is 'egocentric'. For instance: Is the peanut to the right or to the left of me? Is the bigger monkey 'further' to my right? 'Allocentric space', the type of space that we see represented in maps, is itself represented in a different region of the mammalian brain: the hippocampus. Our hippocampi are located within our medial temporal lobes, running along the ventral aspects of both our cerebral hemispheres).

The DLPFC receives additional inputs from the superior temporal convexity, the superior temporal sulcus, and the inferotemporal cortex (Passingham, 1993). Its thalamic afferents originate in the dorsomedial nucleus, the medial pulvinar, ventral anterior nucleus, and the paracentral nucleus of the anterior intralaminar groups. All these nuclei also send projections to ventrolateral PFC (below). Indeed, 'prefrontal cortex' is defined as that cortex which receives its thalamic innervation from the latter's 'dorsomedial' nucleus.

DLPFC sends projections to the PMCs and there are reciprocal connections with lateral and medial areas 6 and 8. DLPFC does not send direct projections to the primary motor cortices (BA 4); hence, its influence must be relayed to this motor output region via intermediaries: the PMC or other, subcortical,

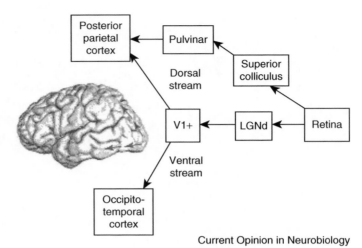

Current Opinion in Neurobiology

Fig. 32 Cartoon showing the organization of the dorsal 'where is it' and ventral 'what is it' pathways of the visual system. The 'where is it' pathway utilizes structures within the parietal cortex to localize a perceived object. The 'what is it' pathway utilizes structures in the temporal lobe to identify the object seen. *Reprinted from Current Opinion in Neurobiology, 14;(2), Goodale & Westwood, An evolving view of duplex vision: separate but interacting cortical pathways for perception and action. 203–211,* © *2004,* with permission from Elsevier Ltd. (See colour plate section).

structures (and these are delineated in more detail in Chapter 4). Descending projections (from DLPFC) target the oculomotor system (supplementing those of BA 8) and the paramedian pontine tegmentum. There are heavy projections to the deep layers of the superior colliculi (again, crucial to visual processing). The latter may also be reached via relays running through the basal ganglia (as may the cerebellum, via relays running through the PMC). Finally, DLPFC sends reciprocal projections to its contralateral homologue, via the corpus callosum, through which it also sends projections to the contralateral inferior parietal lobe.

Hence, to summarize, one notable feature of DLPFC is the rich afferent innervation it receives from the parietal cortex, providing it with visuospatial data concerning the visual world and objects within it (in terms of their coordinates, in egocentric space). The DLPFC also communicates with many other cortical and subcortical 'visual' regions. Another feature is its numerous projections to PMCs (those regions of frontal cortex characteristically concerned with programming actions; above). Hence, the DLPFC is one area that we might expect to be particularly engaged whenever an organism must make its way, or 'choose its steps', through a novel (or hostile) terrain. Hence, we may be reminded of the plight of 'Ralf', a character described in William Golding's novel 'The Lord of the Flies'. At the head of this chapter, we encountered him making his way through a rather forbidding environment:

> Suddenly, pacing by the water, he was overcome with astonishment. He found himself understanding the weariness of this life, where every path was an improvisation and a considerable part of one's waking life was spent watching one's feet.

> The Lord of the Flies

However, DLPFC also has other attributes that make it a prime candidate (region) for involvement in 'determining' what should be done next.

Working memory

The DLPFC is very much implicated in what has been termed 'working memory' (Baddeley, 1986; Goldman-Rakic & Selemon, 1997). The latter refers to those processes supporting the temporary retention of salient information within our conscious awareness, so that it may guide our ongoing behaviour. Classically, working memory retains an average of seven items of data, so it is no surprise that many telephone numbers comprise seven digits! Indeed, a commonly cited example of working memory in action is the scenario enacted by most of us whenever someone tells us a new telephone number. We may hold it 'in our mind' while we use it or write it down. We hold the data 'on line' (actually, we probably rehearse it, through our 'phonological loop', above) as we use it to guide our actions: the right index finger touching the telephone keys in numerical sequence, the precision grip holding the pen, and writing down the salient digits. Again, if we are right-handed, these data (within working memory, reverberating throughout the phonological loop and DLPFC) are being translated into signals that will ultimately impact the motor cortex (the right-hand region, over on the dorsal aspect of the left hemisphere's motor homunculus; Figure 10); then, there will follow that stream of neural activity that we traced throughout the brain and spinal cord in Chapter 1.

Nevertheless, merely rehearsing a telephone number may not necessarily place very great demands upon the DLPFC. The latter is more likely to become engaged if numbers have to be manipulated in some way (e.g. 'now say those seven numbers back to me but, this time, in the reverse order!'). As has been shown in human neuroimaging experiments, there seems to be a lawful increase in activity in DLPFC as working-memory 'load' is increased (see Figure 33). In other words, DLPFC can be shown to 'work harder' as the numerical demands placed upon it are lawfully increased.

Consistent with the above is the finding that, in non-human primates, circumscribed DLPFC lesions are associated with deficits in what are called

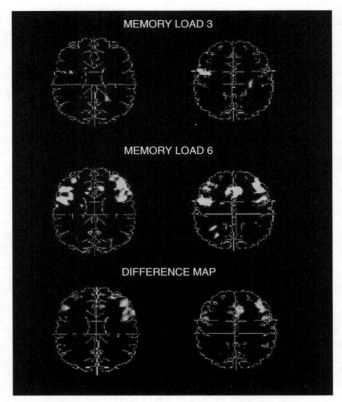

Fig. 33 Data taken from a study by Rypma & colleagues showing that activation within dorsolateral prefrontal cortex increases as working memory load is increased. When subjects are required to recall 6 as opposed to 3 items of information (in working memory) there is greater activity in bilateral dorsolateral prefrontal cortex and also the anterior cingulate cortex (close to the midline). *Reprinted from NeuroImage, 9 (2), Rypma et al. Load-dependent rules of frontal brain regions in the maintenance of working memory, 216–226. © 1999* with permission from Elsevier Ltd. (See colour plate section).

'delayed response' tasks. These are conditional learning tasks in which an animal must choose between spatial locations on the basis of information held within its working memory, e.g. 'where was the peanut?' (Passingham, 1993). Following lesions to the DLPFC, monkeys seem unable to retain spatial memory over the short term. Crucially, the same animals do not evince deficits on tasks that engage memory for object characteristics (see Goldman-Rakic, 1996), serving to emphasize (once again) that there is a distinction between the cortical dorsal stream involved with spatial information (i.e. the putative 'where is it?' pathway) and a ventral stream involved with object information (i.e. the putative 'what is it?' pathway). To reiterate: the monkey with a DLPFC lesion seems to 'know' that he is searching for a peanut, it is just that he 'cannot find it'. He seems to remember the object but not its location.

Notice, also, that this specific deficit simultaneously serves to tell us something rather interesting about the capabilities that are retained while the PMC remains intact. The monkey with a DLPFC lesion (above) may still perform 'actions'; their programming 'mechanism' (PMC) is intact. However, what the animal lacks is a basis upon which to initiate those actions (he does not recall where the peanut is, in space). Hence, he is deprived of an accurate goal. He exhibits a prefrontal deficit (akin to the human beset by a dynamic aphasia, who does not speak, though he can repeat words; above).

'Internal response' generation

Now, many authors have discussed the contribution of DLPFC to response generation and the extent to which there may be functional distinctions between areas 46 and 9, and between these areas and the more ventral prefrontal regions (below). Some have favoured a hierarchical relationship between dorsal and ventral prefrontal cortices (Petrides, 1996), with the former being involved in the 'monitoring' of an organism's responses (including their ability to manipulate and 'self-order' responses, 'on line') while the latter 'actively retrieves' memorized responses from posterior association cortices (including the temporal and occipital regions; see Hagoort, 2007, for the relevance of this latter function to lexical retrieval).

Frith and colleagues attributed 'willed action' to DLPFC on the basis of experiments (conducted in humans) requiring the 'internal generation' of responses in motor and verbal domains (Frith et al. 1991a, b; Table 7). This work involved people choosing 'which' finger to move (in response to a neutral stimulus) or 'which' word to say during a simple verbal fluency protocol (e.g. 'please say any word that you can think of, beginning with the letter "S"'; see Figures 28 and 34). Using both sorts of response modality (finger movement and word generation), it was shown that DLPFC exhibited greater activation during 'self-chosen' responses. (See Figure 35, which demonstrates a similar finding during syllable-generation: the 'La/Ba' experiment).

Novelty, randomness, and repetition

Of course, when we consider the ability of an organism to 'self-order' its responses, especially when there is an added emphasis upon their generating as much 'novelty' as possible (and note: such novelty may comprise both the resulting 'sequence', and/or its component 'items') there will be an 'interaction' between working memory (the ability to hold such components 'in mind',

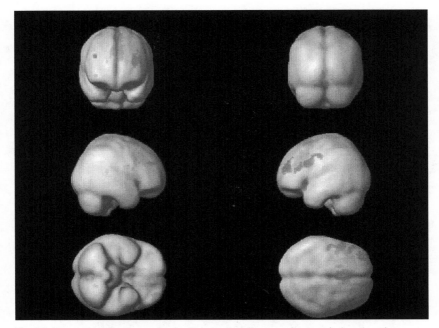

Fig. 34 Data taken from a paper by Spence & colleagues (in press) showing those areas of the brain activated during multiple verbal fluency paradigms. These data were obtained using functional magnetic resonance imaging. Most prominent among the activations are those seen in the left dorsolateral prefrontal cortex, the supplementary motor area and anterior cingulate cortex of the medial prefrontal region and also some activity within the left inferior frontal region. (See colour plate section).

'on line') and the generative ability that the organism is hypothesized to possess, which allows it to manipulate their (the components') order or sequence. What I have just said may seem rather convoluted, so I hope to clarify it through the following example:

Most older children and adults will be able to recite the months of the year in the usual direction, 'going forwards': January, February, March, etc., through till they reach December. This requires minimal working-memory capacity (you just need to keep track of what you've already said so that the stereotypic, over-learned sequence can 'run' by itself, rather like a script or programme).

However, it requires rather greater working-memory resource to recite the months of the year in the reverse order: December, November, October ... and so on back to January. Indeed, it is not unusual to meet adults who cannot perform this task (especially in the context of neurological or psychiatric disease). Therefore, we might consider that we are making the DLPFC and other 'executive' brain regions 'work harder' here, largely because most people's brains will not already

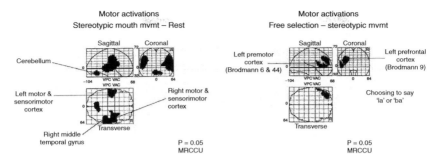

Fig. 35 Data obtained in healthy human males using Positron Emission Tomography. Here, the subjects were called upon to generate the words "la" or "ba" in a fixed sequence or in a sequence of their own choosing. On the left are shown those areas activated when subjects perform the fixed sterotypic sequence (la ba ba la), indicating activity within the premotor and motor regions, corresponding to the face area in the human motor homunculus. There is also prominent activation within the cerebellum (in the midline). On the right is a map showing those areas exhibiting greater activation during the enunciation of a sequence chosen by the subjects themselves compared with activity elicited when they performed the fixed sequence, stereotypic task. There is greater activation within the left dorsolateral prefrontal and also premotor cortices when subjects choose what to say.
These data are taken from studies by Spence et al. 1998

have rehearsed 'saying the months of the year in reverse order', previously; hence, it is not usually a simple case of just 'running the programme'. Most people have probably not spent much time doing this before and so they probably have to construct the programme afresh; they have to think! (Note also, that as well as constructing the 'new' programme they must 'resist' falling into the well-worn, stereotypic, over-learned, sequence; e.g. when they get to 'April', they must follow it with 'March' (going backwards) and not revert to 'May' (as if they were going forwards)).

Now, consider an even worse test of mental function! This time I ask you to recite the months of the year in a random sequence but I stipulate that you must not 're-use' any of them until you have mentioned all of them once. Hence, you must not only randomise the sequence (of 12 items), you must simultaneously keep track of the exemplars that you have already used: January, April, December and so on ... allowing no repetitions at all until all 12 months have been used (spoken) once. This is difficult to do. (For the musically minded, it is rather like being asked to improvise in the style of the Second Viennese School, generating novelty within the constraints of 12-note serialism).

As we make these tasks more difficult, we place greater demands upon working memory ('keeping track of our prior responses' while retaining an awareness of those responses that are currently 'allowed' or 'forbidden'). However, when we introduce an element of self-initiated selection – self-ordering – we stress working memory even further, for, while the subject may 'choose' their response they must also be aware of what they have recently 'chosen'. So, response-generation and working memory are often confounded (i.e. they are often probed concurrently, at the same time) in these sorts of procedures. (To probe 'generation' relatively discretely, in the above case, we might have asked subjects to generate any months, in any order they liked, without worrying about repetitions. In such a scenario, if taken at face value, working memory should have been hypothesized to feature less prominently (though there are caveats; below)).

Now, the extent to which the working memory and 'internal generation' components of such tasks can be adequately differentiated has been a topic of much debate (Spence & Frith, 1999). Can we tease apart those DLPFC regions concerned with 'working memory' and those concerned with 'response generation'? Is this even theoretically feasible?

An insight offered by the primate researcher Patricia Goldman-Rakic (1996) informs this debate; indeed, it also seems to predict the failure of currently available functional neuroimaging techniques to adequately demonstrate such a neat dissociation at the level of relatively large neuronal populations (i.e. within DLPFC). Her insight comes from work in non-human primates, using an 'oculomotor delayed-response task', of the kind alluded to previously, where animals are called upon to remember visuospatial stimuli in order to guide their subsequent motor responses. In other words, in order to be able to move accurately at the next turn, the animal must remember where the salient objects are hidden in their environment; and the item to be recalled is updated on every trial (Goldman-Rakic, 1996). Now, when single-neuron recordings were obtained from the DLPFC (BA 46) during such procedures, multiple classes of neuron were identified and they lay in close proximity to each other: cells engaged in registering the sensory cue, cells engaged in holding the cued information 'on line', and cells engaged in releasing the motor response in the course of an ensuing task performance (whether that task was conducted in the manual or oculomotor domain). Hence:

> [I]n aggregate, DLPFC contains a local circuit that encompasses the entire range of sub-functions necessary to carry out an integrated response: sensory input, through retention in short-term memory, to motor response. Thus, attentional, memorial and response control mechanisms exist within this one area of prefrontal cortex and need not be allocated to separate architectonic regions.
>
> (Goldman-Rakic, 1996, p. 1447)

What this means for the purposes of our journey through the frontal lobes is that it may not be realistic to think that we may discretely localize separate regions of the DLPFC engaged in sensory, mnemonic, and motor components of some voluntary tasks, as they (the cells 'responsible' for subcomponents of such tasks) may be lying in very close proximity to each other. Hence, the sorts of images that we obtain through scanning human subjects may lack the required 'resolution' (spatial discrimination) to tell such areas apart. A technique that can only resolve neuronal populations at the level of several millimetres will not differentiate neurons that are literally lying 'side-by-side'. Hence, it would be difficult to separate activations attributable to 'internal-generation' from those due to 'working memory' using conventional functional neuroimaging techniques (the relevant neuronal populations would be likely to 'overlap').

Goldman-Rakic also goes on to present evidence for the activity of certain DLPFC neurons actually predicting 'failure' on the delayed-response task (when a memory-related activation decays 'too soon'), and for some neuronal circuits being concurrently involved in the initiation *and* inhibition of motor responses. Hence, she posits that the 'central executive' (one of the terms that psychologists have used to describe the higher 'control' processes of the human brain; in a model posited by the British psychologist Alan Baddelely; Table 7) may actually comprise multiple central executives – each 'domain-specific' and anatomically distinct. A 'spatial' central executive might be located in the DLPFC, whereas a central executive involved in 'responses made on the basis of object-related characteristics' might be located in the ventral, orbitofrontal cortex (OFC, utilizing the contribution of the ventral, 'what is it?' pathway; above); and verbal and semantic responses might be generated in infero-lateral prefrontal cortex (BA 45; Goldman-Rakic, 1996).

However, Golman-Rakic's conceptualization of prefrontal executive processes has been questioned by some, including Petrides (1996), who disputes her parcellation of these processes between 'domain-specific' regions of the PFC. Instead, Petrides provides evidence that the DLPFC is implicated in the 'monitoring' and manipulation of responses, independent of their information domain (their content, i.e. whether data are 'spatial' or 'object-related'). Petrides and colleagues have used a 'self-ordering' task to examine DLPFC function, in which the subject determines the sequence in which they select from among given stimuli in their environment. Thus, the selection is 'internally generated' (in Frith's terms, above), but also relies upon working memory for the 'monitoring' of previous responses (since, rather like our third 'months of the year' example, above, the subject may not choose a stimulus twice before all the other stimuli have been selected once). This Petrides task activates the DLPFC.

Furthermore, in humans, there are multiple lines of evidence supporting a role for DLPFC in 'self-initiated' selection, the 'internal generation' of action. Damage to the DLPFC in humans can lead to a lack of spontaneous speech and activity, distractibility by environmental stimuli (implying a lack of cognitive 'control'), and the repetitive, stereotypic use of inappropriate behavioural responses: 'perseveration' (Milner, 1963; here, perseveration refers to the repeated use of a behavioural response that has become contextually inappropriate). Hence, if I ask someone to produce as many words as possible, within 1 minute, beginning with the letter 'S', then I might be pleased to receive the following sequence (Freudians should now avert their gaze):

> Safe, satisfy, sartorial, sadist, smug, sausage, stench, syphilis ...

However, the following pattern would be regarded as perseverative:

> Safe, save, safe, safe ... safer, safest, safe ...

Perseverative responses have also been called 'defaults' by Goldman-Rakic and Selemon (1997). Such phenomena suggest an inability, on the part of the subject, to escape recurrent, habitual patterns of responding, in order to choose or initiate a correct (new) course of action. Hence, the organism falls back on what has gone before; their responses are intrinsically repetitive. Neuropsychological studies have reported such disturbed initiation of action sequences in the presence of left DLPFC lesions in particular (Petrides & Milner, 1982), and experimental studies in primates have provided congruent findings (Passingham, 1993).

In summary, a number of lines of empirical evidence support the role of PFC, and DLPFC in particular, in the initiation of 'novel' streams of behaviour, and the suppression of 'stereotypic', 'default', or 'perseverative' modes of responding. If we are thinking hierarchically, then DLPFC is a candidate region of interest when it comes to considering how a 'normal', 'healthy' subject goes about her daily life, initiating new behaviours, engaging in activities where the ability to produce varied, elaborated responses may be desirable. Consider conversation, elaboration, even exaggeration! Our conversations are potentially 'infinite' in the variety of response-combinations (i.e. word sequences) that they may require of us. Hagoort (2007) notes that our 'attentional control' allows 'individuals to speak while seeing irrelevant objects or hearing interlocutors [in their environment]; to take turns in conversational settings; or, in the case of bilingualism, to select the correct language in a particular communicative setting' (p. 244). We are capable of doing so many things 'at the same time'. Our interactions deteriorate drastically if we are reduced to using single words (e.g. the 'Tan' of Broca's canonical case). Indeed, DLPFC is one of those regions, anterior to 'Broca's area' (i.e. left BA 44/45), where lesions may precipitate dynamic aphasia: a person repeats what others say but cannot initiate spontaneous speech (Figure 29). Hence, DLPFC seems to be very much implicated in 'choice'. (Note: there has been a very recent report of another primate – the 'putty-faced' monkey, *Cercopithecus nictitans* – deploying a very simple choice repertoire, comprising building blocks of just two forms of utterance (i.e. two sounds), to communicate with his conspecifics in their natural habitat. It is interesting to speculate regarding the demands that this mode of communication places upon his cognitive system: in order for its performance to be successful, the monkey requires an ability to recall two items of utterance, an ability to manipulate their sequence, and an understanding of their symbolic meaning, within a 'community' of other monkeys. Apparently, 'pyow-pyow' means that there is a leopard coming! (Arnold & Zuberbuhler, 2008)).

Humans have difficulty avoiding response regularities

Now, if we continue to dissect what the DLPFC is doing during the generation of human 'choice', then much will depend upon our understanding of the 'precise' instructions that were given to experimental subjects at the beginning of each study. For, in the protocols that I have just referred to (above) concerning the 'random' recitation of the months of the year, and the Petrides 'self-ordering' task, subjects were allowed to 'choose' the sequence of their responses, albeit while having to 'bear in mind' those responses that they had already given since they were *not* allowed to repeat themselves until all potential exemplars had been selected (e.g. all 12 months of the year). However, in other protocols, such as the verbal (orthographic, letter) fluency paradigm (above), the subjects were *never* allowed to repeat themselves, though they did have much larger potential 'set' sizes to choose from (e.g. all the words that they might remember beginning with the letter 'S'). To draw a further distinction, there are verbal and motor response paradigms where the constraints upon subjects seem to be much less taxing, where they are called upon to generate 'novelty' albeit without the need to 'worry' about repeating an exemplar, e.g. in the 'La/Ba' protocol (see Figure 35), the finger movement protocol of Frith and colleagues, and the various versions of the joystick protocol reported in the PET literature emerging from Hammersmith Hospital in the 1990s (e.g. in papers by Deiber, Jenkins, Playford, and other colleagues of Passingham; where there were usually four joystick directions to choose from). In these latter cases, one might imagine that the demands upon the DLPFC are actually quite different again (from those stipulated above): the emphasis is upon 're-ordering' and manipulating relatively few exemplars (rather than having to search the whole lexicon for words beginning with the letter 'S' and never repeating them); and it requires only a very short-term recall of what has gone before (in order to facilitate, short-term 'novelty'; Deiber et al. 1991; Jenkins et al. 1992; Playford et al. 1992; and Spence et al. 1997). So, although many of these experimental approaches share superficial similarities (e.g. the required generation of novel sequences of responses), on closer inspection it is clear that subjects must obey rather different rules during each procedure for the generation of such (apparent) novelty.

Now, it has been noted by Baddeley & Della Sala (1996) that the generation of 'truly random' responses 'should' actually place relatively little load upon human working memory because, in a truly random sequence, each successive response 'should' be entirely independent of those preceding it. If you roll a die it does not matter whether a 'six' appeared on the last occasion when you rolled it (or, indeed, the last 20 occasions), there is still a one in six probability that this event may occur again. Two throws of the die are statistically independent events. Hence, a human subject might expect to generate a 'truly' random sequence of responses by deliberately *not* considering what she had just said, rather as if she were throwing a die (or pulling lottery balls from a hat, and 'then immediately replacing those that had been called').

However, though this 'could' and 'should' be the case in theory, it seems, on the balance of empirical evidence, that this is *not* how human beings behave in reality. When humans generate 'randomness' (or, rather, attempt to generate their best approximation of randomness) they can be shown to be utilizing working-memory resources, indeed, to be 'constrained' by the limits of those resources (Baddeley, 1966). They introduce biases into their responses by avoiding (obviously) stereotypic patterns (patterns which, of course, might have arisen 'simply by chance' under 'truly random' conditions, e.g. strings of consecutive numbers: see the work of Jahanshahi, described below). Hence, our actions tend to be 'pseudo-random', at best. In other words, we *do not* behave like random-number generators or lottery machines (even when we are asked to do so), we *are* influenced by the identities of those responses that we have recently made: our actions are *not* truly independent of each other, in time (and we shall return to Baddeley's work in this area; in Chapter 10). So, to be explicit, *the human organism has a limited capacity to produce 'truly' random response sequences because the influence of recent responses impacts the generation of subsequent responses; they are not truly independent events. Hence, we humans evince what might be called 'response regularities'.*

Now, this characteristic of human novelty generation can be further elucidated empirically using 'dual task' protocols, in which subjects are called upon to generate random responses at the same time as performing another cognitive task, one that is known to place extra demands upon working-memory capacity. For instance, one might ask a subject to generate a random sequence of motor responses at the same time as performing a verbal fluency paradigm. So, while the randomness of motor acts, made using a joystick, might have been assumed to have placed very little demand upon working-memory resources (one is, after all, free to 'repeat' recent movements, i.e. there is no prohibition upon repeating oneself), 'randomness' is nevertheless found to be diminished under such dual-task conditions, suggesting that the attempted generation of random responses 'competes' for (working-memory) resources with other non-habituated tasks. Indeed, Passingham (1996) has reported experiments showing that if a novel motor task and a verbal fluency task are performed concurrently, their mutual interference impacts prefrontal (and anterior cingulate) cortical function. Furthermore, such interference is *not* exhibited once one of the tasks has become automated, i.e. routine. (Parenthetically, this concurs with a body of human functional neuroimaging data demonstrating that DLPFC is engaged during the learning of new motor tasks, but no longer engaged when such tasks have become routine (e.g. Jenkins et al. 1994; Passingham, 1997). This also has implications for related neural circuitry (see Chapter 4)). So, although we are not able to generate truly random response sequences we, nevertheless, expend working-memory (prefrontal cortical) resources upon trying to do so. Hence, we might predict that we should be even worse at generating randomness (and by extrapolation, novelty) if prefrontal resources are diverted during dual-task protocols or impaired, in other ways.

Therefore, it is interesting to consider the evidence provided by a study utilizing transcranial magnetic stimulation (TMS), which has demonstrated that the left DLPFC plays a specific role in the 'attempted' generation of random responses (compared with right DLPFC and medial PFC; Jahanshahi et al. 1998). In this study, when healthy subjects were asked to generate random numbers orally, they tended to exhibit certain characteristic response patterns (or regularities) while attempting to comply with 'randomness' (e.g. they tended to avoid producing 'stereotypic' sequences of consecutive numbers, such as '1, 2, 3, . . .'; even though such sequences would have been permissible, as they *could* theoretically have occurred under 'chance' conditions). Hence, these subjects generated a form of 'pseudo-randomness', avoiding what they may have thought of as most obviously stereotypic. However, when TMS was applied over the left DLPFC, to briefly disrupt its function, the effect was that subjects generated *more* of these habitual responses (i.e. they emitted more 'consecutive' number sequences). A simple interpretation of this experimental finding is that TMS briefly 'turned off' left DLPFC. As this effect led to a more habitual pattern of responding, it suggests that left DLPFC was originally implicated in trying to inhibit such routines (habitual patterns), allowing subjects to at least attempt 'randomness' (by suppressing 'obvious' response patterns and thereby generating pseudo-randomness). Thus, when such inhibition was interfered with (transiently, by TMS), the subjects reverted to more habitual patterns of response (consecutive numbers, 1, 2, 3, etc., rather than their former pseudo-randomness).

To produce real 'randomness' is difficult for human subjects (as demonstrated in Baddeley's seminal 1966 experiments, which we shall reconsider in Chapter 10). Indeed, Jahanshahi and colleagues situate their findings within a 'neural network' model of response generation, whereby cues to respond, arising in the external environment, initially activate habitual response patterns but then these stereotypic patterns undergo modulation (i.e. they are made 'less' habitual) by the action of a 'higher' 'controller'. This 'controller' 'tries' to prevent the organism from lapsing into habitual (stereotypic) patterns of response. For random (oral) responses, Jahanshahi et al. (1998) locate their controller in left DLPFC (implicating BA 9; Table 7). Hence, it is not that the DLPFC generates novelty *per se*, but that it suppresses the 'predictable'.

Notice also that the effect of TMS (when applied over left DLPFC) on the attempted generation of randomness is similar to that seen when healthy subjects are called upon to 'dual task' (above), or when patients with Parkinson's disease or schizophrenia attempt to generate randomness (without TMS; see Spence & Frith, 1999): hence, a similar neural substrate and accompanying cognitive deficit (affecting the hypothetical 'controller') may be hypothesized to pertain in each of these cases. If the controller is defective, then the performer (the subject, the actor) may have greater difficulty suppressing stereotypic responses; they may end up resorting to a form of 'default' setting (as posited by Goldman-Rakic & Selemon, 1997; above). (In subsequent chapters we shall examine some salient neuropsychiatric disorders and their respective impacts upon prefrontal function in greater detail).

Furthermore, functional neuroimaging studies of healthy people have demonstrated that placing 'excessive' cognitive demands upon such executive processes may actually 'reduce' prefrontal activity (Goldberg et al. 1998; Figure 36). So, a 'controller' may fail because of disease or because it is required to do 'too much'; i.e. there are finite constraints upon executive resources (a subject that we shall return to in Chapter 10).

A pause, for timing

Now, in many of the studies that we have just described, subjects were allowed to select for themselves 'which' movements or responses to make, although they were 'temporally' constrained by having to make those movements at

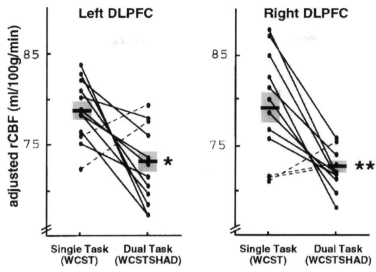

Fig. 36 Data taken from a positron emission tomography study by Goldberg & colleagues. When healthy subjects were asked to perform a single executive task (the Wisconsin Card Sort Test) they increased activation within bilateral dorsolateral prefrontal cortex (DLPFC). However, when they had to perform two executive tasks at the same time their bilateral DLPFC activations were reduced, in most cases. This illustrates an apparent decompensation when executive regions are required to perform more than one task at a time. *Reprinted from Goldberg et al 1998, NeuroImage, 7: 296–303* with permission from Elsevier Ltd.

particular moments in time, e.g. in response to an auditory (or tactile) pacing signal. Hence, although they chose the 'identity' of their response, they did not determine its 'timing'. There is, however, an alternative paradigm (one that is much more akin to Benjamin Libet's experiments; see Prologue) in which subjects are told 'which' movement to make, while being left free (i.e. 'allowed') to make that movement 'whenever they wish'. Jahanshahi and colleagues (1995) showed that when human subjects selected the moment at which they made their movements, this was also associated with activation of the DLPFC (and we have demonstrated a revision of this finding over shorter temporal durations; see Figures 24b and c). Hence, we may conclude that the DLPFC plays a substantial role in the generation of novel movement sequences and that it is activated when there is an element of 'choice'; whether that choice primarily concerns the identity of the movement that may be made or the time at which such a movement may occur (Passingham, 1997).

Indeed, a plausible account has been offered suggesting that DLPFC may help to formulate action 'plans' (or goals), while specific motor commands are 'delegated' to premotor regions for 'programming' (Passingham, 1993; 1997; Jeannerod, 1997). This notion is also compatible with data derived from single unit recordings (in animals) showing that movement-related DLPFC activity actually *precedes* that seen in premotor and subcortical regions (Goldman-Rakic et al. 1992; Passingham, 1993). Hence, the 'higher' 'controller' activates 'first'. However, all these data prompt a further question: By what mechanism does the PFC 'select' only one course of action from among a multitude of potential choices? One possibility (again consistent with the 'randomness' and TMS data described above) is that most behavioural outputs undergo 'inhibition' by DLPFC so that one 'single appropriate act' emerges (Goldman-Rakic, 1987). This formulation is also consistent with the observation that patients sustaining damage to the PFC are often unable to inhibit inappropriate responses to their environment (and I shall say more about this problem when we consider the ventral prefrontal regions; below).

Finally, if we recall our comments towards the beginning of this chapter, concerning the possible existence of a hypothesized 'Will', then we can see that an aspect of that Will, emphasized especially by Locke, and Dilman, was its involvement in 'choice'. Without choice the Will would appear to be redundant. So, while we have not proven the existence of such a Will, and while we should not suggest that DLPFC acts in some kind of neurological vacuum (on its own), we may now postulate that the DLPFC is a region that is implicated in the biology of choice, so that if a 'Will' were to exist, this is one region that could be pivotal to its function. The data that we have just examined (at some length) suggest that DLPFC plays a part in 'choice', especially when there are discernible (behavioural) 'alternatives'.

Anterior cingulate cortex (including Brodmann Areas 32 and 24)

So far, we have devoted a great deal of space to the issue of response selection, to what it is that allows us to choose between response 'alternatives'. However, there is another aspect of action that we have largely neglected: attention to the act itself. How is it that we can be aware of what we are doing, what our choices are, and the consequences of our ensuing acts? The next region that we come to in our progress through the frontal brain – the anterior cingulate cortex (ACC) – is one that is particularly important in this context. Among its other roles, it contributes to attention, response conflict, and error monitoring, and it is implicated in our awareness of pain. It also seems to be pivotally involved in the motivation or drive 'towards action' – a quality that we may relate to that other aspect of the (hypothesized) Will that was mentioned at the very

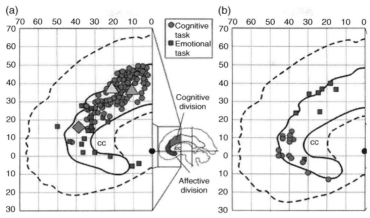

Fig. 37 Diagrams taken from a paper by Bush & colleagues demonstrating the cognitive and affective divisions of the anterior cingulate cortex. The dorsal cognitive division is activated during cognitive tasks (shown on the left, a, in red). During the same tasks there is relative deactivation of the affective division of the anterior cingulate cortex (shown on the right, b, also in red). In contrast, during affective or emotional tasks there is activation of the affective division (shown in blue on the left, a), with accompanying deactivation of the dorsal, cognitive division, (shown in blue on the right, b). Hence there seem to be opposing patterns of activity according to the nature of the task that the anterior cingulate is called upon to 'support'. With permission from Elsevier Ltd.

beginning of this chapter: the Will as some form of 'power' or 'urge' to continue acting, 'Willing'.

The cingulate gyrus comprises a swathe of grey matter running along the medial surface of each hemisphere, above the corpus callosum (that bundle of white matter fibres that we mentioned previously, connecting the cerebral hemispheres with each other; Chapter 1; Figure 7). The cingulum is involved in a great many important processes and exhibits regional sub-specializations. For the present, we shall be mostly concerned with the ACC – that region which is situated ventral (below), rostral (in front of), and dorsal to (above) the anterior corpus callosum (see Figure 37).

In terms of its cytoarchitecture, the ACC exhibits particularly large pyramidal cell neurons in its lamina V (the internal pyramidal layer; Chapter 1; Figure 8), which project into voluntary motor systems (Devinsky et al. 1995). Indeed, the ACC shares functional similarities with the PMC and SMA in that it is involved in the programming of voluntary motor responses. However, the ACC *also* modulates 'autonomic' (involuntary, homeostatic) activity associated with affective (emotional) behaviours and response selection (of which, more below). Furthermore, in human functional neuroimaging studies this area is particularly activated when responses require the subject's conscious 'attention' to action (see Passingham 1996 & 1997 for reviews), and when habitual (or 'pre-potent') responses must be 'suppressed' or inhibited (e.g. Bench et al. 1993). So, almost immediately, we may discern a very different set of capabilities emerging from this pivotal region of the frontal cortex: a mixture of the voluntary and the automatic, the attended to and the suppressed.

Hence, it is of little surprise, that in terms of its connections, ACC 'samples' inputs from more thalamic nuclei than any other cortical region (Devinsky et al. 1995); indeed, this may facilitate its contribution to appropriate response selection. Also, there are strong reciprocal connections between ACC and dorsal, middle, and inferior PFCs; thus, it may be difficult to differentiate the contributions of the ACC and PFC to non-routine behaviours in the brain scanner, as they often co-activate together (e.g. Frith et al. 1991a, b; Spence et al. 2000; reviewed in Passingham, 1996). As it forms a kind of bridge or intermediary between emotional (limbic) and voluntary motor systems, the ACC has also been conceptualized as helping to translate 'intentions into actions' (constituting a place 'where motor control, *drive* and cognition interface'; Paus, 2001; italics added).

In terms of its own organization or structure, one influential classification posits a dichotomy between a ventral, 'affective', component of the ACC, with projections to and from the rostral limbic system, and a dorsal, 'cognitive', component, with projections to and from the voluntary motor system (Devinsky et al. 1995; and see Figure 37). Both these systems may be relevant to the performance of 'willed acts', and, indeed, Devinsky and colleagues (1995) have interpreted the effects of damage to the ACC as constituting reduced 'emotional will power' (see Table 7).

The ACC's proposed 'cognitive' component comprises caudal BA 24 and BA 32 – the cingulate motor areas in the cingulate sulcus and nociceptive cortex (the latter involved in pain processing). These areas project to the spinal cord and red nucleus and have premotor functions. The ACC's affective component comprises BA 25, 33, and rostral 24, has extensive connections with the amygdala and periaqueductal grey, and projects to autonomic brainstem motor nuclei (see Table 2). Focal electrode stimulation of these areas leads to autonomic arousal. The affective ACC is concerned with:

> regulating autonomic and endocrine functions . . . conditioned emotional learning, vocalizations associated with expressing internal states, assessments of motivational content and assigning emotional valence to internal and external stimuli, and maternal–infant interactions.

> (Devinsky et al. 1995, p. 279)

This is certainly a wide-ranging, and complex, portfolio.

Lesions acquired by humans rarely localize so discretely as to fit 'neatly' within this proposed scheme, though the importance of the ACC to action can occasionally be revealed by focal pathology. Patients with ACC lesions may develop 'akinetic mutism'. They are still and silent. If they recover, they may report that at the time of their affliction (i.e. while mute), they had lacked the feeling that they had anything to say. Not only was their mind blank, but they also lacked the 'drive' to communicate. Hence, Damasio and Van Hoesen (1983) report a woman with a left cingulate–SMA lesion who 'felt no will to reply'. In general, such mutism is transitory unless the lesion extends beyond the ACC.

Anterior cingulate cortex lesions can also produce other impairments of action: neglect of hemispace (that half of the external environment contralateral to the ACC affected), the emergence of automatisms (repetitive, seemingly 'unconscious' behaviours witnessed by others during attacks of cingulate epilepsy), 'manneristic' behaviour (the strange or unusual performance of a quasi-purposeful act, which may also be seen during such a seizure, i.e. 'ictally'), and a lack of control over affective responses ('inter-ictally', between seizures). The latter manifests as outbursts of anger, aggression, or violence (Devinsky et al. 1995). Seemingly conversely, lesions of ACC may also reduce responsivity to pain (it may be felt, but not attended to) and can impair social interactions (e.g. maternal–infant behaviours in primates).

Furthermore, if a lesion extends beyond the ACC, into the orbitofrontal PFC (below), then it may have profound effects upon the 'quality' of behaviours that are exhibited by humans. They may become 'sociopathic' or 'socially agnosic', developing a 'blunted' or 'shallow' affect, apathy, impulsivity, disinhibition, sexually deviant behaviour, and a 'lack of judgement or common sense' (Devinsky et al. 1995). Unsurprisingly, their social lives may be radically affected. Indeed, when studied in the laboratory environment, such subjects may evince a lack of 'normal' autonomic responses to emotionally arousing visual images, e.g. those of mutilation. (Damasio et al. 1990; Damasio, 1994).

Hence, it could be argued that the ACC damage (albeit possibly in association with dysfunction extending beyond its anatomical boundaries) precipitates a form of disordered 'Will', both with respect to a failure to generate actions (which fail to be initiated due to a lack of 'willpower') and/or a 'successful' choice of the 'wrong' action (which may be morally deviant, relative to the choices that the same person would have 'made' previously, in health).

So it seems that we have now migrated along a functional, neurological gradient, from the lateral motor systems, where the (pathological) disturbances of function that we noted were very much to do with the 'mechanics' of volition (e.g. the ability to sculpt hand gestures in the dyspraxias, the ability to find the 'right' word, or symbol, in Broca's dysphasia, and the failure to remember where to 'move next' following lesions of the DLPFC), to qualitatively different forms of pathology implicating medial and/or ventral frontal systems, e.g. not having the 'Will', the 'drive', to care to act, or choosing what is morally 'wrong' ('deviant'; Devinsky et al. 1995). Hence, *medial systems seem to bring a new dimension to our considerations of 'choice'*: they seem to imply a tacit neurobiological 'recognition' (at some level) that there is a 'correct' way of behaving, under 'normal' conditions. They seem to suggest that 'normal' biology can code (in some way) for 'norms' of behaviour, and that such 'norms' may be transgressed following focal brain lesions. This is a potentially controversial inference, and we should be careful not to reify social and cultural strictures, or to assume automatically that 'Nature' 'recognizes' the same moral or ethical boundaries that societies do (at any given place and time). Nevertheless, there is no escaping the fact that medial (and ventral) brain lesions affect human behaviour in ways quite different to those occurring after lesions of the more lateral (and dorsal) cerebrum. This is all quite a departure from simply flexing and extending one's right index finger (Chapter 1)!

Orbitofrontal (ventral) prefrontal cortex

If the ACC is implicated in our hypothetical 'Will' (partly as a consequence of 'supporting' some form of energy, willpower, or drive, towards action) then the OFC seems to be particularly relevant to attributing relative 'value' to those objects or targets (in the environment), towards which such a 'Will' might strive. (Hence, it is not so much the drive towards action as the valence of its 'goal' that is pertinent here).

The OFC, lying directly above the orbits of the eyes, and extending medially towards the anterior cingulate, has attracted much interest recently because it has been hypothesized to play a role in the modulation of action by 'reward' and social 'context' (Figure 38). Furthermore, it was among those brain regions probably affected in the famous case of Phineas Gage, a man whose personality was radically altered as a consequence of a railroad construction accident, during which an explosion drove a 'tamping iron' through his head (Damasio, 1994; Figure 39). The iron entered under his left cheek and exited over the vertex of his skull. Remarkably, he survived, although he was said to be 'no longer Gage'. His personality had been affected (see Macmillan, 2000, for an authoritative account of his case). Now, in modern times, it has been suggested that deficits in orbitofrontal and ventromedial PFCs may underlie the cognitive neurobiology of acquired sociopathy (Damasio, 1994; a subject to which we shall return in Chapter 9).

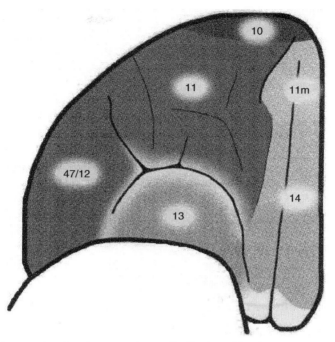

Fig. 38 Cartoon showing the approximate distribution of Brodmann areas on the inferior surface of the right orbitofrontal cortex in humans. Brodmann area 10 is located anteriorally at the frontal pole. Brodmann area 47 is located laterally on the inferior surface of the frontal lobe. Taken from Petrides and Makey (2006; see refs) with permission from Oxford University Press. (See colour plate section).

The OFC includes BAs 13 (caudally), 14 (medially), and 12 and 11 (moving from caudal to anterior along the lateral convexity of the prefrontal lobe; see Figure 38). These areas receive afferents from the thalamus (the dorsomedial, anteromedial, ventral anterior, medial pulvinar, paracentral, and midline nuclei), the amygdala, and other regions within the temporal lobe (carrying information concerning the 'identity' of objects in the external environment). The OFC itself projects to the amygdala and hypothalamus (and is implicated in the control of aggression). Hence, stimulation of the OFC leads to autonomic arousal; and animals will work to receive such stimulation (or a local infusion of drugs; Passingham, 1993). The region receives information regarding all the senses deriving from the temporal lobe. One particularly important aspect of OFC function is its role in learning and reversal (or 'extinction') of stimulus–reinforcement associations, on the basis of reward; a function which is elegantly described with respect to taste, olfaction, and other senses by Rolls (1996).

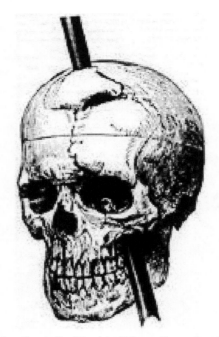

Fig. 39 Image showing the skull of the late Phineas Gage, also demonstrating the trajectory of the tamping iron which entered his skull underneath the left maxilla and exited over the vertex. Hence, maximal damage was probably inflicted upon his left frontal lobe. *J. M. Harlow (1868). Recovery from the passage of an iron bar through the head. One of three figures from Harlow's 1868 paper.*

Indeed, in order to understand what is 'going on' within the OFC, it may be helpful to consider just such an example, and to contrast what we mean by different types of 'taste centre'.

Taste and satiety

A 'primary' taste centre is located within the frontal operculum and insula (Rolls, 1996). Its cells respond to the taste of food, in a way that is unaffected by hunger or satiety. So, no matter what the state of the organism (i.e. whether it is 'hungry' or 'full') food still evokes a specific response in this region. However, in contrast, in a 'secondary' taste area, located within OFC, there are taste neurons whose response is predicated upon the animal's state of satiety: hence, these neurons fire when a taste is presented, *if the animal is hungry*, but not if the taste is presented in the context of satiety. Thus, their activation can be equated with the 'reward' value of a taste currently represented in OFC (Rolls, 1996). There is, therefore, an important distinction between the functions of primary and secondary taste centres, and it may be argued that – from a hierarchical perspective – the latter area is doing something rather more complex and strategically important than the former, in the context of the animal's survival. The secondary taste centre (in OFC) changes its response, not according to the stimulus perceived (in the external environment; after all, a peanut is still a peanut!) but according to the 'internal state' of the organism (i.e. whether or not it is 'hungry'). Hence, if other sensory (and hedonic) systems were to function in a similar manner, then the OFC would be ideally adapted towards supporting 'contingent' behaviours: activities that change according to the 'desires', wants, and rewards pursued by the organism (the agent or actor).

As already noted, the OFC receives information from the ventral, 'what is it?' data stream – information to be processed according to the reward-value of the object represented. Visual and taste information converge upon common neural populations and the neural response to a shape, associated with a certain taste, may be rapidly changed if that taste changes (hence, eliciting a change in reinforcement). Cells in the OFC are specialized for rapidly acquiring stimulus–response associations, relating external objects to their reward-value, and also for detecting a change to 'non-reward' states. The latter demand a change in behaviour. Activation of 'non-reward' neurons (of which there are different types) is also likely to lead to behavioural extinction or reversal (Rolls, 1996). Put more prosaically: when you are no longer hungry, it is time to put down the peanuts. ... Values change, rewards are inherently transient.

Changing contexts

The OFC projects subcortically to the ventral head of the caudate nucleus and other components of the ventral striatum, and lesions in all these regions (OFC, caudate, striatum in general) may impair behavioural reversal (another example of 'diaschesis' in action; above). Rolls (1996) suggests that projections to the striatum (involved as it is in 'movement') provide a means via which the animal's 'behaviour' may be altered when the reinforcement contingencies in the environment change (and we shall return to this proposition in Chapter 4). Indeed, the ventral striatum is also demonstrably responsive to 'reward' (as evidenced by stimulation and local infusion experiments; Passingham, 1993).

Humans with orbitofrontal lesions perform worse than control patients with other frontal lesions on tests of 'discrimination reversal' (Rolls, 1996). Their impairments are highly correlated with socially inappropriate and disinhibited behaviours and also the patients' subjective ratings of their own emotional impairments. Such patients may be impaired at detecting the emotional valence of facial or vocal expressions in others (these are potentially dissociable deficits; Rolls, 1996). Hence, they may have difficulty 'reading' others and changing their own response strategies accordingly, i.e. they may perseverate, persisting in making the same errors even though they may be able to explain, intellectually, what they 'should' have done in a given context (Rolls, 1996). Thus, in 'real life', OFC pathology may cause perseveration of responses among people rendered 'insensitive' to changing environmental contexts (Fuster, 1980). Such patients may do very badly in social situations despite the preservation of their intellect.

'Values'

There is something that may be said about the integrity of the OFC and its involvement with what we might call 'values'. For instance, it can be shown that there are neurons in the OFC that change their firing pattern according to the relative merits of two external stimuli. Hence, while one stimulus may be preferable to begin with, another stimulus may become more attractive, incrementally (for instance, a pleasant flavour may be presented to the organism at steadily increasing concentrations), whereupon both the cells and the organism may change their response profiles. Crucially, the cells are firing according to the reward value of a stimulus, not its visual appearance or its position in space (Padoa-Schioppa & Assad, 2006). Furthermore, there is a demonstrable distinction between the contributions of OFC and ACC to the pursuit of pleasurable rewards (at least in animal models): while OFC lesions impact upon the delay (duration) for which an animal will defer an anticipated reward, ACC lesions impact the energy or drive with which it will pursue that reward (Rudebeck et al. 2006). Hence, while OFC lesions may precipitate impulsivity (a failure of restraint, a radical decrease in 'waiting' time), an ACC lesion may precipitate apathy (i.e. giving up 'too easily'; see Chapter 6).

Within healthy human subjects, there is also the suggestion that some aspects of 'value' may be differentially represented, or coded for, across the OFC. In a review of multiple neuroimaging studies, Elliott and colleagues (2000) discerned the following regularity: where studies reported 'activation' of the medial OFC, there was often a requirement that the subjects 'keep track' of possible reward values pertaining to specific action outcomes (under conditions of reward uncertainty), while in studies eliciting activation of lateral OFC there was often a requirement that subjects 'change' their responses, 'suppressing' a previously rewarded response. Hence, as a rule of thumb, the medial OFC coded for sustained contingencies (values) while the lateral OFC was implicated in deleting or cancelling contingencies. All of this may have obvious ramifications for other systems of preference or value or hierarchy that are perceptible to humans (below).

Furthermore, Dolan (2007), in a more recent review, re-emphasizes the consequences to humans of OFC lesions: changes in behaviour, disinhibition, poor decision-making, overeating, indeed, even the consumption of unusual objects. In essence, humans (and other primates) with OFC lesions lose their powers of 'discrimination'. Their social conduct may become coarsened in various ways: facetious comments, bawdy humour, and indiscreet remarks. Such a change in a person's (apparent) 'personality' may be especially marked in the early stages of those dementias that target the frontal lobes (i.e. the fronto-temporal dementias).

Hence, once again, if one is interested in what it is that might comprise a subject's (hypothetical) 'Will', then the contribution of the OFC would seem to be critical, not so much to the successful performance of an 'act' (although impulsivity, post-OFC lesions, might of course impact the latter) but mainly through the identity of, and the value placed upon, such behaviour. Orbitofrontal cortex impairments seem to impact 'values'.

So, as we predicted at the opening of this chapter, there *is* a discernible gradient across the frontal lobes, extending from the defective 'performance' of volitional acts, consequent upon dorsolateral cortical lesions, to the disturbed 'motivations' underpinning those behaviours exhibited by humans sustaining medial and ventral prefrontal lesions. In the latter case, it is the value (maybe even the 'wisdom') of the behaviour that may seem radically flawed.

Therefore, if we return to the three miscreants, whom we sketched out earlier (above) – the serial adulterer, the malingerer, and the manipulative manager – then one might conjecture that they do *not* manifest behaviours indicative of any impairment, abnormality, or deviation from the 'norm', with respect to the 'performance' of their lateral frontal systems. There is no evidence that they cannot perform volitional acts normally when they 'want' to. So, *if* they have a problem (and it is a big 'if'), then their behaviour implicates their ventromedial systems. Now, I am *not* suggesting that adulterers, malingerers, or Machiavellian managers necessarily evince brain abnormalities, but I am suggesting that when a behaviour is well executed but 'wrong', or at least wrong in the eyes of some of the population, then we might hypothesize that the 'discrepancy' between those who 'do' and 'don't' regard the behaviour as acceptable, may well be a matter of 'values', and such values might be hypothesized to implicate the ventral prefrontal brain. Note, I am *not* claiming that one group is necessarily 'abnormal' *per se*, but that differences across a group, a community or a population in terms of the values and valences they accord behaviours might be differentially represented in these key areas. The reader

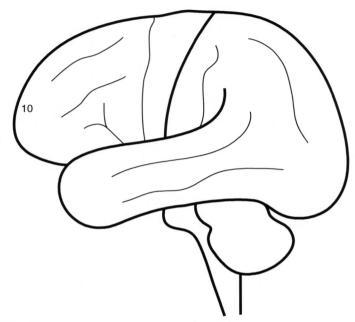

Fig. 40 Cartoon showing the approximate position of Brodmann area 10 at the frontal pole of the human brain.

may think that this is highly unlikely. However, would you think differently about the issue if you knew that 'pathological liars' exhibited abnormalities within their OFCs? (We shall meet this group in Chapter 8).

Towards the poles: frontopolar cortex (Brodmann Area 10)

Throughout this chapter, we have made our way across the frontal lobes, moving ever more anterior, away from the primary motor cortices (BA 4) and towards the very 'front' of the brain. As we have seen, the types of information – pertaining to action – that different frontal regions process vary radically from the simply mechanistic performance of a gesture to the motivated and 'driven' pursuit of a perceived reward. If we want to know 'why' a primate chooses one action over another, then the answer (if a single answer may be momentarily entertained) is likely to be found (and may well be 'distributed') among the brain regions that we have just described. Thus, remembering 'where' to point requires the DLPFC's contribution to working memory (specifically: 'spatial' working memory); the gesture of the finger itself invokes not only the precise control arising from its contralateral motor cortex (i.e. from the 'hand area') but also a 'programme' running in the PMC (itself 'liaising' with parietal regions). If the action was not elicited by events in the external environment, but instead 'internally initiated' then we are likely to posit the involvement of medial premotor systems (e.g. SMA). And, what if an act has been driven by reward expectation? Well, in such a case we might invoke the role of orbitofrontal regions, in order to fully understand the contribution of motivation to such behaviour. Would the monkey move the lever, to obtain the peanut, if his stomach was 'full' and his 'secondary taste area' altered its 'firing'? No, not necessarily: he might defer his movement until he felt hungry once more.

In a sense, our progress over the frontal cortex has involved our 'painting ourselves into a corner' and the remaining region that we have yet to paint, to describe, is the very front of the frontal lobe: the 'rostral prefrontal' or frontopolar cortex (BA 10; Burgess et al. 2007). This is a region that in the not-so-distant past might have been described as 'silent' (as if the brain would have evolved to support and sustain centres that were somehow redundant, without function). However, as we have implied in the case of Phineas Gage (above), it is very unlikely that the most rostral (anterior) regions of the PFC are simply without significant functions. Nevertheless, it may be that their mode of function is so abstract, so 'super-ordinate' within our hierarchical neurological systems that we shall have considerable difficulty in 'understanding' what it is that they 'do'. Indeed, this may be one of those situations in which we must invoke the comment of Ken Hill:

> If the brain were simple enough for us to understand it, we would be too simple to understand it.

> (Cited by Buzsaki, 2006, vii)

Hence, if what the frontal poles actually contributed towards behaviour were simple enough for us to understand, then we should probably be incapable of such understanding. In other words, an organism that is capable of introspection is likely to be a very complex organism, yet its ability to understand 'itself' is necessarily limited by its own processing constraints. Furthermore, only a very simple organism is ever likely to be fully 'understood' by others!

Now, as we have noted, BA 10 lies at the very front of the frontal lobes; hence, it is medial to the dorsolateral and ventrolateral PFCs (above), superior to the OFC, and anterior to the ACC and neighbouring medial prefrontal regions. It receives thalamic afferents from the dorsomedial nucleus, the medial pulvinar, and the paracentral nuclei. It has reciprocal connections with the anterior temporal pole, the anterior OFC and DLPFC.

This area (BA 10) is structurally interesting for a number of reasons. First, it is the largest single architectonic region of PFC; indeed, it is relatively larger in humans compared with any other animal. Second, it is late to 'myelinate' in humans (i.e. in this region, axonal sheaths develop relatively late); and is regarded as the last region within the adult human brain to 'mature' (Burgess et al. 2007). Hence, there are several reasons for positing that BA 10 might be contributory to 'higher' aspects of human cognition. Furthermore, this area has a relatively low cell density in humans, suggesting that it may have 'more space' available for connections with other higher order association areas (Burgess et al. 2007). Indeed, BA 10 is the only PFC region that is almost exclusively connected to supramodal areas in PFC and elsewhere (above).

Isolated lesions of BA 10 are not often described in the neurological literature. It would be unusual to observe a discrete tumour or stroke here. Additionally, because signs of their presence may be very subtle, any such tumours that do arise may present relatively 'late', by which time they may have already extended beyond the confines of area 10's anatomical boundaries. Nevertheless, when Paul Burgess and colleagues, at London University, examined the available neurological literature, concerning this problem, they concluded that people with lesions of BA 10 emerge remarkably unscathed on formal tests of cognitive function and IQ. In other words, they seem to be very well 'preserved'. However, this does not prevent their lives from being adversely affected, for what seems to 'go wrong', in such cases, is that patients lose the ability to 'multi-task': they cannot seem to keep multiple goals in mind so that they might execute a series of procedures, one after another. Hence, patients with BA 10 lesions exhibit deficits in shopping experiments (when they have been asked to move between different outlets, to obtain different classes of item, in the most time-efficient manner possible); they cannot sequence multi-stepped tasks, such as those involved in running 'multiple errands' (see Burgess et al. 2007).

Now, at this point it may be helpful to pause, to expand our terminology somewhat.

The complexities of cooking

When I am engaged in a multi-staged task, such as cooking a meal, I may have a number of future projects that must be borne 'in mind', i.e. kept 'active' neurologically. The tasks that I have yet to perform may be called 'delayed intentions', and my ability to 'picture' or project what I shall do in the future may been termed 'prospective memory' (Fuster, 1980); a 'memory of the future' (Ingvar, 1985). So, for instance, if I am cooking a meal of several components, two of which happen to be potatoes and peas, then I know from experience that the potatoes on the hob will need to boil for about 20 minutes whereas I shall not need to boil the peas until very close to the end, literally within minutes of serving them. Therefore, while I engage in sorting out the potatoes, my 'delayed intention' to prepare and boil the peas is 'somewhere' in my prospective memory. Some people think that BA 10 is pivotally involved in such prospective memory. Some have called this ability to 'take a break' from ongoing plans (i.e. cooking the peas) – to deal with something imminent (i.e. preparing the potatoes) – 'branching' (Koechlin et al. 1999). The idea is that I can literally interrupt my contemplation of a longer-term goal while I execute shorter-term goals, in my immediate environment. However, crucially, the longer-term goal (the prospective memory) is not 'lost'; it is still 'there', somewhere within my mind and brain.

In a sense, all of this speculation opens up a potential vista – a temporal hierarchy of delayed goals – ranging far off into my own projected future: the things that I 'know' I shall do tomorrow, next week, next year. Of course, I do not actually 'know' any of these things for certain; for these are virtual events. I might well change my mind!

Burgess's account

Now, to cease such speculation and return to the empirical realm, Paul Burgess's studies of healthy subjects, using functional neuroimaging, have also suggested another rather subtle role for BA 10 in health. Burgess posits that frontopolar regions are implicated when subjects are required to move (in their minds) between processing external stimuli (data in their immediate environment) and internal stimuli (data that are subjectively available to them; Burgess et al. 2007). He calls these phenomena 'Stimulus-Oriented' (SO) and 'Stimulus-Independent' (SI) attending, respectively:

> Examples of [stimulus oriented] attending range from performance of vigilance tasks, to reading, watching the television, listening to a conversation and so forth. By contrast, [stimulus independent] attending is the attending behaviour required to effect either self-generated or self-maintained thought.

> (Burgess et al. 2007, p. 891)

Furthermore,

> Self-generated thought is cognition that goes beyond the over-learned associations or semantic memories provoked by currently available stimuli ... By contrast, self-maintained thought is where one deliberately maintains a representation in the absence of the stimuli that provoked it.

> (*ibid*, p. 891)

Finally, if we want to know what moving between SO and SI attending would be like in 'real-life', then here is an example:

> ...[W]here one is trying to concentrate on a rather dull lecture (SO attending) versus imagining what one might do [this] evening after the lecture (SI attending).

(*ibid*, p. 892)

Clearly, boring lectures have elicited far more from our 'higher' brain centres than we might ever have imagined!

Burgess and colleagues tested such theories in the laboratory, using functional neuroimaging techniques. On a range of tasks, using very different stimuli, and different types of information, they required their subjects to 'switch' between actions based upon external stimuli (i.e. involving SO attending; above), and ongoing 'internal' plans and intentions (implicating SI attending). Burgess suggests that it was this 'switching', between the 'external' and the 'internal', which maximally implicated the contribution of BA 10 (especially lateral BA 10). Nevertheless, his hypothesis is still preliminary, and further careful work will be required to characterize the contributions of this most subtle of brain regions.

Integrating prefrontal systems

Moreover, there are other accounts of BA 10's possible contribution to human thought and action. Koechlin and Hyafil (2007) present one such formulation, again based upon an interpretation of many varied cognitive neuropsychological and functional neuroimaging experiments performed upon humans. Crucially, they posit an interaction between BA 10 and two other prefrontal areas that we have already surveyed (above): DLPFC and OFC. Furthermore, they suggest that there is a constraint upon cognitive processing within the PFC so that, faced with any set of alternative behaviours, these 'higher' centres can really only support (i.e. maintain) two 'plans' at one time: one 'in' BA 10, the other 'in' DLPFC. The currently preferred behavioural plan is coded within DLPFC (it forms the basis of ongoing action) its possible alternative is coded within BA 10. So, what is it that determines 'preference' here? Well, that task takes us back to the OFC. If the OFC attributes (and revises attributed) 'value' to these perceived behavioural alternatives then:

1. It may influence which one of them gains preferential access to the DLPFC (to become the currently preferred 'behavioural plan'), and

2. It may cause one or both alternatives to be displaced or deleted if/when an emergent third behavioural plan assumes greater value.

Notice again, BA 10 is implicated in 'holding a response', in a kind of 'buffer', so that it might return to the DLPFC if/when it acquires sufficient salience or value.

Notice also that this model hinges upon an attribute of frontal systems that we have identified previously: a limit, a constraint upon processing capacity. What is so interesting about the Koechlin and Hyafil model is that it offers a possible explanation of how behavioural choices could emerge, within such a processing system of limited capacity, and how they might change according to 'value/preference'; it also, intriguingly, manages to proffer a fluid understanding of neural hierarchies. For, while BA 10 is, in some sense, 'downstream' of DLPFC (it is posited to act as its 'buffer'), the function of both these regions is influenced by the OFC. So, if 'values' ('in' OFC) were to be disturbed, then the functions of these other executive regions would be insufficient to 'save' the organism from 'bad' decisions. A man might be able to hold two behavioural plans in his mind/brain, to perform them (adequately) in sequence; however, if their essential valences were abnormal, then these actions might be very 'wrong' indeed (to choose an emotive exemplar: such a man might be very good at organizing train timetables and logistics, without ever questioning their destination).

Hence, an agent inhabiting a complex environment requires all three of these prefrontal centres to be working well, and in harmony, for it to be able to behave efficiently and 'appropriately'.

So, when we begin to consider the frontal pole of the human brain, we encounter a region that is currently at the very limit of our ability to characterize its 'functions'. Nevertheless, what we can say is that they seem very likely to be pivotal to the maintenance of an independent existence (in a world where we must engage in complex, multi-staged tasks and may, occasionally, contemplate our own futures).

Will, choice, and changing the future

Throughout this chapter, we have been concerned with understanding what it is about the brain – specifically about the frontal regions of the brain – which allows a human actor to make and execute choices, to exercise their 'Will'. The regions we have examined are hierarchically 'superior' to primary motor cortex, yet it is probably obvious by now that the functions that we regard as 'normal' rely upon a host of frontal (and other) brain regions acting in assembly; combining their particular response attributes in order that a coherent action might emerge. I shall not reprise the list of foci all over again, but I hope that I have shown that there are certain regularities in the way that the frontal cortex is organized, that we might expect certain of its regions to be particularly involved (implicated) in certain types of responses, and that lesions of specific foci may tend (though not necessarily 'uniquely' nor absolutely 'always') to reveal related patterns of dysfunction. In other words, the architecture of human choice is potentially tractable, understandable.

However, this is not all. For this chapter has also taken us a little further towards understanding what it is that allows an organism to 'change' its immediate future situations. A passive primate would be entirely 'driven' by external events and contingencies (see Chapter 5). A truly passive, mute, and immobile animal would probably not survive for very long. Fortunately, however, the architecture of the primate brain features regions that appear to be evolutionarily adapted for bringing about change, e.g. those medial systems capable of initiating 'responses' in the absence of external cues; those orbitofrontal regions that alter their response profiles according to an organism's internal state; and the frontal poles, which may allow us to structure 'events' in our futures, events that have yet to occur (in 'real time', in 'real life'). If we can 'imagine' different futures then, logically speaking, we may pursue them. Hence, our actions may, potentially, change the world.

Chapter 3

The timing of intentions

Our data suggest that people's awareness of initiating action relates to preparing a *specific* movement, rather than a general abstracted state of intending to perform an action of some kind.[7]
I just play what comes into my mind.[8]

Our journey thus far has led us to rather an interesting contradiction. On the one hand, as we have just seen (at the close of Chapter 2), there are brain regions (located at the frontal poles) that seem to support an awareness of future possibilities, of events and actions that we have yet to see instantiated, in the 'real world'. These regions may allow us to structure a future comprising multiple, virtual undertakings (e.g. the sequence of shops that we might wish to visit while out shopping or the ingredients that we might need to prepare during the cooking of a meal). On the other hand, at the very beginning of this book (in the Prologue), we considered the implications of Benjamin Libet's experiments, concerning the onset of our subjective awareness of an intention to act when performing a very simple task, work that led us to the somewhat disquieting conclusion that subjective awareness arises only *after* a train of neural activity has been set in motion (leading ultimately to a physical act).

The implications of this finding for 'freedom' seemed to be profound: we are only aware of our actions *after* they have 'begun' (Spence, 1996). Hence, on the one hand, we seem to be able to 'see into the future' (or, more accurately, to see into a *possible* future), but on the other hand, when it comes to enacting our plans, we actually acquire an awareness of our activity only *after* its initiation has commenced. We seem to be a most curious breed of dysfunctional clairvoyants, looking forward to the theoretically possible while only becoming

---

7   From P. Haggard and M. Eimer. On the relation between brain potentials and the awareness of voluntary movements. *Experimental Brain Research* 1999; 126: 128–133 (quote is taken from p. 131).

8   Thelonious Monk, quoted in *Jazz at Ronnie Scott's*, 1979.

aware of what we have actually embarked upon (our veridical physical acts) once they have already started.

Now, it may be that this apparent contradiction tells us something interesting about the 'uses' of consciousness (yes, we have lapsed into teleology, again). Certainly, at first pass, it seems to favour the view, propounded by some psychologists and philosophers, that consciousness provides a kind of 'workspace' (Baars and McGovern, 1996), a virtual space in which future scenarios may be played out; a safe space perhaps, for it allows us to 'think the unthinkable' without actually acting upon it. We shall return to this question at other points in this text. However, for now, we shall refocus on our intentions—the timing of what it is that is happening when we *believe* we are initiating an act.

What Libet left 'unresolved'

Of course, when we considered Libet's work (in the Prologue), we did not address the issue of what it was that constituted the 'beginning' of an act, what it was that actually gave rise to the signal that Libet described (the *Bereitschaftspotential* [BP] or 'readiness potential' [RP]). Also, we did not inquire too deeply as to whether the presence of this signal was *sufficient* for an act to occur: in other words, if an RP is detectable, does it necessarily mean that an action is going to go ahead? Is the actor fully 'committed' to acting? Now, there were technical reasons why this 'had' to be the case in the Libet experiments because of the means by which his data were acquired: by retrospectively examining event-related signals, electroencephalograph (EEG) patterns were 'tagged' ('time-locked') to an actual act (a movement) that had already occurred (as verified by electromyography [EMG]).

However, it is possible to imagine that under different circumstances such a signal might arise and not necessarily be played out as a manifest movement. Indeed, we saw that Libet himself favoured the possibility that action was not already fully determined by this stage (the appearance of an RP), and that consciousness retained an ability to 'veto' what 'it' did not wish to 'see' proceed. (We have noted previously the difficulties that arise when we start to divide our 'selves' in this way [what is the 'it' that decides and what does 'it' anticipate is going to happen?] and the very real problems for Libet's conscious power of veto [there being good grounds for suspecting that conscious qualia are themselves the products of preceding neural activity; hence, the 'veto' experience itself comprises a post hoc reconstruction].)

So, how should we proceed? What should we do next? Well, at the end of the Prologue, we posited that there are two scientific responses to such a problem. The first is to walk 'backwards in time', from the moment of our awareness of an intention, to find out what it is that initiates an ensuing act. Hence, we should explore the neurology of volition. On the other hand, our second response should be to walk 'forwards in time', to discover what it is that gives us the 'impression' that we are acting freely, and what it is that seems to 'bind' us to our acts.

Therefore, in Chapters 1 and 2, we went some way towards examining the first of these options, in that we described a 'machine' for volition: what it is that constitutes the bare minimum of a voluntary motor system within the human brain. We saw that there are several hierarchies of neural architecture implicated in the performance of even a very simple act: the motor cortex 'controls' fine finger movement (Chapter 1) but is itself subordinate within a wider, extensive network of systems, instantiated at the level of the cerebral cortex, a network which imbues actions with their 'plans' and 'programmes' (Chapter 2). Hence, we now have a web of areas, 'structures', which are pertinent to action planning and its performance. So, the time has come to return to 'process'—to the timing of actions and intentions, and to discerning how it is that such structures interact with one another in the course of volition.

In this chapter, I hope to provide a finer-grained account of the *timing* of voluntary processes and to develop a deeper understanding of 'when' it is that an intention coheres. (I might also note that my own ideas have changed somewhat as I have confronted these matters. I started out by believing that the prefrontal cortex was the area of primary concern, the cerebral centre where 'the action is', literally. However, as time has gone by, and as we shall see demonstrated later, it has become increasingly apparent that we are actually heavily reliant upon our premotor regions: it is these areas that seem pivotal to both the enactment of volition and the 'binding' of what it is that emerges into our awareness, when we 'own' a given act. I wonder also whether they [the premotor cortices] may be what the jazz musician or improviser 'calls upon' when he is in the midst of a performance (Chapter 10). It is little use having a 'plan' or a 'goal' ('in' one's prefrontal cortex) if the toolbox at one's disposal ('in' the premotor cortex) lacks the necessary, skilled performance programmes to 'save' the situation. As we shall see later on in this book, there is much to be said for 'owning' the *correct* automatic responses.)

Volitional processes

The crux of Libet's contribution lay in his discovery that the BP (or RP) arose earlier than a subject's awareness of their intention to perform a specified 'freely chosen' act. In Libet's account, the potential concerned was maximal over the vertex of the skull and, as we speculated in Chapter 2, a likely source for such a signal, close to the brain's midline, was the supplementary motor area (SMA; Brodmann area [BA] 6), a region of the medial premotor cortex (present in both cerebral hemispheres). We also saw that in the non-human primate literature, summarized by Dick Passingham (1993), the SMA was pivotal to allowing a monkey to initiate tasks that were not prompted (or 'cued') by events in its immediate external environment. Hence, the SMA seemed necessary for the performance of 'internally initiated' acts. Indeed, lesions of the SMA and neighbouring midline structures (such as the anterior cingulate cortex [ACC]) could render an animal mute and lacking in spontaneous activity, though he might still respond to prompts (such responses, to cues in the external environment, reflecting the contribution of his preserved *lateral* premotor system). Thus, if we return to considering humans, then there would seem to be good grounds for positing that the BP tells us something about what is happening within our own *medial* premotor systems.

Now, of course, the literature has developed since the time of Libet's experiments and there are a number of clarifications that may be added, concerning both the structure of the potential itself (its shape and the different elements contained within it) and the implications for its physiology of those deviations from 'normal' that are observed under specific pathological conditions. Indeed, we saw that Libet himself had already remarked upon the effects of certain phenomenological features of the subject's mental state (upon BP): if they allowed themselves a period of 'planning' prior to action, then the BP seemed to appear rather earlier and exhibited a shallow gradient, whereas if they acted 'truly' spontaneously, then it seemed to arise much later and to be more acute or steep in its profile (Figs. 3 and 41). More recently, in a paper published in 2006, Hiroshi Shibasaki and Mark Hallett of the National Institute of Neurological Disorders and Stroke, Bethesda, have usefully summarized further developments in the BP literature. Here, we borrow their analysis of what it is that is now known about this significant signal (Fig. 41 and Table 8).

First of all, it is important to note that the BP is now clearly described as comprising two components, one early ('early BP') and one late ('late BP'). These components may be distinguished on direct observation of the EEG trace and exhibit rather different onset times and gradients. The *early* BP can be seen to arise as much as 2000 ms prior to a spontaneous act, whereas the *late* BP arises later, at around 400 ms prior to the act. Also, the characteristics of these components may be altered by prevailing conditions and differently so in some instances. So, if the agent attends to their intention, is learning a new task, or uses greater physical force, then the early BP is larger. If they prepare for the task, then this early BP also arises earlier (again, consistent with Libet's reported observations). In contrast, when movements require precision, 'discreteness' of distal muscular group involvement (e.g. 'Please move "just" your middle finger now and not any of the others'), or complexity of sequencing, there is an increase in the amplitude of the late BP (Table 8). This suggests that the late BP may be more indicative of

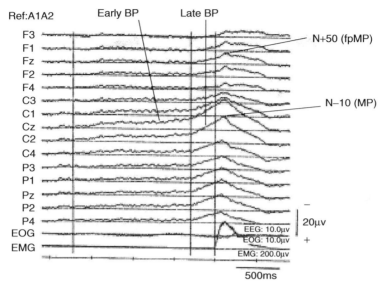

Ref:A1A2   Early BP   Late BP

F3   N+50 (fpMP)
F1
Fz
F2
F4
C3   N−10 (MP)
C1
Cz
C2
C4
P3
P1
Pz
P2
P4   20µv
EOG   EEG: 10.0µv
EMG   EOG: 10.0µv   +
        EMG: 200.0µv

500ms

Fig. 41 Electroencephalograph EEG data demonstrating the early and late phases of the *Bereitschaftspotential* (BP; i.e. readiness potential) prior to spontaneous action. The C leads demonstrate activity over the vertex of the skull. The early BP increases gradually over some seconds prior to action whereas the late BP is represented by an increased gradient closer to the point of explicit activity (as indicated by the EMG trace at the bottom of the figure). Reprinted from Shibasaki H. and Hallett M. (2006). What is the bereitschaftspotential. Clinical Neuropsychology, 117; 11, with permission from Elsevier Ltd.

finer tuning, occurring relatively late in the course of action generation (in other words, it is located relatively 'downstream' in the execution process.)

Where does the BP originate? As we posited earlier, the medial premotor system is clearly important though as successive data sets have accrued a greater understanding has evolved of the BP's neuroanatomical sources. Although the early BP is now thought to emerge from the 'pre-SMA' (that region of the SMA lying anterior to a vertical line passing vertically upwards through the anterior commissure; Chapter 2; Fig. 26) and the SMA proper (where there is a somatotopic representation of the motor system, with the head lying rostrally and the contralateral leg lying caudally), more recent investigations of its sources have also implicated the cingulate motor system (lying lower down on the medial surface of the frontal lobe).

In very detailed functional magnetic resonance imaging (fMRI) studies of humans, examining single brain slices (in order to be able to acquire many scans at high frequencies, i.e. at short time intervals), Cunnington and

Table 8 Movement-related cortical potentials

Potential	Characteristics
Early *Bereitschaftspotential*	Emerges ~2000 ms prior to action.
	Maximal over the midline (vertex).
	Sources: pre-SMAs, SMAs (exhibiting a somatotopic distribution).
	Increases with intention; exhibits earlier onset with planning.
	Reduced amplitude in Parkinson's and cerebellar disease.
	During praxis, early components are detected in parietal EEG leads.
Late *Bereitschaftspotential*	Emerges ~400 ms prior to action.
	Maximal over the hemisphere contralateral to movement.
	Sources: primary motor cortex (somatotopic distribution) and lateral premotor cortex (also evincing a somatotopic distribution).
	Increases if precision or complexity required.
	Smaller in cerebellar disease and dystonias.
	In some literatures, the late Bereitschaftspotential is also termed the 'lateralized readiness potential' (LRP).
P–50 (Pre-motion positivity)	Emerges ~50 ms prior to action.
	Maximal over the hemisphere ipsilateral to movement.
	Source: unknown.
N–10	Emerges ~10 ms prior to action.
	Maximal over a small area of the primary motor cortex contralateral to the moving limb.
	Source: corresponds to movement site on motor homunculus.
	Thought to reflect activity of pyramidal tract neurons in primary motor cortex (BA 4).
N+50	Emerges ~50 ms post movement.
	Maximal over frontal regions.
	May represent kinaesthetic feedback from distal action.
P+90	Emerges ~90 ms post movement.
	Maximal over the parietal cortex contralateral to the moving limb.
	May represent kinaesthetic feedback from distal action.
N+160	Emerges ~160 ms post movement.
	Maximal over the parietal cortex contralateral to the moving limb.
P+300	Emerges ~300 ms post movement.
	Termed the 'reafferente Potentiale' by Kornhuber and Deecke (1965).

SMAs, supplementary motor areas; BA, Broadmann area.

Source: Adapted from Shibasaki and Hallett (2006).

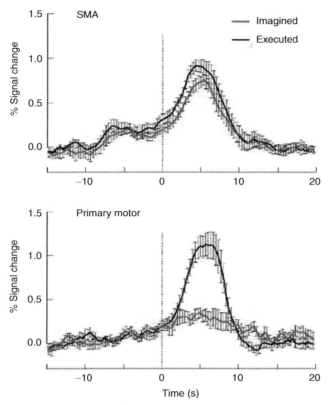

Fig. 42 Graphs showing a blood oxygen level-dependant response in the primary motor cortex and supplementary motor areas (SMAs) during motor activity in healthy humans, acquired using functional magnetic resonance imaging. Note that activity increases in the primary motor cortex during executed movements but not during imagined movements. In contrast, activity in the SMA increases during executed and also imagined movements. Hence, the SMA appears to be involved in the planning of movements whereas the involvement of the primary motor cortex is restricted to the final execution of an explicit movement. (From Cunnington et al., *Human Movement Science* 2005; 24: 644–656 with permission from Elsevier Ltd.) (See colour plate section).

colleagues (2005) have systematically shown that, during the performance of an act, the pre-SMA activates *prior to* the primary motor cortex. Indeed, they have also demonstrated that this area of the SMA is active during *imagined* movements, and those periods when humans observe the movements of another (Fig. 42). Hence, Cunnington and colleagues (2005) suggest that the pre-SMA 'generates and encodes motor representations which are then maintained in *readiness* for action' (p. 644, emphasis added). So, an activation of the pre-SMA, manifest as it might be through the appearance of an *early* BP signal, might not necessarily 'commit' an agent to action, because this region is engaged in a 'readiness' for action, a readiness that extends to actions that the agent, herself or himself, may never actually perform (e.g. when they are simply imagined or observed being performed by others; Fig. 42).

In contrast, the late BP signal implicates the primary motor and lateral premotor cortices, contralateral to the hand that is about to move. The later (BP) elements also exhibit a more specific localization: that is, if it is a finger that is about to move, then it will be the finger area, the somatotopic representation of that finger in the primary motor cortex, that manifests the late BP.

However, we should also add some more detailed points of clarification:

1. Because of the way that EEG signals are detected from the brain, its surface folding and undulating beneath the skull, the detected point of a maximum signal need not necessarily follow the 'rules' that we might anticipate. Hence, although a finger movement (on the right) will be associated with an EEG signal (a late BP) that is maximal over the contralateral finger area (in the contralateral, left, cerebral hemisphere's primary motor cortex), a right foot movement might actually exhibit its maximum EEG correlate ipsilaterally (i.e. over the vertex of that side of the skull [the right] that lies on the same side of the body as the moving foot). This is not because the ipsilateral motor cortex is 'moving' the moving limb. It is because of the spatial orientation of the active, contralateral 'foot area', in the contralateral (left) hemisphere's motor strip: its signal is projected, at right angles, from a region of the homunculus that is 'bending' over the medial lip of the activated hemisphere (the motor homunculus; see Fig. 10, and Brunia and van Boxtel, 2000, p. 519). Hence, although it is *generated* within the left hemisphere, this signal *projects* to the right of the skull's midline (i.e. across the midsagittal plane).

2. Furthermore, if the movement to be executed is part of an everyday gesture (rather than a 'simple' finger movement), then the early BP actually commences over the parietal regions (see Shibasaki and Hallett, 2006, p. 2345; this is of interest because it converges with what we know about the role of parietal regions in the planning of *skilled* movements and those deficits that arise in the dyspraxias; Chapter 2). Hence, the character of a movement has an impact upon the early correlates of its preparation.

Similarly, different forms of pathology have different effects on the early and late components of the BP. Parkinson's disease is associated with a reduction in the amplitude of the early but not the late BP (Note: this seems to point to greater disruption of the *medial* premotor system; Chapter 2). Unilateral hemiparesis (e.g. that following a 'stroke') has an effect on the late but not the early BP (hence, its impact seems to be upon that part of the signal that is most connected with the movement's execution, at the level of the primary motor and *lateral* premotor cortices). In contrast, cerebellar disease reduces the amplitude of both BPs. Indeed, in animal models, destruction of the cerebellar dentate nucleus abolishes the BP in its entirety. This suggests that cerebellar function contributes to both BP components; its impact on the late BP component is certainly consistent with its modulation of the primary motor cortex via projections relayed through the thalamus, and originating within the dentate nucleus (Brunia and van Boxtel, 2000, p. 514). Dystonic movements (abnormal involuntary movements) have no effect on the early BP but are associated with smaller late BPs (hence implicating the involvement of the primary motor and lateral premotor cortices). In general, it is very unusual for an 'organic' (i.e. a verifiably pathological) movement disorder to be associated with an entirely 'normal' BP (throughout both its early and late components; Shibasaki and Hallett, 2006).

Mirror movements

Indeed, there is a further pathological condition the impact of which on the BP may actually shed light upon the organization of the cortical motor system. Under certain conditions, the latter allows the 'release' of so-called 'mirror movements' to occur; these are unintentional movements of one (purportedly relaxed) limb that accompany, and coincide with, the purposeful movement of the opposite limb.

> 'The examination requires the examiner only to observe both hands during voluntary fine finger movements of each hand in turn; for example, sequentially pressing each finger against the thumb of one hand whilst the other hand is relaxed. Mirroring occurs when there are visible involuntary movements of the "relaxed" hand that appear to replicate the timing and type of movement being carried out by the voluntary activated hand.'

> (Farmer, 2005, p. 1330)

Such movements may be normal in early childhood, but they have usually ceased by about the age of 11 years. These early movements probably reflect the initial immaturity of the motor system and a transient inability of the *active* hemisphere to inhibit its contralateral neighbour (e.g. if the left motor strip is initiating movement of the right hand, then the corresponding region of the right motor strip 'should be' inhibited, via transcallosal fibres; indeed, Serrien et al. [2006] refer to such mirror movements as 'defaults' that need to be inhibited by the dominant hemisphere; see Table 9). If mirror movements have not

Table 9 Proposed hemispheric contributions to motor activity (in a right-handed subject)

Left hemisphere	Right hemisphere
Asymmetrical (larger) representation of the cortical hand area; larger primary motor cortex (BA 4) and descending corticospinal tracts.	Less extensive (and less well-defined) motor representation.
Lower threshold for excitability (elicited movements) on transcranial magnetic stimulation.	
Implicated in skilled behaviours; parietal lesions render the contralateral hand dyspraxic.	May be implicated more in exploratory movements in novel situations (hence, its contribution may have been underestimated in laboratory-based, brain-imaging literatures).
More active during complex movements.	More implicated in spatial functions, spatial attention, and monitoring functions.
Because of proposed temporal processing attributes, more involved in *sequential* behaviours, tool use, and bimanual coordination.	
Control of 'open-loop' aspects of movement: movements based on well-established motor programmes.	Implicated in 'closed-loop' aspects of movement, where sensory feedback guides behaviour.
More involved in limb trajectory.	May be more involved in maintaining limb position and posture.
Open-loop specialization may be limited to feed-forward specification of limb dynamics.	Closed-loop, sensory-mediated, mechanisms implicated in the control of final limb position.
More involved in processing 'local' features of a stimulus (intensification of high spatial frequency favours information processing at a local level).	Preferential encoding of global features of stimulus (low spatial frequency data).
Relatively greater inhibition of the *right* hemisphere during unilateral movements (to counteract production of 'default mirror movements' [p. 163]).	Relatively greater involvement *early on* in the acquisition of new skills (later the skill becomes 'represented' on the left.)
More active when movement is run according to 'internal' representations.	More implicated when movement is run according to external environment.

The control of the left hemisphere over the right need not be exclusively inhibitory: it has been noted that after section of the corpus callosum, left hand movement may cease temporarily (suggesting that the left hemisphere may also facilitate the right hemisphere's control of the left hand).

Source: Modified from Serrien et al. (2006).

disappeared in the course of childhood, then their persistence may be indicative of certain congenital medical conditions (e.g. X-linked Kallman's syndrome, Klippel-Fiel syndrome, and congenital hemiplegia; Farmer, 2005). Alternatively, mirror movements may 'return' in later life as a consequence of acquired pathology (e.g. hemiplegic 'stroke', dystonic movement disorders [where mirror movements arise in the affected, abnormal limb], or asymmetrical Parkinson's disease [where they may arise in the relatively normal, minimally affected limb]). How might such movements arise? From a strictly neurological perspective, there are two possible ways in which a mirror movement might emerge:

1. It could be that there is an abnormal degree of connectivity between the 'normal' motor cortex that is generating movement in the contralateral 'normal hand' (of course, both hands are anatomically 'normal'; it is their movements that differ) and the innervation of the ipsilateral 'abnormal hand' (the one that manifests mirror movements). Hence, in congenital conditions, mirroring may indicate the abnormal persistence of *ipsilateral* corticospinal pathways to the ipsilateral limb.

2. Alternatively, and especially in the acquired syndromes, an abnormal, 'mirroring' limb might offer an indication that its 'own' (contralateral) hemisphere's motor strip is not subject to adequate inhibition by its neighbour (the hemisphere ipsilateral to the 'abnormal' limb). In other words, if the left hand is exhibiting mirror movements, then this may be because the right motor strip is not being inhibited (as it 'should be') by the left motor cortex, during normal movements of the right hand. In this case, it may be that a primary pathology has interrupted the ability of the 'normal' primary motor cortex to inhibit its homologue in the contralateral hemisphere (e.g. through a disruption of callosal fibres).

Now, it follows that these two modes of pathology would have different implications for the structure of premovement cortical potentials (especially the late BP). For, in the first case, the congenital persistence of abnormal corticospinal pathways, we should expect the 'normal' motor cortex to exhibit a late BP. This would be associated with its normal generation of movements in the contralateral hand. In contrast, its neighbour, the primary motor cortex innervating the 'mirror hand', would *not* manifest a late BP (because it is *not* the source of that hand's movements). As it is the 'normal' motor cortex that is responsible for the movements of both hands, it is solely the 'normal' motor cortex that generates a late BP.

In contrast, in an acquired condition, where mirror movements are attributable to an abnormal (disinhibited) activation of the motor cortex contralateral to the mirror hand, we should expect to see late BPs over *both* motor strips—the 'normal' one generating the 'normal' movement (in its contralateral hand) and the abnormal one reacting in a disinhibited manner to its homologue's activation (and there is some evidence in favour of this; Maegaki et al., 2002).

By way of being counterfactual, mirror movements also tell us something rather interesting about the 'normal' state of affairs (neurologically), suggesting that a motor cortex (specifically, the dominant motor cortex; Table 9) usually inhibits its neighbour during the course of action generation. That such a train of events is likely to occur in the 'normal' situation (i.e. that the initiation of action by one motor strip is accompanied by inhibition of its homologue) is elegantly demonstrated in the advanced EEG analysis reported by Vidal and colleagues (2003). They showed that during a motor task requiring alternating use of either hand, activity in the SMA preceded that seen in the 'active' motor cortex (as indexed by a signal similar to the late BP: the 'lateralized RP'). However, the active motor cortex's late BP was also accompanied by a synchronized and inverted signal over the contralateral motor cortex (see Figs. 43 and 44). Hence, they concluded that during such motor behaviours, 'an inhibition of the primary motor cortex contralateral to the non-responding hand is implemented' (Vidal et al., 2003, p. 796). This is something that will be of particular relevance when we come to consider some of the ways in which the control of hand actions can 'break down' (in Chapter 5).

The source of the signal(s)

Therefore, in summary, with respect to the BP, we can say that the emergence of a voluntary act does indeed implicate the early contribution of the medial premotor systems, and that the sequence of BP signals seems to implicate the SMA and other medial premotor structures first (in the generation of the early BP), and *then* the primary motor and lateral premotor cortices (in the generation of the late BP). Also, although general preparatory factors (such as prior intention and learning) seem to modulate the early BP, it is the precision and specific location of the final movement that modulate the late BP. In other words, there appears to be a connection between the increased specificity of the later signal in terms of its motor correlate (e.g. the cortical representation of a specific finger) and the precision of an ensuing act. The late BP seems to be a marker of pyramidal tract involvement (hence, movement precision). Indeed, this is consistent with a view (endorsed by both Brunia and van Boxtel [2000], and Shibasaki and Hallett [2006]) that the BP is actually a correlate of postsynaptic potentials arising at the apical dendrites of cortical pyramidal cells (see Chapter 1).

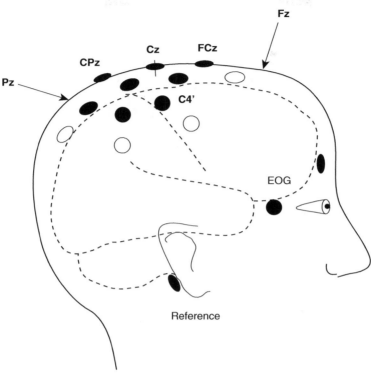

Fig. 43 Cartoon showing the approximate placement positions of electroencephalograph (EEG) leads over the human skull. Notice that lead Cz is located over the vertex. (From Vidal et al., *Psychophysiology* 2003; 40: 796–805)

Hence, we now have a view about where the BP 'comes from'. We have a picture of the 'early' antecedents of action. But where does this leave us with respect to our subjective awareness, our 'intention to act'? At what point in this stream of neural events do we become aware that we are about to, 'intend to', perform a specific act? Having 'walked backwards' in time to study the emergence of the early BP, we now need to turn around again and 'walk forwards' in time, in order to assay our own subjectivity.

Awareness of volition

If the BP were linked to conscious awareness, as is implicit in Libet's work, if it constituted the cerebral process that 'eventually' gave rise to a subjective 'intention' to act, then the moment of onset of the BP (whether it occurred relatively early or relatively late) *should* exhibit a temporal relationship, a correlation, with the onset of that (paired, corresponding) 'intention'. In other

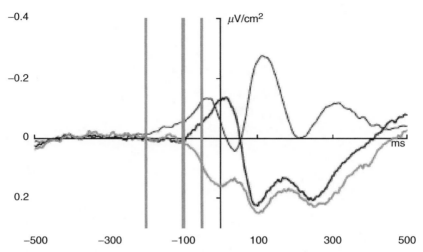

Fig. 44 Electroencephalograph EEG data showing the amplitude of the surface Laplacian estimation as a function of time, over the supplementary motor area (SMA, shown by the thin black line), for the sensory motor cortex contralateral to the responding hand (the bold black line) and the sensory motor cortex ipsilateral to the responding hand (in the lower bold grey line). At time 0 (midway between −100 and 100 ms), the responding hand moves, as indicated by electromyography EMG. At this point, the sensorimotor cortices' signals are in antiphase. These data are consistent with the view that there is an inhibition of the sensorimotor cortex ipsilateral to the responding hand. In other words, the SMA and the sensorimotor cortex contralateral to the responding hand are involved in the initiation of such movement while the sensorimotor cortex ipsilateral to the response is suppressed. (From Vidal et al., *Psychophysiology* 2003; 40: 796–805)

words, if the BP were the *causal* initiator of intentions, then we should expect to see intentions arise at a certain regular interval *after* 'their' BPs had commenced. I note that this is implicit in Libet's work because his studies provided two remarkable findings:

1. That intentions arise only *after* the BP has commenced (Libet et al., 1983); and

2. That a period of 'neuronal adequacy' is required for a subjective experience (in philosophical language, a qualia; see the Prologue) to arise (Libet et al., 1964).

Hence, one might have deduced that it is the BP that 'causes' a conscious intention to arise (albeit rather late).

However, there are problems. For we have already noted on several occasions that the duration of an antecedent BP is highly variable (depending on the preparation of the subject, their pre-existing intentions, etc.) and we have just described a distinction between 'early' and 'late' BPs (Shibasaki and

Hallett, 2006). So, if a neural signal is causally related to the onset of an intention, if it is the process that (somehow) constitutes 'neuronal adequacy', then which BP is it? Is it the early one or the late one? Indeed, can we be sure that either one of them contributes to our 'awareness' as such?

It is here that we turn to an interesting recapitulation of Libet's work, in a series of intricate experiments conducted by Patrick Haggard and his colleagues at the University of London. Haggard has taken the Libet paradigm (the 'internally initiated' generation of actions, while keeping track of subjective time by reference to a clock face; Fig. 4) and augmented it in order to dissect the subcomponents of the cerebral signal in increasingly fine-grained detail. This work has greatly enriched our understanding of Libet's findings and their implications for 'freedom'.

In a paper published in 1999, Haggard and Martin Eimer described an experiment in which they asked subjects to make finger movements while noting the times of their intentions to move (and, on other occasions, the moment of the perceived movement itself). However, in their version of this (Libet) task, Haggard and Eimer additionally required subjects to choose whether to move the left or right index finger. Hence, as well as their EEG equipment allowing them to discern (retrospectively) the time of onset of the early BP, it also enabled them to determine when the electrical signals specific to the ensuing movement became lateralized—that is, the point at which it became the *left* primary motor and lateral premotor cortices that were specifically involved in a movement of the *right* index finger (as opposed to their respective, contralateral, homologues). Through their use of event-related EEG, time-locked to the moment of ensuing movements, Haggard and Eimer (1999) were able to differentiate such lateralized signals (similar in composition to 'late BP'), occurring relatively 'late' in the emergence of a movement, from the 'earlier' onset ('early') BP. They also made specific predictions that are crucial to their experiment's interpretation:

1. If the early BP is involved in the generation of an 'intention to act', then the onset of the early BP and subjective recognition of an intention should covary in time (i.e. if the early BP's onset is relatively 'late', then the subject's conscious intention should also arise relatively 'late');

2. However, if the early BP is not implicated in the genesis of intentions, then such covariation in timings should not arise.

What did they find? They found that the time of onset of the early BP and the time of onset of subjective intention were not related: they did *not* covary in time. Instead, it was the time of onset of the lateralized signal (akin to the late BP) that covaried with subjective intention. If the lateralized signal arose earlier, then so did the subject's awareness of their 'intention to act'; if the lateralized signal was relatively delayed, then so was their subjective awareness.

The implications of these findings for our concept of agency are important to note. The lateralized signal occurs *later* in the course of action generation than the early BP; it occurs 'closer' to the time of action (it is, after all, a variant of the 'late' BP). Hence, by definition, it is a signal that arises relatively *late* in the volitional process. Yet, it is this signal that exhibits a temporal correlation with the onset of subjective 'intention'. So, what this means is that our subjective awareness of an intention to act arises even *later* in the volitional scheme of things than Libet had originally proposed (Libet et al., 1983). It appears that by the time that our subject becomes aware of her intention to act, the electrophysiological antecedents of that act have already progressed beyond the *medial* premotor system, beyond the temporal limits of the 'early BP'; they are closer to the processes of movement specification and execution, located within the primary motor and lateral premotor cortices, 'downstream' from the SMA. In other words, *awareness of an intention to act arises even later than we had previously thought.* Indeed, according to Haggard and Eimer (1999), awareness of an intention arises '*after* the stage of movement selection' (p. 131, emphasis added).

However, there is more, for Haggard and colleagues have also examined how our experiences of prior intention and voluntary movement might themselves be 'moved' in time: that is, how they might be forced earlier or later, relative to the onset of veridical action. How have they done this? Two lines of work are informative. The first concerns our awareness of 'movement' (c.f. 'intention').

The serial nature of motor programming

To adequately understand this first line of work, we need to pause to consider a theoretical account of action planning, one that particularly applies to automated, overlearnt activities (Sternberg et al., 1978). How is it that my brain programmes a sequence of linked motor events when 'I' must perform a chain of actions? Does the brain (i.e. the premotor cortex) 'begin' to programme the sequence, 'allow' me to commence my performance (prior to programme completion), and then make up the *rest* of the sequence as I go along, or does it programme the *whole* sequence before it 'allows' me to start 'in the first place'? One can see that there may be pros and cons to either procedure here and that it may be that these alternatives are theoretical 'extremes': that is, the 'real answer' lies somewhere in the middle (although it might be expedient to 'get on and do things', it would also be advantageous to be able to modify ongoing motor acts 'live' if new contingencies were to arise mid-sequence).

Nevertheless, there is a body of work that favours the latter version of motor programming: there are data suggesting that a programme is 'written' before its action correlate is 'released'. This finding originates in work by Sternberg and colleagues (see Sternberg et al., 1978; and Haggard et al., 1999). If subjects are presented with short and long chains of action sequences to be performed (e.g. sequences of letters to be typed, by touch typists, highly practiced in those actions which they are then called upon to perform), it can be shown that their response times (i.e. the times it takes for them to *commence* their action sequences) exhibit a correlation with the length of the ensuing sequences. Hence, the data suggest that the length of a sequence impacts the length of time required for that sequence to be programmed (as a series of movements); only *after* the sequence is programmed does the action commence. So, rather than starting an act, in the midst of its programming:

Programme: Movements 1, 2, 3,

Then

Act: Movements 1, 2,

Then

Continue programming: Movement 4, 5, end.
Act: Movements 3, 4, 5, end

The sequence is instead fully programmed before its performance begins:

Programme: Movements 1, 2, 3, 4, 5, end

Then

Act: Movements 1, 2, 3, 4, 5, end

Now, if this is the case, at what point does the agent become aware of 'her' movement? Does awareness arise before or after the sequence is programmed? We might predict that awareness of an actual movement (rather than its pre-ceding intention) *should* arise relatively late in the process. After all, it should relate to a veridical event, something that actually impacts upon the external world. So, it might arise very late. Indeed, if awareness relied upon *peripheral* feedback for its data (i.e. the responses of muscles and afferent, sensory, nerves to movements arising at the periphery), then movement awareness might actu-ally arise post hoc, after the movement had occurred.

However, it seems that this is not the case and, as was actually also demon-strated by Benjamin Libet, most subjects become aware of their 'movement' *before* the movement itself is enacted (or at least evidenced in the form of an EMG trace from the relevant muscle group). This suggests that our awareness of movement is related to 'central' processes, processes occurring within our brains, rather than those emerging at the periphery of our bodies (and there are other convergent literatures that support this point of view; see Jeannerod, 2006). So, we tend to 'anticipate' our movements (i.e. we perceive them as occurring *earlier* than they actually do in time), even though we experience our intentions relatively late within the process of volition (i.e. we experience them *after* the brain has initiated causation.) This point is worth emphasizing because it provides another example of how our voluntary processes depart from what we should expect on the basis of everyday phenomenology and classical (Cartesian) philosophy. While the latter imposes the following sequence on our actions:

INTENTION → BRAIN EVENT → MOVEMENT → AWARENESS VIA FEEDBACK

The work of Libet, Haggard, and others points in this direction instead:

BRAIN EVENT → INTENTION → 'PERCEIVED' MOVEMENT→ 'ACTUAL' MOVEMENT

Now, we have seen that work by Haggard and Eimer (1999) served to 'push' awareness of *intentions* later in the volitional process, these experiences exhibiting a temporal correlation with the onset of lateralized motor signals (not 'early BP'). Therefore, awareness of intentions appears to be related to motor programming (it is 'downstream' of the SMA) *after* the point of movement selection (according to Haggard and Eimer, 1999). But when do we become aware of 'movement'? Is this also linked to motor programming?

To answer these questions, Haggard and colleagues (1999) devised another variant on the Libet experiment. They had touch typists prepare to type (nonword) scripts of varying lengths, which they subsequently typed while performing a component of the Libet task (this time noting the time of onset of their own typing *movements*). As expected (on the basis of the foregoing literature), longer scripts were associated with longer response times (i.e. the onset of action performance took longer to appear when the subsequent movement sequence was going to be longer). This is in keeping with the Sternberg notion that motor programming is 'serial': a sequence is selected one movement at a time, from a store of possible movements; then, the response begins (so that longer sequences take longer to 'write', prior to movement). However, the experimenters' additional finding is really quite remarkable. Haggard and colleagues found that the longer the sequence of ensuing action, the *earlier* the onset of awareness of movements in their subjects. Hence, response time and onset of awareness were inversely correlated: the longer a sequence of acts, the later its onset in 'real' time (i.e. the longer the response time), but the *earlier* the subject's awareness of her impending movements. This finding suggests that awareness of movement is somehow linked, or 'tagged', to a moment *before* the specification of an action sequence. Haggard and colleagues (1999) say that it is 'generated upstream of the locus of complexity effects' (p. 300).

Hence, awareness of movement (a movement that has not actually occurred yet) is, in some way, 'pulled' further forward in time, even earlier than the onset of the veridical action, when that action sequence takes longer to programme. So, it isn't that awareness of movement is yoked to the *content* of motor programming; it is that movement awareness is linked to the *onset* of motor programming (and the earlier this arises in time, prior to action, then the earlier the 'movement' is perceived by its 'author').

Now, the reader may have already noticed an interesting contrast coming into focus here:

1. The onset of an 'intention' is linked not to the early BP but to the later, lateralized RP, and hence to the *programming* of specific features of an act (e.g. the laterality of the finger to be used; Haggard and Eimer, 1999).

2. However, the onset of awareness of the ensuing 'movement' is linked not to the content of programming but to its time of *onset* (Haggard et al., 1999), the beginning of action programming.

On first pass, this seems rather incongruous (to me). It is as if awareness of intention and awareness of ensuing movement have somehow 'passed each other by', in time. Intention is 'tagged' (in some sense) to a later process (the *content* of action programming) than is awareness of the movement itself (tagged, in some sense, to the *onset* of action programming). It is as if awareness of intention and awareness of movement are 'pulled' closer to each other, across time (see Fig. 45).

Disrupting motor preparation with TMS

Now this leads us to yet another clever experiment conducted by Haggard's group. In this case, in a further elaboration upon Libet's clock experiment, Haggard and Elena Magno (1999) used transcranial magnetic stimulation (TMS) as a means of disrupting local neuronal activity. They applied TMS over the left primary motor cortex and the SMA of healthy subjects who were using the Libet clock face to estimate the moment of onset of their own movements (specifically, movements of the *right* index finger during a reaction-time experiment; see Fig. 46). The experimenters found that stimulation over the left primary motor cortex significantly delayed the onset of ensuing movement (as reflected in the response time) but did not substantially affect the *perceived* time of movement onset (i.e. its perception by the subject, looking at the clock

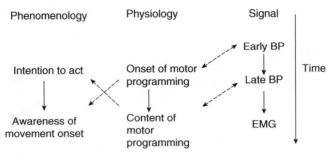

Fig. 45 Schematic showing the relationship between phenomenology, physiology, and electroencephalograph EEG signals during the emergence of a spontaneous motor act. From a phenomenological perspective, the intention to act precedes our awareness of movement onset. However, from a physiological perspective, the onset of motor programming precedes the finalization of the content of such motor programming, yet these components are related to apparently contradictory elements within subjective phenomenology. The content of motor programming is temporally linked to subjective awareness of an intention to act, while the onset of motor programming is temporally related to subjective awareness of movement onset. Note also that the content of motor programming is related to the late phase of the *Bereitschaftspotential* (BP) or readiness potential (RP). These data are derived from the work of Benjamin Libet, Patrick Haggard & colleagues.

face). However, although stimulation over the SMA was associated with less of a delay in action onset, it *did* precipitate a delay in the *perception* of movement. Hence, Haggard and Magno (1999) concluded:

> '[O]ur awareness of movement is at least partly an awareness of premotor processes occurring prior to the activation of motor cortex.' (p. 107).

So, this finding suggests yet another interesting contrast: whereas 'intentions to act' are associated with activity in the primary motor and lateral premotor cortices (as evidenced by their temporal relationship to the emergence of the lateralized RP), the subjective recognition of an ensuing movement may be disrupted by TMS over the *medial* premotor system, specifically the SMA. Again, the earlier phenomenological process ('intention') implicates the later neurological event (lateralized RP, late BP), and the later phenomenological event (awareness of a 'movement') implicates the earlier ('upstream') neurological event (arising within the medial premotor cortex, the SMA; a source of the early BP; and, indeed, as we know from the work of Cunnington and colleagues [2005], an area that undergoes activation *prior* to the primary motor cortex in the genesis of an 'internally initiated' movement). Hence, there is a kind of temporal overlap or interdigitation (see Fig. 45).

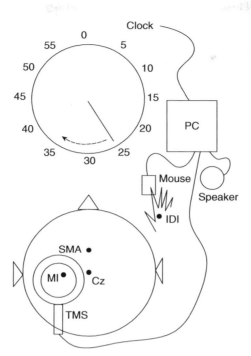

Fig. 46 Cartoon demonstrating the experimental apparatus used by Haggard and Magno. Subjects were required to look at a Libet clock face and to make movements using the right index finger (IDI). They were also subjected to transcranial magnetic stimulation (TMS), which was applied over the left primary motor cortex (M1) or the supplementary motor area (SMA). (From Haggard and Mango, Experimental Brain Research 1999; 127: 102–107, with kind permission from Springer Science and Business Media).

Now, it is hard to overemphasize how strange this series of findings is, for it seems to commit us to the following account of volition: our awareness of our own movement is temporally related to a neural process that commences prior to the (neural) process that is related to our (subsequent) awareness of our intentions. If all of this is true, then not only do 'intentions to act' arise later in the volitional process than even Benjamin Libet had specified but also the neurological processes that somehow 'anchor' our intentions in time arise later than those that 'anchor' our awareness of our own movements. Hence, we are, in a sense, doubly 'late': our intentions are late not only in real time (because they are related to the lateralized RP) but also in biological processing terms (because they are anchored to the *content* of action programming, whereas our awareness of movement is anchored to the *onset* of action programming). Another way of stating this difference might be to say that our intention is bound to the identity of a movement (i.e. it arises 'post-selection'), whereas our awareness of movement is bound to the emergence of movement per se (it is tagged to the *onset* of selection).

The 'binding' of action

Adding yet another level of complexity to this state of affairs, there is a further paper by Haggard and colleagues (2002), in which the authors go some way towards explaining why such 'binding' of phenomenological correlates might have arisen. Again, they studied healthy subjects engaged in finger movements, but this time they asked them to estimate both the timing of their movements *and* the timing of environmental sounds linked to those movements. Sometimes the subjects pressed a key and an audible tone followed, at an interval; sometimes hand muscle movements were elicited from the subjects by TMS applied over their motor cortices (and again followed by a tone). When the subjects were themselves responsible for making the movements that precipitated these sounds (in a Libet experimental setting), they seemed to experience their own movements as arising relatively 'late', whereas the resultant sounds were experienced relatively 'early' (i.e. these phenomenological correlates, self-generated movement and sound, were said to be 'attracted' in time). In contrast, when the subjects' movements were elicited not by voluntary means but by TMS, then their movements were perceived as arising relatively 'early' in time whereas the associated sound was perceived as arising relatively 'later' than in the index condition (a so-called 'repulsion effect').

The authors suggest that under normal circumstances our awareness of our voluntary actions is 'bound' to their consequences, in time. In other words, if we cause something to happen, then our conscious processes 'bind' the action to its outcome (they bring them 'closer' together, in time). In contrast, where involuntary movements occur in the context of other environmental stimuli, we perceive the former's onset at an enhanced temporal separation from any, subsequent, spurious consequences 'out there' in the sensory environment. Hence, we have a potential means of differentiating the endogenous from the exogenous among the consequences of bodily movement, a way of distinguishing voluntary actions from externally 'caused' events (Haggard et al., 2002).

These are complex data and they deserve careful consideration. They also require replication and some conclusion as to their ubiquity: are these effects true in everyone? In some of their papers, Haggard's group point out that not all their subjects 'behave' in these ways. Might some of us be wired differently? It is too early to say. Nevertheless, these findings seem to imply an interesting evolutionary development (in most 'healthy' human subjects): complex brains evolved not only to possess systems for action generation but also systems for distinguishing the internally initiated act from involuntary events, externally induced associations of phenomena within the sensory environment. Implicit in this evolutionary process there seems to be a tacit acknowledgement (though 'what' or 'who' is acknowledging it I cannot say) that certain forms of brain will generate new behaviours 'internally', and that at some level within such brains there will be a 'requirement' to differentiate the 'internal' from the 'external', the 'willed' from the 'caused'. Indeed, as we shall see in later chapters of this book, and as we have already seen in the case of SMA activation occurring while other agents are observed in action (e.g. the work of Cunnington and colleagues), when we pursue the cognitive neurobiological architecture of volition, we find representations of not only our 'own' acts but also the actions and intentions of others.

I am not sure that this necessarily brings us any closer to an understanding of what it is that Bernard Schlink described as the 'it' (in our Prologue), the complex 'selector' of behaviours that (at times) seems to run counter to our intentions, that is the author of those reversals of intention that we somehow seem capable of, the times when we 'do what we have to do' (even though we had thought we wouldn't). Nevertheless, it does seem to point to the importance of medial premotor systems in both the generation of our self-initiated actions and our awareness of their timing. Indeed, before we leave these references to the work of Benjamin Libet behind, there is one further element that we shall find addressed in a later paper by Patrick Haggard.

Free won't

The reader may recall that in his attempt to defend the concept of 'free will', Benjamin Libet invoked the possibility that our conscious awareness of our intentions might (somehow) accrue and retain the power of veto over undesirable actions in the course of their genesis. So, even though we might become aware of our intentions to act somewhat 'late', at some finite delay *after* the emergence of a specific action's neural antecedents, we might nevertheless be able to suppress what was about to happen, before it emerged as an act. Now, we argued in the Prologue that there were logical reasons for doubting whether such a conscious veto was any more 'free' than a conscious intention as both were likely to comprise the (late) phenomenological correlates of antecedent neural events; nevertheless, we acknowledged that there were strong phenomenological (and commonsensical) grounds for believing that such a veto exists (indeed, we experience something like it whenever we 'change our minds'.) So, what is interesting is that Patrick Haggard has again described what it is that Benjamin Libet envisaged in neurophysiological terms.

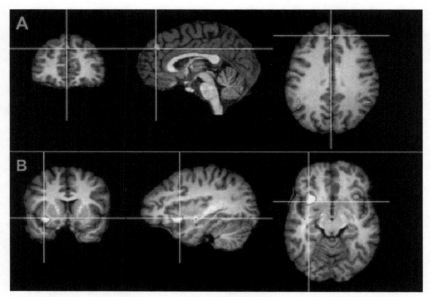

Fig. 47 Data showing those areas of the brain exhibiting greater activity when subjects cancelled their intentions to act. 'A' shows brain slices through dorsomedial frontal cortex; 'B' shows slices through anterior insula. (From Brass and Haggard, *Journal of Neuroscience* 2007; 27: 9141–9145). (See colour plate section).

In a recently published functional neuroimaging study, Brass and Haggard (2007) described yet another variant of the Libet paradigm. This time they required healthy subjects to prepare to move, while watching the Libet clock face, and some of the time they were to generate voluntary acts and some of the time they were to 'cancel' such acts (post-intention but prior to movement). Under each condition, they were asked to note the time at which their intentions arose. The authors found that intentions to act arose at approximately 140 ms prior to veridical acts, and that (as expected) action performance was associated with activation of the primary motor cortex (and cerebellum). When subjects experienced intentions to act, they activated the pre-SMA and medial premotor structures (whether or not these intentions were subsequently acted upon; this is consistent with the work of Cunnington and others).

However, when subjects *cancelled* their intentions, when they 'decided' not to act, they exhibited additional activation in an area of the prefrontal cortex, 'higher' up on the medial surface of the frontal lobe than the SMA ('dorsomedial' frontal cortex [BA 9]; a region of the prefrontal rather than the premotor cortex). Hence, the authors posit that this medial prefrontal region is implicated in 'self-control', in *stopping agents* from enacting intentions. Therefore, in a sense, Brass and Haggard have located Libet's focus of 'free won't' (see Fig. 47). It doesn't mean that we are 'free' (in the libertarian sense), but it does suggest that there is a neural correlate of our 'changing our minds'.

Summary

In this chapter, we have examined some very detailed and elegantly designed experiments, which have required great attention to fine distinctions. We have examined 'intentions' and the subjective awareness of 'movement'. Latterly, we have touched upon 'vetoes', cancelled intentions. All these studies serve to enhance our understanding of what it is that happens while 'freely chosen' intentions and 'internally initiated' acts are generated (or not generated, cancelled) in the healthy human brain. We have clarified the timing of some of those components that constitute the cerebral motor response and we have identified patterns of association pertaining between subjective phenomena (i.e. our experiences of intention and movement, volition) and the cognitive, neurobiological processes that underpin action. We have demonstrated the pivotal contribution of the medial premotor systems to action generation and medial prefrontal systems to action suppression (the 'cancelling' of intentions, self-control).

The reader who has persevered thus far, moving step by step through this important body of literature, may now like to consider taking a break, perhaps making a cup of tea. She may already have decided to make one. Indeed, she may have put the kettle 'on'. Alternatively, she may have just cancelled that intention.

Chapter 4

Volitional architectures

A cortico-basal ganglia network is a functional group comprising different cortical, striatal and pallidal components, in addition to the various cell groups (for example, dopaminergic) in the midbrain that constitute the brain's value system, as well as associated diencephalic structures (for example, the thalamus and the subthalamic nucleus). The integration of various physiological processes in these components results in the output of the network – that is, behaviour.[9]

[A]ll would like to follow the thread of their own actions' consequences; but the more they sharpen their eyes, the less they can discern a continuous line ...[10]

At the beginning of this book, in chapters 1 and 2, we were particularly concerned with delineating the structures that 'support' our apparent capacity for volition, for our 'internally initiated' voluntary behaviours. At that time, our emphasis was very much upon identifying such structures and studying the paths via which they might communicate with other structures, also engaged during the performance of purposeful, volitional activity, e.g. in the movement of a right index finger (Chapter 1). Furthermore, in order to delineate the components of a (hypothetical) 'Will' (in Chapter 2), we dwelt upon the specific contributions of defined areas within the frontal lobes, their cytoarchitectures, their patterns of projections, and the characteristic effects upon humans (and non-human primates) of lesions located within their defined fields. All this was necessary in order for us to be able to achieve an awareness of the 'major players' – the most important regions of the brain – engaged in

[9] From H.H. Yin and B.J. Knowlton. The role of the basal ganglia in habit formation. *Nature Reviews Neuroscience* 2006; 7: 464–476 (quote is taken from p. 471).

[10] Italo Calvino. *Invisible Cities* (translated by William Weaver). London: Vintage, 1997 (first published in Italy as *Le cita invisibili*, 1972), p. 142.

supporting human action. However, it also risked engendering a rather naive view of the brain's function – as if it were merely comprised of a series of component (cortical) modules 'talking' to each other; as if each module or component pursued its 'own' project while being capable of isolation from its neighbours; as if (one day) it might be taken out and 'replaced', rather like a faulty transistor in a radio or television. In this chapter, we attempt to remedy this situation. Rather than dwelling upon specific foci we move, instead, towards a consideration of 'circuits', the distributed processes that support human action. Indeed, we consider a series of different forms of circuitry, in order to see what it is that each may contribute to our understanding of voluntary behaviour.

However, before we do all this, I wish to recount a moment from 'real life'. I do this because it serves to highlight the seriousness of our undertaking. It points the way towards some of the doors that we could be opening, were we *really* to comprehend the neural basis of human behaviour.

Night time in the factory

Some years ago, I attended a scientific meeting at a former monastery in a European country. It was an honour to be invited, and I was very pleased to attend. There were some famous speakers on the faculty and I was looking forward to hearing what each of those invited had to say. So it was only after we had arrived, when all of us had convened for dinner on the first evening, that we were informed of the history of that place, our venue. It had been a hospital of sorts during the period of National Socialism, under the reign of the Nazis, at the height of the Second World War, and many people with psychiatric diagnoses had been murdered there. Our venue had once been a centre for so-called 'euthanasia'.

Now, it was in this rather incongruous setting, among beautiful architecture and tranquil gardens, and with a growing awareness of a terrible (though invisible) past, 'behind us', that I heard one of the philosophers in the party make his presentation. He was talking about the impossibility of 'Free Will' and was admonishing psychologists and neuroscientists for their rather hesitant steps towards ejecting this archaic remnant of 'folk psychology' from the human brain. Successive writers and experimenters, he said, had been too fond of retaining some 'supervising' entity within the central nervous system, some 'control' process that kept all the other functions in check. All this was unhelpful because, inevitably, it led to an infinite regress: if there really were control processes in the brain, sitting at the head of a neural hierarchy, then what was perched at the top of that hierarchy? What was in control of the 'controller'? We always seemed to return to the myth of the homunculus, a little man sitting in a control room, making decisions inside the human brain. That was a problem because, inevitably, there would need to be another little man sitting in the control centre of the homunculus' brain, and inside that little man's head another little man, and so on and so forth, *ad infinitum.*

What was the solution to this intractable problem? The reader will be disappointed to learn that the philosopher did not provide an answer! However, he did tell us how we might recognize such a solution if ever we were to find one. *We would have 'explained' human action when our model of the brain resembled a factory turning over at night.* We would have solved the mystery of human volition when we had described a mechanism that ran 'by itself'. We 'should' be able to walk around such a model, inspect its machines and systems, and see it all working and fully functioning *without* the necessity for any 'human' presence. However, while our models of the brain retained a 'controller', while there was still within that nocturnal factory a little man (or woman) in a white coat tinkering with the controls, or even only very occasionally pulling a lever, then we would *not* have explained human action. What we were aiming for was a machine that ran without 'us'; and there was no room for a ghost in that machine.

Now, there are several emotional responses that one might have experienced in the face of such an account of the human condition. Indeed, I must admit that I found it especially bleak in view of the setting in which it was expounded. We were enjoined to compare ourselves to machines while sitting in a factory of other people's deaths. We were systems that 'should' be running on a kind of 'automatic'. Any remaining control process was really just a cop-out.

However, there is a critically important point at the heart of the philosopher's rhetoric. How *does* the brain initiate, modulate, and terminate action, in the absence of a controller – a little man sitting in his little white room, pulling at all the levers? If there is no control room, then what is it that is 'calling the shots'? And can we find any way of thinking past the ubiquitous homunculus? As we have already seen, in this book, even the most eminent neuroscientists have invoked the language of 'control' when speaking of primate actions. We saw in Table 7 (Chapter 2) just some of the many terms that have been used to convey the concept of an 'executive', a 'controller', a 'supervisory' attentional system, modulating motor function; the terms evolve but the concept remains familiar: there is 'something' that is in 'control', in the primate brain. However, to our philosopher, this is precisely the problem. It is all unnecessarily mysterious. We need to do away with the controller; we need to evict him!

So it is that in this chapter we offer one route out of this apparent impasse. We examine the 'circuits' that contribute to our cognitive neurobiological function and we describe how they circulate information. With circuits – re-entrant

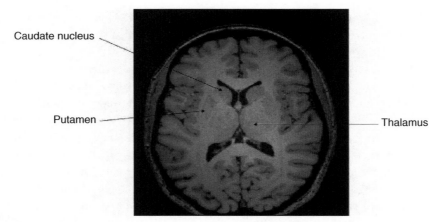

Fig. 48 MRI scan showing transverse section of the healthy brain: the arrows indicate the larger structures of the basal ganglia.

loops in which information is recurrently re-cycled, in trajectories that are (ultimately) circular – there need be no 'top' and no 'bottom'. Hence, there might be no need for us to identify (and retain) a ghostly central 'controller'. Perhaps. Maybe. We shall see.

Basal ganglia circuits and parallel 're-entrant' 'loops'

On several occasions, in the course of this book, we have mentioned the basal ganglia and referred to their role in the control of movement. Now we shall address these structures in greater detail, with a particular view to identifying the circuits that run *between* them. Such circuits actually form intermediate pathways within much longer circuits (the so-called basal ganglia-thalamo-cortical 'loops'), running between the cerebral cortex, basal ganglia, and specific thalamic nuclei, whence they project *back* to the cortex. These circuits are said to be 'semi-closed' because they each exhibit open, relatively widespread origins (distributed across connected cerebral cortical regions), their projections condensing upon a series of relays within the loops themselves and, subsequently, via the final relay, to a specific region of the cortex, which effectively 'closes' each loop. Hence, in the 'motor' loop (below) the supplementary motor area (SMA; BA 6) comprises the cortical region that contributes to the wider origin of the loop while also constituting its final destination, its point of closure.

Now, at the level of the basal ganglia themselves, each loop bifurcates between two alternate routes, each of which is of great importance: the so-called 'direct' and 'indirect' pathways (below). These pathways have different and potentially 'opposing' effects upon the 'output' of discrete basal ganglia-thalamo-cortical systems, enhancing or suppressing their thalamic transmissions to the frontal cortex. As noted, such a pairing of potentially opposing local networks is repeated across each of the loops or 're-entrant' circuits, to which the basal ganglia contribute (five are most often described, though there may be more).

Overall, such loops derive their varied origins from throughout most of the cerebral cortices; they then 'target' specific regions of the basal ganglia via their projections (a funnelling of axonal information, akin to that seen within the *corona radiata*; Chapter 1), whence they proceed to connect the latter, via the thalamus, with specific regions of the frontal lobes; as implied (above), these 'targets' give the loops their names (e.g. the supplementary motor area is the focus of the 'motor' loop) and help us in elucidating their functions (below). Thus, information seems to be condensed from across wide swathes (of interconnected areas) of the cerebral cortex, and re-focussed upon relatively specific regions of the 'premotor' and 'prefrontal' cortices, via these basal ganglia-thalamo-cortical circuits, before being potentially 're-circulated' within their 'loops' (below).

Now, the basal ganglia, by definition, comprise a group of grey matter structures ('ganglia') located towards the bases of the cerebral hemispheres. As alluded to (above), their current definition and conceptualization places an especial emphasis upon their contribution to the control of movement, hence, all those structures that we are about to describe share in this function. Historically, however, and from a strictly neurological perspective, we 'might' have included certain other nuclei among their number, nuclei that also comprise grey matter and reside within the hemispheric white matter, but which are *not* thought to be pivotal to the control of movement; hence, the claustrum and the amygdala have tended to be excluded from current accounts of these structures. Therefore, as the term is currently applied, the 'basal ganglia' specifically refer to nuclei that are pivotal to the control of movement, though it has also become increasingly apparent that these same nuclei make important contributions to motivation and cognition (below). Hence, the nuclei of the basal ganglia, as currently defined, are:

1. The 'striatum': predominantly comprising the caudate nucleus and the putamen (though also including the nucleus accumbens, a part of the limbic system). The caudate and putamen develop from the same embryonic 'telencephalic' structure (Table 10) and, as a result, are composed throughout of the same cell types (the most common, comprising approximately 75% of the total, are 'medium-sized' neurons with 'spiny' dendrites). The caudate and putamen are also fused anteriorly. These components of the striatum form the 'input' nuclei of the basal ganglia.

2. The 'pallidum' (or globus pallidus): derives from the embryonic 'diencephalon' (Table 10), and lies medial to the putamen and lateral to the internal capsule (see Figure 49). It comprises two components: one termed the lateral (GPL) or 'external' (G Pe) segment, and the other the medial (GPM) or 'internal' (G Pi) segment. The latter has a midbrain extension known as the *pars reticulata* of the substantia nigra (SNpr); this is pale in appearance and resembles the pallidum cytologically; it contains only pure 'GABA' neurons (inhibitory neurons containing the amino acid neurotransmitter gamma amino butyric acid). The globus pallidum and the SNpr may be considered a single functional entity (though they are physically divided by the 'internal capsule'; Figure 13, Chapter 1); together, they constitute the major 'output' nuclei of the basal ganglia.

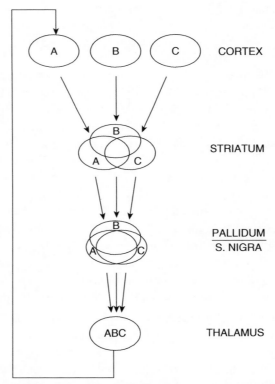

Fig. 49 Cartoon showing the generic organization of the basal ganglia-thalamo-cortical loops. Projections run between the cortex, striatum, pallidum, and thalamus before projecting back to the cortex. The loops are semi closed in that multiple cortical areas project to the lower levels within each loop, but the loop is closed by its thalamic projection back to a specific cortical focus (as indicated by A in the figure).

Table 10 Principal divisions of the adult brain

Division	Components
Telencephalon	Cerebral cortex, basal ganglia, and olfactory bulbs
Diencephalon	Thalamus, hypothalamus, and epithalamus
Mesencephalon	The midbrain, including structures around the cerebral aqueduct, superior and inferior colliculi, and cerebral peduncles
Metencephalon	Pons and cerebellum
Myelencephalon	Open and closed medulla

"In early development, the brain and spinal cord arise from the neural tube, which greatly expands at the front end of the embryo to form the main divisions of the brain." (Woolsey et al., 2008, p. 8).

3. The 'subthalamic nucleus' (STN): as the name implies, lies below the thalamus, at its junction with the midbrain. It is unique among the basal ganglia in that it utilizes the excitatory neurotransmitter glutamate (an amino acid). The STN's contribution to motor control will be addressed presently (below).

4. The main pigmented component of the substantia nigra, known as the *pars compacta* (SNpc) lies dorsal to the *pars reticulata* and is comprised of dopaminergic neurons whose cell bodies contain neuromelanin. The latter, a dark pigment, gives the substantia nigra its name (i.e. substantia nigra = 'black substance' in Latin). The SNpc comprises about 400 000 neurons, nearly all of which project to the striatum via the 'nigrostriatal' pathway (below). Each nigral neuron forms more than a million varicosities (beads), which make synaptic contact with the 'spiny' dendrites of GABAergic neurons (the 'medium-sized' neurons, referred to above). The predominant effect of dopaminergic activity in the striatum is inhibitory (especially upon the enkephalin-containing GABAergic cells projecting from the striatum to G Pe, as part of the 'indirect' pathway; below). Dopamine is a catecholamine neurotransmitter (below).

Nuclei within the thalamus are also implicated in basal ganglia function: the ventral anterior (VA) nucleus and the anterior part of the ventrolateral (VL) nucleus. In addition, the dorsomedial nucleus is involved in the three 'prefrontal' (i.e. 'higher') loops that we shall describe (the dorsolateral prefrontal, lateral orbitofrontal, and anterior cingulate circuits; below).

Circuit patterns

In general, the following patterns recur within each of the (five or more) loops running through the basal ganglia:

1. To begin with, the cortical 'input' to the striatum is excitatory, comprising glutamatergic corticostriate neurons conveying information from the

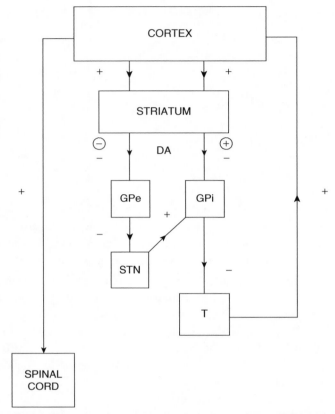

Fig. 50 Cartoon demonstrating the organization of basal ganglia-thalamo-cortical loops in relation to the motor system and also the influence of the neurotransmitter dopamine. Within each loop there is a direct and indirect pathway. The direct pathway facilitates cortical activation via excitatory projections between the thalamus and cortex. Dopamine (DA) facilitates the functioning of the direct pathway (as indicated by the + in the figure). Meanwhile, the indirect pathway reduces output to the cortex. The indirect pathway is inhibited by dopamine (as indicated by the minus sign shown in the figure). (See colour plate section).

cortex to the caudate or putamen. These inputs derive from small pyramidal cells in cortical laminae V and VI (see Chapter 1). For each loop, the contributory cortical areas are regions that tend also to be interconnected with each other (hence, the primary motor, primary somatosensory, lateral, and medial premotor cortices (PMCs) each contribute to the 'motor' or 'SMA' loop, below).

2. The striatum itself houses excitatory cholinergic 'internuncial' neurons (which are 'aspiny') and inhibitory GABA-containing internuncials. It receives

(inhibitory) dopaminergic innervation via the nigrostriatal pathway (from SNpc, above).

3. From within the striatum, there emerge inhibitory pathways, utilizing GABA and expressing certain other neurotransmitters (i.e. substance P, dynorphin, and enkephalin) to communicate with structures 'down-stream' of the striatum.

4. As noted, there are two forms of pathway 'down-stream' of the striatum (within each basal ganglia 'loop' system):

   (i) A 'direct' pathway, conveys inhibitory tone from the striatum to the G Pi (via neurons utilizing GABA, substance P, and dynorphin); whereupon a second inhibitory pathway relays inhibitory tone from the G Pi to the thalamus (via neurons utilizing GABA; above). This 'direct' pathway, therefore, comprises a sequential 'inhibition of an inhibition' so that its ultimate effect is to 'facilitate' thalamic transmission to the cortex (i.e. the next stage in each 'loop'). (Note: neurons within the first leg of the direct pathway, which express genes coding for substance P, also express dopamine receptors of the D1 family. Though predominantly inhibitory in its effects, dopamine serves to 'excite' the direct pathway.)

   (ii) An 'indirect' pathway, conveys inhibitory tone from the striatum to the G Pe (via neurons utilizing GABA and enkephalin); whereupon another relay conveys inhibitory tone between the G Pe and the sub-thalamic nucleus (via neurons utilizing GABA); whence a further relay conveys excitatory tone (utilizing glutamate) from the subthalamic nucleus to the G Pi (which, of course, then sends a further inhibitory relay to the thalamus, the latter utilizing GABA). Hence, this 'indirect' pathway exhibits a rather more complex architecture than the direct pathway (above). Ultimately, however, its role is to 'inhibit' thalamic transmission to the cortex. Therefore, its effect is in opposition to that of the direct pathway. (Note also: neurons within the first leg of the indirect pathway, which express genes coding for enkephalin, also express dopamine receptors of the D2 family. Dopamine tends to 'inhibit' the indirect pathway.)

5. Finally, each 'loop' pathway closes with thalamic projections, returning to the cortex. These are excitatory in nature (utilizing glutamate as their neurotransmitter). For each loop, a 'different' frontal region constitutes its output target (see below).

An understanding of the direct and indirect pathways will be very important when we come to consider how cortical activity is modulated, both by endogenous neurotransmitters (e.g. dopamine) and also by exogenous substances (e.g. the amphetamines, cocaine, and antipsychotic medications). Though the circuitry is complex, it is a useful 'rule of thumb' to regard the direct pathway as facilitating thalamo-cortical transmission (hence, as increasing cortical 'activation'), while the indirect pathway reduces thalamic output (thereby reducing cortical activation).

The basal ganglia-thalamo-cortical loops

As noted (above), there are several different 'loops' running through the basal ganglia and, at the time of writing, five have been described, albeit in varying detail (see Figure 51). We set out their main features below; then we focus upon those aspects of their structure and function that are germane to the problem of volition. The five 'loops' we describe are those originally delineated in a classic paper by Garrett E. Alexander, Mahlon R. DeLong, and Peter L. Strick (in 1986):

1. The 'motor' circuit: This loop of re-entrant projections takes its origins from across the primary motor, primary somatosensory, lateral, and medial PMCs and passes through the putamen, the globus pallidus interna (G Pi), and then on, through the VL nucleus of the thalamus, before projecting back to the SMA (BA 6). While other loops derive their origins solely from the ipsilateral cerebral cortex, the motor loop is different in that the primary motor cortex (BA 4) projects to both 'its own' (ipsilateral) putamen (and associated loop) and its contralateral neighbour (i.e. the 'other' loop). Hence, each motor loop 'condenses' data from across both hemispheres. Also, at the level of the basal ganglia, within these motor circuits, there is a somatotopic distribution of three groups of projections: those relating to the movements of the contralateral leg, represented relatively laterally (in the case of the putamen, this involves its dorsolateral sector), the contralateral arm, represented centrally, and the face, represented relatively medially (in the putamen, this implicates its ventromedial sector). Hence, this pattern provides yet another example of a somatotopic representation occurring within the motor system (as evidenced in primary motor and medial PMCs; chapters 1 & 2).

2. An 'oculomotor' circuit: This takes its origins from the frontal eye fields (BA 8; Chapter 2) – dorsolateral prefrontal and posterior parietal cortices. It passes via the caudate nucleus and substantia nigra pars reticulata to the VA nucleus of the thalamus and then projects back to the frontal eye fields (thereby closing the loop). SNpr also sends an inhibitory GABAergic projection to the superior colliculus, where it synapses on cells controlling saccadic eye movements. Hence, the oculomotor circuit is well

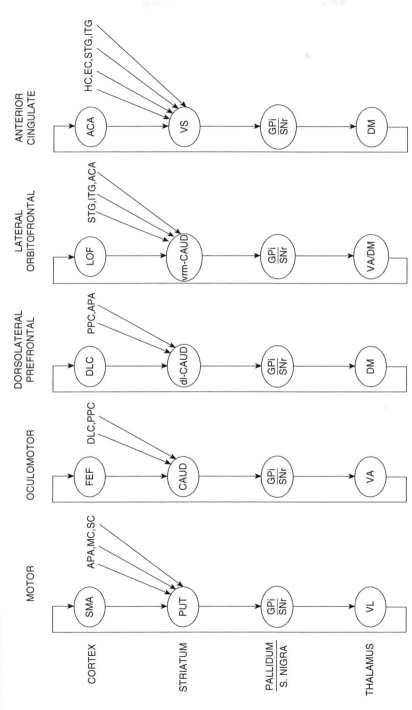

Fig. 51 Cartoon demonstrating the five basal ganglia-thalamo-cortical loop circuits described by Alexander & colleagues in 1986.

placed to contribute to the modulation of eye movements and gaze in a way analogous to the motor circuit's modulation of limb and face movements (above).

3. A 'dorsolateral prefrontal' circuit: Here, the dorsolateral caudate nucleus receives excitatory inputs from the 'association' cortices, including dorsolateral prefrontal cortex (DLPFC) itself, posterior parietal and lateral premotor cortices, then it relays them via the pallidum and the VA and dorsomedial nuclei of the thalamus. These thalamic nuclei project back to the DLPFC. Hence, this circuit is very likely to be implicated in cognitive functions such as working memory, visuospatial cognition, and new learning (e.g. of motor routines, especially those that are reliant upon external environmental cues).

4. A 'lateral orbitofrontal' circuit: In this case, projections from the lateral orbitofrontal cortex (OFC), and the auditory and visual association cortices of the (superior and inferior) temporal lobes, target the ventromedial caudate nucleus, and are then relayed via the pallidum to the VA and dorsomedial nuclei of the thalamus, whence their returning projections target the lateral OFC (i.e., closing the loop). This network is implicated in behavioural 'switching' and response 'suppression': bilateral lesions of the lateral OFC and ventromedial caudate can each precipitate perseverative behaviours (manifest when an animal can no longer suppress those responses that have become contextually inappropriate and, therefore, un-rewarding; Chapter 2).

5. An 'anterior cingulate' circuit: This loop takes its origins from among certain of the 'limbic' areas, including the cingulate gyrus, the amygdala, and other temporal lobe regions. The latter project to the nucleus accumbens (part of the 'ventral' striatum; above) and the ventral pallidum, whereupon relays pass to the dorsomedial nucleus of the thalamus before returning to the anterior cingulate (thereby closing the loop). This combination of limbic (emotional, motivational) information and the cingulate's access to motor circuits (above) suggests that this loop is ideally suited to 'bridging' the limbic and the motor systems. Hence, some authors have argued that the anterior cingulate loop is likely to be implicated in the (motor) expression of emotions, such as smiling and gesturing, and adopting aggressive and submissive postures. Remember also that lesions of the anterior cingulate region are implicated in causing akinetic mutism, lack of 'emotional will power', and the extinction of maternal–infant bonding behaviours in primates (as we saw in Chapter 2). Hence, this circuit is likely to be contributory to some very important (and complex) social behaviour (and see Chapter 6).

Clearly, these are complex systems and such an account provides only a thumbnail sketch of their most significant putative contributions to behaviour. Indeed, I shall address certain of these circuits in more detail below. However, first I wish to mention certain 'other patterns' that are discernible at the level of the striatum, and which may be hypothesized to impact basal ganglia-thalamo-cortical circuit function:

1. It is readily apparent that a distinction may be drawn between the innervation of the 'dorsal' and 'ventral' regions of the striatum. While the former, largely comprising the putamen, derives its projections from motor and association cortices (consistent with its being pivotal to the modulation of 'movement'), the latter, largely comprising the caudate (and nucleus accumbens) derives its projections from orbitofrontal, limbic, and temporal lobe structures (hence, it is more likely to be implicated in 'motivation'). Thus, it would be unsurprising if the dorsal and ventral striatum facilitated different aspects of voluntary behaviour.

2. Putamen and caudate also receive different (intralaminar) thalamic innervations: the centromedian nucleus projects to the putamen, conveying relays from the cerebellum and the pallidum; while the nucleus lateralis projects to the anterior striatum (especially the caudate nucleus), again conveying relays from the cerebellum.

3. There is a discernible neurochemical gradient instantiated across the striatum, with the rostral (anterior) regions being particularly rich in dopaminergic, substance P, and acetylcholinergic inputs, while the caudal (postero-inferior) regions are relatively rich in serotonin and glutamic acid decarboxylase (the enzyme catalysing the formation of GABA; below).

4. Such neurochemical tone modulates the response of the striatum to cortical and thalamic afferents (above).

5. The origin of such tone also varies across the striatum. Whereas the relatively dorsal striatum (in this case, the caudate and putamen) derives its dopaminergic innervation from the nigrostriatal (or 'meso-striatal') pathway, originating in the SNpc (with an additional input from the retrorubal nucleus), the relatively ventral striatum (in this case, the nucleus accumbens) derives its dopaminergic innervation from the ventral tegmental area (VTA or 'paranigral' nucleus) and the medial SNpc (a 'mesolimbic' pathway, which also projects to the septal nuclei, hippocampus, amygdala, and prefrontal and cingulate cortices, via the 'medial forebrain bundle'; Standring, 2005).

6. However, both the dorsal and ventral striatum derive their serotonergic innervation from the dorsal raphe nuclei, and their noradrenergic input from the locus coeruleus (below).

Understanding voluntary movement

Clearly, the 'motor' circuit (described above) will be central to our understanding of voluntary movement, volition. Indeed, as we have already seen, it provides structural links between some of the key regions implicated in motor function, e.g. those projections running between the primary motor cortex, SMA, and putamen. However, we also know that this circuit may be distinguished from another, which we have outlined in Chapter 1: the 'pyramidal' tract (running from the primary motor cortex, via the internal capsule and the medulla, to the ventral horn of the contralateral spinal cord; Figure 12). Hence, we may speculate that it is likely that the 'motor' circuit makes its contribution to motor control via some 'modulation' of this other (pyramidal) tract. Indeed, it is in keeping with this hypothesis that the SMA, the cortical target of the motor circuit ('loop'), is located 'upstream' of primary motor cortex, both in terms of its anatomy (in that it lies 'anterior' to the primary motor cortex) and its function (in that it comprises medial 'premotor' cortex; i.e. a hierarchically 'superior' tier within the cortical motor system; Chapter 2). Furthermore, as we have learned from the work of Libet, Haggard, Cunnington, and others (reviewed in Chapter 3), the SMA is activated (and thereby implicated) during the emergence of an 'internally initiated' voluntary act at a time *prior to* the activation of the primary motor cortex. So, if the motor circuit serves to modulate function at the level of the SMA (via thalamo-cortical projections), then it is very likely to have implications for the 'early' stages of an 'internally initiated' act.

Indeed, all this is congruent with evidence that we have already encountered concerning certain pathologies of voluntary movement – those that implicate the 'motor' circuit, 'below the level of the SMA', i.e. at the level of the basal ganglia. For instance, in Parkinson's disease, a deficiency of dopaminergic transmission at the level of the putamen causes akinesia and bradykinesia (absence or slowness of movement, respectively), muscular rigidity, and tremor. *Self-initiated, 'internally initiated'* movement is impeded; the early component of the *Bereitschaftspotential* is diminished; in other words, there is a problem with the 'medial' premotor system, including the SMA. How might this have arisen?

Well, a central feature of Parkinson's disease is the degeneration of the substantia nigra *pars compacta*, the source of the dopaminergic nigrostriatal pathway. Such degeneration leads to a loss of nigrostriatal terminals within the striatum, and reduced levels of dopamine. (Dopamine 'receptors' remain; however, they are located on the GABAergic (medium spiny) neurons constituting the striatal origins of both the direct and indirect pathways. Hence, whereas D1 receptors occupy the GABAergic/substance P/dynorphin relays from the striatum to the globus pallidus interna (in the direct pathway), D2 receptors occupy the GABAergic/enkephalin relays from the striatum to the globus pallidus externa (in the indirect pathway; above).) The effect of such a local loss of dopaminergic tone (at the level of the striatum) is, therefore, understandable if we consider what dopamine normally 'does' in this region. We saw that through its activity at D1 and D2 receptors (above) dopamine acts to specifically 'excite' and 'inhibit' the direct and indirect pathways, respectively. Hence, dopamine normally has a 'dual action' at the level of the striatum.

So, when dopaminergic transmission is reduced, as a consequence of SNpc degeneration in the context of Parkinson's disease, the effect is to remove excitation from the direct pathway and to remove inhibition from the indirect pathway. Less tone in the direct pathway lessens the drive to the thalamo-cortical projections (thereby, potentially reducing cortical, SMA, activation). Meanwhile, the indirect pathway is 'disinhibited'. Hence, 'downstream', within this (indirect) pathway, the subthalamic nucleus is 'released' from its own 'inhibition' (by the G Pe) thereby allowing its increased 'excitation' of G Pi to precipitate excessive 'inhibition' of the motor nuclei within the thalamus. Therefore, bearing in mind that the indirect pathway normally serves to 'inhibit' thalamo-cortical transmission, the outcome in Parkinson's disease is likely to be an 'exaggeration' of such inhibition (i.e. a marked diminution) of transmission within the affected basal ganglia-thalamo-cortical circuits. Hence, in the case of the 'motor' circuit, there will be a reduction of excitatory (glutamatergic) transmission to the SMA.

So, it is unsurprising that when people with Parkinson's disease are studied, using functional neuroimaging techniques, while they attempt to produce voluntary movements, they are found to exhibit relative hypofunction of the SMA and other motor regions (e.g. Playford et al. 1992); indeed, such hypofunction is susceptible to 'reversal' through the use of dopamine agonists (such as apomorphine; see Jenkins et al. 1992).

Hence, an understanding of the 'motor' circuit and dopamine's potential modulation of its function enables us to understand some pathological, 'avolitional' states, and to specify the steps that might be taken, therapeutically, to reverse (or at least ameliorate) their behavioural consequences.

Thus, substances that 'facilitate' the function of the direct pathway, such as dopamine (the synaptic levels of which may be increased through the administration of its precursor molecule, L-dihydroxyphenylalanine, i.e. 'L-DOPA'), dopamine agonists (e.g. apomorphine), the amphetamines (which cause an increased release of endogenous dopamine into the inter-neuronal synapses), cocaine (which prevents the 're-uptake' of that dopamine once it has entered the synapse; thereby leading to heightened stimulation of dopamine receptors), and opioids, cannabinoids, and nicotine (all of which lead to increased firing of dopaminergic neurons), 'should' have a 'positive' influence upon cortical function ('positive' in the sense that they will 'increase' thalamic transmission, though of course the effects of 'excessive' transmission may be far from positive in life, e.g. amphetamine-induced psychosis). Therefore, the administration of dopamine precursors and agonists may be therapeutic in Parkinson's disease, enhancing SMA function and restoring self-initiated movement (and this may be demonstrated empirically: see Jenkins et al. 1992).

Furthermore, knowing *which* elements of the direct and indirect pathways are perturbed in Parkinson's disease has also allowed neurosurgeons to intervene specifically to lesion or stimulate targeted foci. Lesions to subthalamic nucleus and the globus pallidus interna may have therapeutic consequences, as may implantation of stimulating electrodes (i.e. 'deep brain stimulation') in these same foci (Pereira & Aziz, 2006).

Finally, and as a counterfactual, it is worth considering what happens to patients who take 'classical' antipsychotic drugs (e.g. haloperidol and chlorpromazine, used in the treatment of schizophrenia), agents that 'antagonize' (i.e. 'block') dopamine D2 receptors. Until very recently, all the available proven antipsychotics exhibited such D2 antagonism (i.e. this is what they all had 'in common'); indeed, their therapeutic (antipsychotic) potency correlated with their affinity for these same receptors (Seeman & Lee, 1975; Creese et al. 1976). Clearly, if such drugs block D2 receptors, then they can impede the inhibitory influence of dopamine on the indirect pathway (normally exerted upon those GABAergic neurons that also express enkephalin; above). If the indirect pathway becomes disinhibited, then it serves to relay excessive inhibition to the motor thalamus (as in Parkinson's disease), and one should expect that motor function will be impaired among those receiving such medications. Indeed, this is what happens. One of the major side effects of antipsychotic medications (especially the older, 'first-generation', or 'typical' antipsychotics) is their production of iatrogenic, 'extrapyramidal' side effects; i.e. patients may be rendered 'parkinsonian' (Barnes & Spence, 2000).

Fortunately, these effects may be countered via the administration of 'anticholinergic' medications. (Note: the effect of the latter is to oppose the actions of acetylcholine (an excitatory neurotransmitter within the striatum; itself contributing potential opposition to dopamine's role as an inhibitory neurotransmitter, also at the level of the striatum). Reducing the impact of (excitatory) acetylcholine, at the level of the striatum, offsets the interruption of (inhibitory) dopaminergic function produced by haloperidol or chlorpromazine; hence, parkinsonism may be reversed. Thus, we can make clinical use of the apparent antagonism pertaining between dopamine and acetylcholine, and of that between dopamine receptor antagonists and anticholinergic medications, at the level of the striatum.)

To summarize, we now have an insight into *how* the motor circuit helps to support voluntary behaviour and how its support may be modulated by dopamine and deficits of dopaminergic neurotransmission. A dysfunction within the motor circuit impacts the SMA at the level of the cortex, and SMA dysfunction impacts the ability of the organism – the person – to generate 'internally initiated' acts.

The moment of action

Nevertheless, apart from modulating the function of SMA, what is it that actually happens 'within' the basal ganglia during the course of a specified act?

Well, in order to answer this question, we first need to recognize that the basal ganglia are the focus of 'continued' activity even when the organism is at 'rest'. For instance, the nigrostriatal pathway is 'spontaneously active' at all times. Hence, given that dopamine (delivered via that pathway) is an 'inhibitory' neurotransmitter, the implication seems to be that nigrostriatal tone is constantly 'silencing' the striatum (Fitzgerald, 1992). Moreover, both sets of pallidal neurons – the G Pi and G Pe – are *also* spontaneously active at rest, at levels sufficient to 'silence' the VL nucleus of the thalamus and the subthalamic nucleus, respectively. Hence, one interpretation is that when we are 'at rest' our 'brakes are on'.

However, during an emerging movement, the 'pallidal' neurons, residing within the appropriate somatotopic representation (e.g. that corresponding to the right arm) become active, thereby 'disinhibiting' the motor thalamus, whereupon excitatory transmission to SMA (and motor cortex) increases. Furthermore, it is thought that the 'putamen' influences the direction of such ensuing movements, scales the strength of muscular contractions, and 'collaborates' with SMA in organizing the sequence of excitation of cell columns occurring within the primary motor cortex (i.e. those regions of the motor homunculus implicated in the emergent act; Chapter 1). However, it is also worth noting that during the performance of a specific voluntary movement, activation of cells within the basal ganglia occurs 'after' that seen in cortical pyramidal neurons, i.e. basal ganglia activation 'follows' the cortex, suggesting that the former contribute to the control of movements via 'modulatory' effects impacting their direction, amplitude, and velocity. In other words, the basal ganglia do not seem to 'initiate' actions, they serve instead to modify or facilitate them (and see Fitzgerald, 1992).

Furthermore, as I have already intimated several times (above), it is clear that the basal ganglia also make 'wider' contributions to behaviour (and cognition), beyond the purely motoric, and that these are readily apparent (as counterfactuals) when things 'go wrong'. For instance, people affected by Parkinson's disease exhibit not only slowness of movement ('bradykinesia'), but also slowness of thought ('bradyphrenia'); moreover, they may be subject to severe emotional disturbance (depression is common). These symptoms may be understood to constitute the manifestations of disturbances occurring within different basal ganglia-thalamo-cortical loops. Nevertheless, is there any 'deeper' way of understanding what it is that is 'going wrong' 'within' a specific loop, when the basal ganglia cease to function properly? Is there any way of understanding how such a 'local' dysfunction might impact 'wider' brain performance?

Well, in a fascinating theoretical paper, Brown and Marsden (1998) offer a potential solution. They suggest that under 'normal' conditions the basal ganglia facilitate the 'synchronization' of cortical activity during 'the selection and promulgation of an appropriate movement, or indeed an appropriate sequence of thought' (p. 1803). Hence, the role of the basal ganglia is hypothesized to be very much to do with the 'timing' of activity within and across circuits. The central problem is one of 'synchronized' cell firing. So, in order to be able to understand such a theory in more detail, it may be helpful to pause to consider what it is that is happening 'across' the brain (i.e. 'above' the level of the basal ganglia) when we are 'at rest' and *not* engaged in action.

We have already seen (in the Prologue) that electroencephalography (EEG) may be used to interrogate brain states when human beings engage in actions. However, it can also reveal intriguing data concerning the activity of our brains when they are engaged in 'rest' (a highly questionable concept: is the brain ever truly 'resting', is it ever 'quiet'?). What is happening when a human subject sits with her eyes closed, feeling subjectively 'relaxed'? Well, on the EEG such a state coincides with a widespread, and rather regular, pattern of 'brain waves' oscillating at a frequency of approximately 8–13 cycles per second (Hertz, Hz). This pattern, termed the 'alpha rhythm', suggests that widespread regions of the brain are somehow 'in phase'; i.e. that despite their separation from each other in physical (brain) space their electrical activities are correlated in time (i.e. synchronized). This alpha rhythm is something that we may access on a regular basis prior to sleep (and perhaps at exceedingly boring lectures). However, during 'active' wakefulness, when we are alert and attending to our environment, we oscillate in the 'beta rhythm', cycling at around 14–25 Hz. Slower rhythms emerge during sleep (and also during coma; see Zeman, 2002, pp. 78–91 for an accessible review).

Now, immediately prior to an act, or when we are called upon to attend to a salient environmental stimulus, our EEG undergoes 'desynchronization' in those regions of the brain that are functionally implicated. Hence, in motor circuits (just prior to and during an act) a rhythm is established that is synchronized at a much higher frequency, of between 25–100 Hz, across mutually engaged brain regions. This rhythm has been termed the 'gamma frequency' and it is thought by some to have particular relevance to conscious awareness. Crucially, the gamma frequency indicates that linked areas are firing at high frequency, in phase with each other. Hence, it may be via such a synchronization that distributed brain regions cooperate, to 'support' emergent behaviours.

Brown and Marsden posit that a kind of 'attention' is achieved while we are 'in' the gamma frequency range (note, however, that this is an 'attention' that does not necessarily need to be fully 'conscious', since it also arises during rapid eye movement (REM) sleep – that portion of our sleep during which we dream; below). Such a form of attention binds 'input to output by making activities related to each coherent' (p. 1802). In this context, coherent means synchronous, in phase.

Now, it is interesting to note that these gamma frequency oscillations are reduced in Parkinson's disease and that they are restored by the administration of L-DOPA. Hence, dopamine seems to be implicated in their maintenance. Furthermore, these cortical oscillations have an apparent correlate in the so-called 'Piper rhythm' discernible at the level of voluntary musculature. The latter describes the tendency of motor units to 'beat', more or less synchronously, at a frequency of 30–50 Hz. This, in turn, is interesting as the primary motor cortex exhibits the same rhythm, suggesting that the Piper rhythm may be centrally driven. Again, the Piper rhythm is lost in untreated Parkinson's disease and is restored with L-DOPA therapy (see Brown & Marsden, 1998). So, once again, dopamine (and its impact upon the basal ganglia) is implicated in the maintenance of rhythmic activities across the brain – electrical rhythms that are pertinent to the preparation and performance of movements.

Furthermore, this central idea, that the basal ganglia are acting to 'coordinate' distributed neural activity, and that some form of 'attention' is contributory to their success, is congruent with what we have alluded to previously concerning the ability of Parkinson's disease patients to suddenly produce a motor response, despite the severity of their motoric impairment, should an environmental stimulus be surprising or compelling enough:

> That some defect of attention is important in diseases of the basal ganglia is revealed by the observation of paradoxical kinesis, in which patients with Parkinson's disease so akinetic that they can barely move, may deftly sidestep an oncoming car or flee from a fire.

> (Brown & Marsden, 1998, p. 1802)

The implication here is that while the basal ganglia 'should' *normally* facilitate the binding of information from across the brain (into a coherent signal), if these nuclei are dysfunctional (as in states such as Parkinson's disease), and an 'emergency' arises, then 'lower' centres (actually the 'reticular activating system' of the brain stem) may suddenly 'take over' and impel the organism towards survival. In other words, the patient avoids the car or the fire because 'his' reticular activating system intervenes, doing what 'his' basal ganglia 'should' have done, had they been 'healthy'.

Moving between circuits, in the course of learning

Finally, before we leave behind the architecture of the basal ganglia-thalamo-cortical circuits, it is appropriate to consider those circumstances under which information may be 'transferred' between them. A suitable example is provided by the case of motor learning.

We saw, in Chapter 2, that the neural substrates of volitional activity might vary considerably according to whether a specified movement was novel or routine (i.e. over-learned), 'internally initiated', or elicited in response to an external stimulus. We saw then that certain cortical regions were particularly implicated by the drawing of such distinctions:

1. Some cortical regions are particularly activated during the early acquisition of a new motor routine and reduce their activity when that routine has become automated (e.g. DLPFC; see Jenkins et al. 1994);

2. There is a shift from more 'anterior' to more 'posterior' motor regions being implicated in the performance of a motor sequence as that sequence becomes automated;

3. At the level of the cortex, this shift is exemplified by less prefrontal (and anterior premotor) activation and more (posterior premotor and) primary motor cortical activation. At the level of the basal ganglia, this shift is exemplified by less rostral, striatal activation within the caudate nucleus and increased activation within the putamen (see Jueptner et al. 1997a,b);

4. However, while we have previously conceived of such a 'shift' as occurring from 'anterior to posterior', it is now apparent (having considered the basal ganglia-thalamo-cortical circuits in some detail) that the shift may also be conceived of as being more 'lateral' in nature, i.e. one that occurs between successive 'loops': from the earlier involvement of the dorsolateral prefrontal (or 'associational') loop to the later involvement of the motor loop (targeting the SMA; Yin & Knowlton, 2006; Figure 52).

Indeed, Yin and Knowlton (2006) hypothesize that, in the course of new learning, information is shared by the DLPFC circuit with the SMA 'motor' circuit and

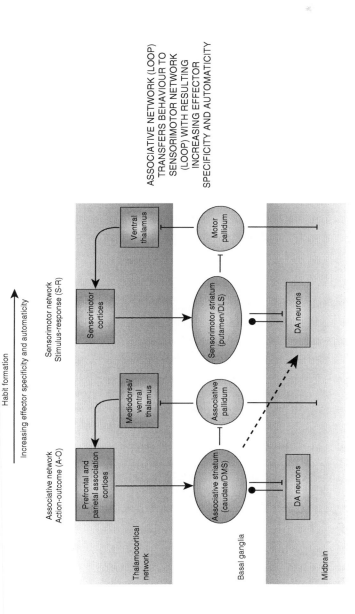

Fig. 52 Cartoon taken from a paper by Yin & Knowlton (2006) illustrating how information passes between the associative (dorsolateral prefrontal cortex) loop and the sensorimotor (supplementary motor area) loop in the context of motor learning. Information orbits the associative network during the early stages of motor learning. However, as learning becomes consolidated there is a transfer of information to the sensorimotor network. This transfer of information is associated with increasing effector specificity and also automaticity. This may be described as habit formation. Reproduced with permission from Macmillan Publishers Ltd., *Nature Reviews Neuroscience*, The role of the basal ganglia in habit formation, Yin HH and Knowlton BJ, 2006.

that, at the level of the striatum, caudate activity gives way to an involvement of the putamen. Furthermore, there are phenomenological consequences upon such automation:

1. 'Effector specificity' increases: This means that early on in the acquisition of a new motor skill, different limbs, fingers, or other 'effectors' might have performed the new task equally well, each retaining a potential to take the behaviour forward. However, as a skill becomes automated, so it 'focusses' upon a given effector, e.g. the right hand. Hence, at a later stage in the process, other effectors can no longer simply 'take over'. Therefore, if we lose or damage the favoured 'effector' (the implementer of our learned 'routine'), then the skill must be re-learned. Yin and Knowlton suggest that the relative flexibility of effector deployment exhibited early on in the learning process is attributable to 'higher' prefrontal regions being involved and having access to 'multiple' neural mechanisms via which to realize such a performance. In other words, a 'plan' at the level of DLPFC might be implemented via multiple 'solutions' (programmes) at the level of PMCs. However, later on in the process (i.e. following 'learning'), one (specific) programme is (routinely) 'run' to perform the task. In other words, as a consequence of automation, it has become consolidated upon a much more restricted neural substrate (effector).

2. Early in the acquisition of a new skill, 'higher' centres are being engaged and so their resources are synchronously utilized, temporarily 'tied-up'. Hence, if the actor is called upon to perform a second, competing, novel, or complicated task at the same time, then 'interference' will arise: i.e. trying to perform an 'executive' task at the same time as acquiring a new motor sequence may impair performance of both tasks (we saw this in Chapter 2, in the example provided by Dick Passingham, when human subjects attempted to perform verbal fluency at the same time as learning a novel motor sequence). However, when automation *has* occurred, when the new motor sequence has become 'over-learned', then there should no longer be any decrement detectable during subsequent synchronous performance of an executive task (since the executive's resources are no longer deployed on the first task, they are not required to be split, or 'divided', when the second task comes along).

3. Finally, although the motor sequence becomes automated (and hence, no longer primarily requires the engagement of 'higher' centres), it may still be subjected to 'renewed' scrutiny (i.e. attention), at a later date; the actor may decide to deliberately attend to their actions once more, whereupon 'higher' circuits will become 're-engaged' (i.e. activated; and this has be demonstrated empirically; Jueptner et al. 1997a, b).

Closing the loop

Now it is time to summarize. We have delineated a series of neural circuits (or 'loops'), each of which passes through the basal ganglia and each of which appears to have characteristic cortical targets and behavioural salience. As we have been concerned, for the most part, with the execution of voluntary acts, we have focussed for the time being upon the motor circuit. However, we shall return to this and other circuits at later stages in this text (especially in Chapter 6). The central point of this exposition has been to demonstrate one means by which the brain may act in concert, to link the activities (and thereby processing contributions) of distant, though connected, neural regions in action. Moving a finger may well rely very heavily upon the integrity of the pyramidal tract, but the smooth functioning of that system owes a great deal to another, extrapyramidal, system, which targets its influence upon the SMA. Furthermore, while these circuits may be quite sufficient for the modulation and execution of finely tuned, overly learned, well-rehearsed motor routines, there are other circuits similarly pivotal to other kinds of behaviour. We have seen that the DLPFC circuit is especially likely to be contributory during the early stages of motor skill acquisition, and it seems very likely that an anterior cingulate circuit may be similarly implicated when we engage in 'emotional' behaviours, doing those things which seem to manifest the contributions of limbic, 'affective' regions of the brain through motor acts (e.g. in the course of 'maternal' behaviours). Behavioural anatomy begins to look rather more complex. It is harder to define a hierarchy, a 'top' or a 'bottom', within such processes.

Now we shall continue, with a consideration of other forms of circuitry and how these might impact voluntary behaviour.

Neurochemical architectures

In the foregoing sections, we delineated one means whereby an 'architecture' might be imposed upon the primate brain: namely, in terms of its anatomical circuits, e.g. the re-entrant 'loops' running through its basal ganglia and serving to modulate activity within specific PMC and PFC regions. Hence, in those sections of the text, anatomy was very much the determining principle while neurochemistry was afforded only incidental significance, contingent upon the various relays of the circuits that we were then attempting to describe. So, while dopamine appeared critical to the modulation of striatal output, glutamate constituted a rather more ubiquitous neurotransmitter, comprising the substrate for many important 'links' in our 'chains': from cortex to striatum, from subthalamic nucleus to G Pi, and from thalamus back to cortex. Now, in this section, we are changing our approach. Here, it will be the neurochemistry that defines architectural form; and we shall confine our account to those neurotransmitters that are most likely to impact voluntary behaviour, as it is currently understood.

I might add that I have written 'as it is currently understood' for an important reason. For, although we are going to focus our account of volition upon certain 'predictable' neurotransmitters, e.g. dopamine and serotonin (below), we are doing this largely because we have most data concerning these molecules and their neuronal instantiations. However, we should acknowledge that there are numerous neurotransmitters within the human brain (e.g. the neuropeptides alone currently number more than 60; Gartside & Marsden, 2006), so that any understanding we may profess (now) is highly likely to be conditional upon further, future discoveries. Nevertheless, there is currently quite a disparity between what is known about the five or six best-understood neurotransmitter systems and the rest, so we are more likely to be 'accurate' in our present account if we focus upon the former.

Dopamine

Dopamine is an example of a 'catecholamine' neurotransmitter, i.e. its molecule comprises an organic compound with a catechol nucleus (a benzene ring with two adjacent hydroxyl substitutions) and an amine group (Figure 53). It is the product of successive enzymatic modifications of the amino acid tyrosine and, under normal conditions, the 'rate-limiting' step in its production is that carried out by the enzyme tyrosine hydroxylase (Figure 54; Deutch & Roth, 1999).

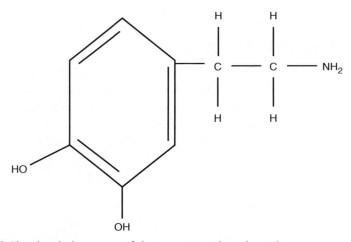

Fig. 53 The chemical structure of the neurotransmitter dopamine.

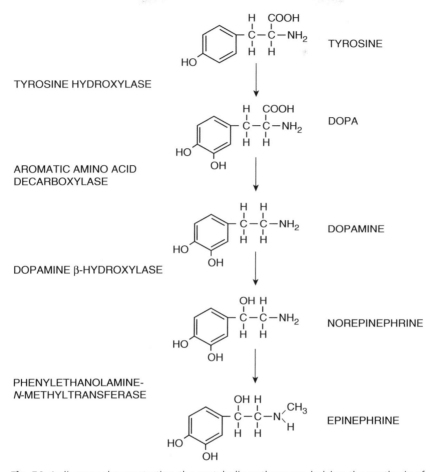

Fig. 54 A diagram demonstrating the metabolic pathway underlying the synthesis of the neurotransmitters dopamine and noradrenaline (norepinephrine, in the figure).

Dopamine is found in the midbrains of most vertebrate species. However, in humans, there are four main pathways that are of particular behavioural (and medical) significance (Figure 55):

1. The 'nigrostriatal' dopamine pathway projects from the substantia nigra pars compacta to the striatum, and is implicated in the control of movement (above).

2. The 'mesolimbic' dopamine pathway projects from the VTA of the midbrain to the nucleus accumbens (in the ventral striatum), and is implicated in many reinforced behaviours, such as those pursuant upon pleasurable experiences, and the 'powerful euphoria' of drugs of abuse (Stahl, 1999).

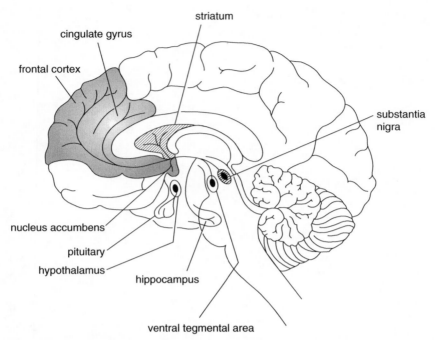

Fig. 55 Cartoon showing the distribution of the dopamine pathways within the human brain. Note that while the substantia nigra is particularly implicated in motor function the ventral tegmental area is particularly implicated in reward and motivation.

3. The 'mesocortical' dopamine pathway also originates within the VTA, but projects to the limbic cortex. It is particularly implicated in the likely genesis of psychotic symptoms (e.g. delusions and hallucinations).

4. The 'tuberoinfundibular' dopamine pathway projects from the hypothalamus to the anterior pituitary gland (where dopamine acts to inhibit prolactin release, having a role in the systemic modulation of hormonal function).

Though this is a very simple description of four complex systems, one may immediately discern that the influence of dopamine upon human behaviour (and hence, volition) is likely to vary according to those of its systems being targeted. Hence, a disturbance within the nigrostriatal pathway might impact the 'mechanics' of voluntary behaviour (as we saw with Parkinson's disease and 'parkinsonism', above), rendering one's movements 'slow' and difficult, while dysfunction in other systems may have rather more impact upon 'higher' aspects of volition, e.g. the disturbed reasoning that may have generated the 'goal' behind an abnormal act carried out during a psychotic episode (as when a young man jumps from a building, believing that he can fly; a putative consequence of mesocortical dysfunction) and the execution of 'immoral' acts (such as theft and prostitution), deemed 'necessary' by an addict in order to sate her desire for an addictive substance (largely impacting her mesolimbic system). Thus, one molecule (dopamine) has multiple potential impacts upon human conduct, according to whether it is present in excess or relative deficiency, according to whether its presence impacts a 'purely motor' system or one with implications for higher 'orders' of cognition and behaviour (e.g. impacting that which is 'rational' or 'enjoyable').

Furthermore, a feature of dopamine projections, which comes into focus when they are compared with those of other neurotransmitter systems, is their targeting of the frontal brain. There is a relative lack of dopamine in 'posterior neocortices' (i.e. those cortical association areas posterior to the Rolandic fissure; Arnsten & Robbins, 2002).

At the level of the cortex, the function for which there is most evidence of dopaminergic contribution is working memory – a process that we have already identified as implicating the DLPFC. Such a contribution is mediated via receptors of the D1 family. Hence, in animal models, stimulation of D1 receptors may enhance working-memory function: manifest as improved performance on certain 'delayed response' tasks (see Chapter 2). Conversely, reduced levels of dopamine (or the presence of a D1 receptor antagonist) may impair working-memory performance. However, there appears to be an optimal level of dopaminergic activity, so that too little or too much D1 stimulation leads to a decrement in performance. This is consistent with the Yerkes–Dodson principle – that there is an optimal level of arousal required for the performance of a given task (Arnsten & Robbins, 2002); if arousal fails to reach such a level, or indeed it goes 'beyond' it, then performance is rendered 'sub-optimal'. Such a response curve is exemplified by an 'inverted-U', as shown in Figure 56, which may be demonstrated most readily in 'animal models', where D1 agonists and antagonists have been used to elicit quantifiable variation in dopaminergic tone and consequent levels of task performance. Indeed, there is a further crucial subtlety, which may impede the 'straightforward' therapeutic modulation of PFCs (when we come to 'treating' humans). As is shown in Figure 56, 'different' prefrontal regions may have 'different' dose–response profiles ('inverted-Us') describing their responses to dopamine (and, by implication, other substances). So, whereas a given dose of a specified drug may be beneficial for the response dynamics of one or more regions, it might be too little or too much for those of others. This leads Arnsten and Robbins to conclude:

> In other words, different operations possibly mediated by distinct regions of the [prefrontal cortex] may have differing neurochemical needs in terms of the modulatory functions provided by the midbrain [dopamine] system.

(Arnsten & Robbins, 2002, p. 59)

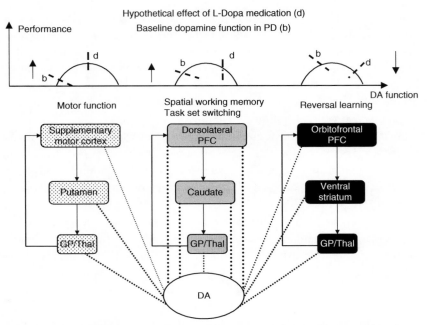

Fig. 56 Cartoon taken from Arnstein & Robbins (2002) demonstrating the different hypothetical effects of L-dopa medication upon the function of different frontal regions in the human brain. While an increase in dopamine may lead to improved motor function, instantiated through the substrate of the motor (supplementary motor area) loop, and improved spatial working-memory performance, as instantiated through the cognitive (dorsolateral prefrontal) loop the same increase in dopamine may lead to a deterioration in function within the orbitofrontal loop. Hence, the level of a transmitter which permits optimal functioning in some brain regions may be associated with suboptimal functioning in other brain regions. This poses something of a problem for therapeutic interventions. With permission from Oxford University Press.

Now, some flavour of this impact of (variable) dopaminergic function upon cognitive performance is discernible among studies of humans. Consider the following example.

Given what we have stated (above), we may posit that within the PFC higher levels of dopamine might be relatively 'good' for cognitive function, indeed, that the latter might be relatively 'enhanced'; conversely, if there were to be lower levels of dopamine, then cognition might be relatively 'impaired'. Now, within the cortex, the principal process via which dopamine is removed from the synaptic cleft (following neurotransmission) is through its metabolism (i.e. its breakdown or 'catabolism') by the enzyme catechol-O-methyltransferase (COMT).

So, theoretically, whether COMT 'works' slower or faster might be expected to have an impact upon intra-synaptic dopamine levels and, hence, upon cognitive performance. Well, it so happens that in the human brain the efficiency of COMT (i.e. whether it catabolizes dopamine relatively slowly or quickly) is influenced by a functional polymorphism of a gene coding for its synthesis (i.e. the production of COMT). This polymorphism consists of two 'co-dominant' alleles ('Val' or 'Met') at codon 158 (in exon 4 of the COMT gene, on chromosome 22q11.1–q11.2; Hosak, 2007). The Met allele gives rise to a relatively inefficient form of the COMT enzyme, which therefore metabolizes dopamine relatively slowly (in the PFC). In contrast, the Val allele gives rise to a relatively efficient form of COMT, which therefore metabolizes dopamine relatively quickly. Thus, any dopamine that is released into the prefrontal synapses of a Met/Met (homozygotic) brain is likely to remain 'longer' in those synapses than dopamine released into the PFC of a Val/Val (homozygotic) brain. Indeed, the difference in COMT activity between these homozygotic states (genotypes) is estimated to be three- to fourfold (with heterozygotic individuals, i.e. 'Val/Mets', manifesting intermediate COMT activity; Hosak, 2007).

Now, this enzymatic effect 'should' have quantifiable cognitive consequences and it does. In one study by Egan and colleagues (2001), using a complex cognitive task called the Wisconsin Card Sorting Test (WCST), the authors found that not only did the 'Met/Mets' perform better than the 'Val/Vals' but that 4.1% of the variance in task performance (actually, in 'perseverative errors') across groups could be explained by this single difference in genotype. Hence, a single functional polymorphism, impacting prefrontal dopaminergic metabolism, has a discernible effect upon cognitive performance in healthy humans. Those who are homozygotic for the Met allele at codon 158 (of the COMT gene) appear to have an 'edge' when it comes to performing the WCST.

Hence, it may be of interest to consider what it is that the WCST actually tests. The task was described by Grant and Berg (1948) and was the subject of an influential study by Milner (1963). It is certainly a complicated procedure. The protocol is that the test subject is confronted with a pack of cards, upon which there are symbols of varying design, colour, and number. On the table, in front of them, the examiner sets out four exemplar cards, each of which differs from its neighbours in terms of their three characteristics (symbol design, colour, and number; Figure 57). The subject is invited by their examiner to 'sort' the remaining cards according to a rule of their own devising. Hence, they might sort the deck, one card at a time, according to numbers, e.g. all the cards with one symbol being placed in one pile, all the cards with two symbols going into another, and so on (up to four; Figure 57). Alternatively, they might

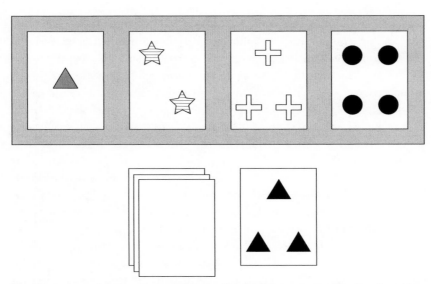

Fig. 57 Cartoon showing the materials used in the Wisconsin Card Sorting Test. The subject is presented with a pack of cards exhibiting different symbols, in different colours, and in different numbers on each card. They are asked to sort the pack, one card at a time according to a scheme of their own devising. They are then told whether or not each placement of a card is 'correct' or 'incorrect'. Only the examiner knows the correct rule.

sort the pack according to colour: all the cards with red designs going in one pile, all the greens going into another, etc. (there are four colours). The point is that the rule is arbitrary and, crucially, only 'known' to the examiner. In essence, the subject must 'guess' what the rule is that currently applies, and sort the cards accordingly. She receives feedback after the sorting of each (individual) card. If she has guessed correctly, then she repeats the process (applying the same rule to the placement of the next card), if she has guessed incorrectly, then she must change her rule immediately. So, for instance, if the numerical rule turned out to be wrong (i.e. if the examiner said 'no, that was not correct') then the subject might swap to using a colour rule instead.

This is a tricky task to undertake; one is essentially trying to arrive at an abstract rule in rather under-constrained circumstances. Furthermore, if and when the subject gets the answer 'right', then the examiner will 'change' the rule after a set number of correct responses (e.g. 10). So, having been told that she is correct, over a sequence of successive card sorts, our subject is then confronted with a seemingly arbitrary change in feedback (i.e. what was 'right' has suddenly become 'wrong'); she has to 'unlearn' her own previous rule and rapidly apply another.

Clearly, such a complex task is likely to tap into multiple cognitive domains: one needs adequate visual and motor function, one requires attention and some degree of abstract reasoning; one must be able to 'internally generate' new rules when the current rule is deemed 'incorrect' or when the feedback changes; one must be able to suppress the over-learned response – the rule that was formerly correct but which is now 'contextually inappropriate'. The test is scored according to how many correct categories subjects achieve within a set period (i.e. at how many points did they generate what was temporarily the 'right' answer) and how many perseverative errors occur (i.e. how many times did subjects fail to heed a negative result and repeat an incorrect sorting rule). As we saw (above), Egan and colleagues found that these latter, perseverative, errors were the ones that exhibited a relationship with the COMT genotype. Just over 4% of the variance in perseverative errors was attributable to the Val/Met polymorphism.

This suggests a substantial relationship between the state of prefrontal dopamine metabolism and the ability of a subject to cease performing 'contextually inappropriate' responses in order to change their behaviour. This is a rather more complex (higher level) impact upon volition than that evinced in the limb movements of someone suffering from Parkinson's disease. Through COMT, we begin to see how neurochemistry might actually impact quite complex shifts in behavioural strategy (i.e. in changing the subjective rule applied during an arbitrary experimental task) in contrast to a much more 'mechanical' impairment consequent upon degeneration of the substantia nigra *pars compacta*.

Serotonin

Serotonin (5-hydroxytryptamine, 5HT) is a monoamine neurotransmitter (Figure 58) that also has effects upon voluntary behaviour, although these

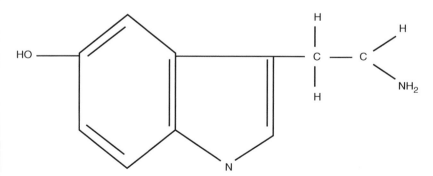

Fig. 58 Diagram showing the chemical structure of the neurotransmitter serotonin (5-hydroxytryptamine, 5HT).

effects seem rather more pervasive (less 'focussed') than those of dopamine. Serotonin is the product of successive enzymatic modifications of the dietary amino acid tryptophan – the latter entering the brain via a 'transporter' mechanism, at which it must compete with other 'large neutral amino acids' (Gartside & Marsden, 2006). Hence, it is possible, for experimental purposes, to manipulate (dietary) amino acid intake so that tryptophan is 'excluded' from transporter uptake (by competing amino acids), whereupon brain serotonin is subsequently diminished. In other words, it is possible to study the effects of radically reducing serotonergic tone in the human brain, *in vivo* (below). However, under 'normal' physiological conditions, the rate of serotonin production is correlated with tryptophan uptake, since the relevant 'rate-limiting' enzyme, tryptophan hydroxylase, is unsaturated (therefore, in essence, the enzyme can 'cope with' whatever amount of tryptophan is normally taken up, so that the latter determines the amount of serotonin subsequently synthesized; Gartside & Marsden, 2006; Deutch & Roth, 1999; Figure 59).

Synthesis of serotonin occurs within a group of cells located in the midbrain and brainstem 'raphe' nuclei. Rostrally, at the level of the pons, the dorsal and

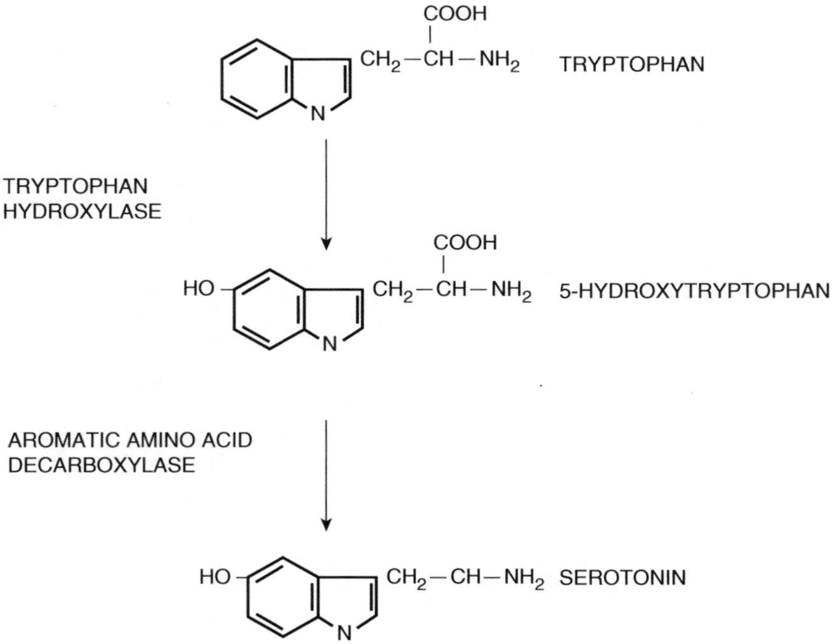

Fig. 59 Diagram showing the metabolic pathway for the production of serotonin (5-HT).

median raphe nuclei send projections to the forebrain (Figure 60; below). Caudally, at the level of the medulla, the obscurus, magnus, and pallidus raphe nuclei send descending projections to the spinal cord. Hence, serotonergic projections may be conceptualized as targeting five important systems:

1. The prefrontal cortex;
2. The basal ganglia (including the striatum);
3. The limbic cortex (extending to the hippocampus and the amygdala);
4. The hypothalamus; and
5. The spinal cord (specifically, the dorsal and ventral horns).

While dorsal and median raphe projections may overlap, there are some regional specificities – e.g. the frontal cortex receives predominantly 'dorsal' raphe inputs, while the dorsal hippocampus receives predominantly 'median' raphe innervation.

Given its widespread distribution, it is unsurprising that serotonin has been regarded as a 'modulator' of many complex functions: 'mood and emotion, sleep/wakefulness and regulation of circadian functions, control of feeding and sexual behaviours, body temperature, perceptions, and emesis [vomiting]' (Gartside & Marsden, 2006, p. 16). Furthermore, this might 'explain' why there are so many classes of serotonin receptor (14, according to one recent

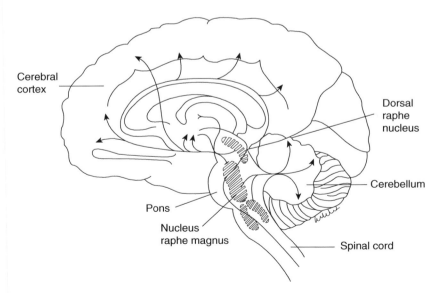

Fig. 60 Cartoon showing the projections of the serotonergic system within the human brain. See text for details.

review: Gartside & Marsden, 2006), possibly lending some regional specificity to its functions.

From the point of view of our interest in 'volitional architectures', serotonin innervates three structures that are of especial salience: the PFC (where it seems particularly pertinent to orbitofrontal (OFC) function; below); the basal ganglia (where it may impact motoric activity); and the spinal cord (where its dorsal innervation inhibits pain transmission, while its ventral input regulates lower motor neuron output).

As mentioned, at the level of the cortex, serotonin seems preferentially implicated in OFC function, as opposed to that of the DLPFC. The latter hypothesis is borne out by experiments inducing tryptophan depletion (above), whereupon humans exhibit selective deficits in reversal learning and certain 'gambling' tasks, procedures and deficits that usually reflect OFC function and dysfunction, respectively (Arnsten & Robbins, 2002). Indeed, while lesions of OFC may render humans impulsive, it seems likely that disturbance of serotonergic function may do something rather similar, e.g. there is an association between impulsive violence of various types and reduced cerebrospinal fluid (CSF) levels of a serotonin metabolite (5-hydroxy-indoleacetic acid; 5-HIAA; Linnoila & Charney, 1999). Some historically pivotal findings include the following:

1. A correlation between CSF levels of 5-HIAA and the risk of suicidal behaviours among patients with (unipolar) depression (Asberg et al. 1976);

2. A correlation between CSF levels of 5-HIAA and scores on a scale of aggression, indexing lifetime antisocial behaviours, among young navy recruits (Brown et al. 1979, 1982); and

3. A relationship between CSF 5-HIAA levels and mode of offending among those remanded to a forensic psychiatric facility (Linnoila et al. 1983): those whose violence was *not* premeditated exhibited 'lower' 5-HIAA levels, and the latter were lowest of all among those who had previously attempted suicide.

Hence, the conclusion from a large body of empirical evidence (extensively reviewed by Linnoila & Charney, 1999) is that there is a link between reduced levels of serotonergic function and impaired impulse control.

Furthermore, one of the most prescribed classes of 'antidepressant' medication currently available is that of the selective serotonin re-uptake inhibitors (SSRIs); drugs that specifically interfere with the 're-uptake' of serotonin from the synapse, thereby allowing it to remain physiologically active for longer. Obviously, these drugs are used to treat depression, but they are also used to explicitly control certain dysfunctional 'behaviours', e.g. bingeing and vomiting in bulimia nervosa, obsessional ruminations and compulsive rituals in obsessive compulsive disorder and certain other dysfunctional 'habits' (as outlined in a seminal publication by Kramer, 1993, *Listening to Prozac*). While this does not 'prove' that a (primary) disturbance of serotonergic function underlies all these complex psychopathologies, it does suggest that certain complex behaviours are susceptible to modulation by changes in serotonergic tone. In other words, increasing serotonin levels can help to restore an element of 'control'.

However, 'too much' serotonin might also prove problematic; it can cause a certain kind of 'purposeless' activity manifest in the clinical condition 'akathisia'. The latter describes an unpleasant sense of 'motor restlessness' that may occur in some psychiatric disorders, and as a consequence of certain of their treatments. A patient may feel acutely distressed, being unable to relax or to cease moving. They pace up and down; they rock to and fro; having to sit still in order to eat or converse during an interview may be intolerable for them. They cannot watch the television or listen to music without getting up to walk about. Sadly, there is an increased risk of attempted suicide, such is the distress caused by this condition.

Two contrasting forms of medication may cause akathisia:

1. Treatment with 'older', 'typical' antipsychotic drugs, especially those that have a high affinity for dopamine receptors. Thus, they seem to cause akathisia via some consequence of dopamine receptor blockade (antagonism).

2. Treatment with SSRIs, especially those that have a short 'half-life', e.g. paroxetine, where blood levels rise and fall rapidly. Thus, it appears that an acute increase in serotonergic tone may (somehow) precipitate motor restlessness.

Notice again how two neurotransmitters seem to be implicated in a form of pathological imbalance or neurochemical 'seesaw', as was the case with the parkinsonism caused by antipsychotic medications and alleviated by anticholinergics (above). In the present case, a blockade of dopamine neurotransmission and enhanced levels of serotonin *both* seem to cause akathisia. Furthermore, although the precise mechanism of this distressing state is unknown, some of its treatments implicate further neurochemical systems, i.e. akathisia may be ameliorated by the use of beta-blockers (drugs that antagonize noradrenergic neurotransmission) and benzodiazepines (drugs that are GABAergic in their impact).

Indeed, there is another contrast between serotonin and dopamine that is also of interest, especially in the context of volition. Notice how a deficit of serotonin transmission seems to 'release' certain behaviours; 'impulsivity' implies a failure to control, to constrain responses. This seems to be particularly the case for violent acts. However, some difficulty with the balance of control is also implied by the presence of obsessional ruminations, an inability to refrain from compulsive acts, and the emergence of recurring patterns of damaging behaviour (e.g. bingeing, vomiting, overdosing, and self-cutting); all these states are treated with SSRIs (i.e. the elevation of serotonin levels). Therefore, at an albeit simplistic level of analysis, low levels of serotonin transmission seem to be linked to problems with 'restraint'. Conversely, dopamine depletion (as exemplified by Parkinson's disease) leads to a reduction of behaviour; fewer 'internally initiated' responses. If anything, there is too much restraint. So, these two molecules (serotonin and dopamine) have different structures and different neurological architectures (projections); and they sometimes impact different types of behaviour; however, when they impact at the 'same' level of volition (e.g. the emergence of 'purposeless', stereotypic behaviours, such as those seen in akathisia), they seem to have 'opposing' effects. Hence, we seem to be approaching a kind of neurochemical 'balance', underlying behaviour.

Indeed, we might envisage a kind of 'response space' – a range of behaviours that an organism might (potentially) perform, one that is impacted from different 'directions' by different neurotransmitter systems; some serving to 'expand' the response space (as is the case when dopamine facilitates 'internally initiated' action) some serving to 'constrain', or 'restrain', it (as is the case when increasing serotonin neurotransmission seems to reduce impulsivity). This notion of a 'space of responses' is something that we shall return to later in this book (in Chapter 10). (Indeed, I shall argue that it is pivotal to any continued notion of 'freedom'.)

Finally, before we leave serotonin behind (for the time being), we should also mention that some authors have called this neurotransmitter the 'social status hormone' (*sic*, Wilkinson, 2005). Indeed, it is striking that serotonin can be shown to have a relationship with the way that primates (and some other species) organize their 'societies'. In non-human primates, the dominant male at the head of a hierarchy can be shown to have higher serotonin levels than his subordinates, and their 'pecking order' may be 'adjusted' by boosting the serotonin levels of the latter or depleting those of the former (Raleigh et al. 1984, 1991; and see Wilkinson, 2005, for a broader consideration of social status and inequality). So, upon reflection, one might be tempted to propose that serotonin is normally something of a 'counter-revolutionary neurotransmitter'! Usually, it correlates with the *status quo*.

Now, of course, hierarchies are complex social arrangements, and their maintenance, no doubt, relies upon a range of 'social' behaviours and relationships enacted among all of those concerned. Nevertheless, it is interesting to note, once again, how a consideration of serotonin neurotransmission takes us towards an entirely different order, or level, of animal 'behaviour': the means via which primates maintain their 'status'. Indeed, some authors have even tentatively suggested a correspondence between behavioural/social neurochemistry and Freudian notions of the mind: if the primitive 'Id' – the energetic seeker of pleasure – is supported by the dopaminergic system (that substrate for the 'euphoria' elicited by illicit intoxicants; Stahl, 1999; above), then the 'Ego', that 'rational' controller of social behaviour, resembles a serotonergic response to the constraints of communal living (see Fink & Taylor, 2003, p. 191). As bald a notion as this seems, we have already seen how, through their perturbations, the neurochemical systems reveal what might be called (albeit teleologically) their 'design features'. Too little dopamine, and we may not act; too little serotonin, and we may lose 'control'.

Noradrenaline

We have already encountered noradrenaline (or 'norepinephrine', as it is known in the United States of America; above); it is a catecholamine neuro-transmitter, the product of dopamine's metabolism by the enzyme dopamine beta hydroxylase (Figure 54). Noradrenaline-containing cells are found within the pons and medulla, and the former is the location of the 'locus coeruleus': the origin of a group of neurons projecting to the forebrain, brainstem, and spinal cord (Figure 61; Deutch & Roth, 1999). However, noradrenergic cells in

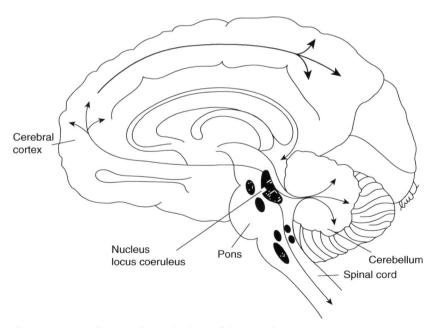

Cerebral cortex

Nucleus locus coeruleus

Pons

Cerebellum

Spinal cord

Fig. 61 Cartoon showing the projections of the noradrenergic system within the human brain. See text for details.

both the pons and medulla also project to the ventral forebrain and diencephalic regions (including the thalamus, hypothalamus, and limbic areas such as the amygdala, hippocampus, and septum). Hence, rather like serotonin (above), noradrenaline exhibits extensive projections, suggesting that it has widespread influences throughout the brain. Its own origin (the locus coeruleus) is subject to modulation by DLPFC, a means via which levels of 'attention' may be regulated (Arnsten & Robbins, 2002).

Now, Arnsten and Robbins (2002) suggest that noradrenaline acts as a 'chemical switch' at the level of the cortex. Hence, when it is present at lower levels it preferentially enhances PFC function (as might be manifest through improved working-memory performance), but when it is present at higher levels it preferentially enhances the function of the 'posterior brain'. An effect of the latter would be to preferentially enhance or promote processing of incoming sensory data (at the expense of 'higher' cognitive operations). Such a shift in cortical activity might be elicited under conditions of extreme stress. One implication is that the subject may be able to attend more closely to their environment though they may be less able to perform complex cognitive tasks. (Consider what it may be like to be plunged into the heart of a crowded foreign city, where one does not speak the language, and cannot understand what other people are saying. Sensory 'overload' becomes obvious and taxing. Then consider attempting to claim 'asylum' there.)

Prefrontal cortical function, in the form of working-memory performance, is enhanced via the activity of noradrenaline at post-synaptic α_2-receptors (see Arnsten & Robbins, 2002). Hence, in lesioned monkeys PFC function may be ameliorated by the administration of α_2-agonists (e.g. clonidine and guanfacine). Such agents are especially good at enhancing performance in distracting situations. Indeed, at higher doses they also improve orbitofrontal functions. Conversely, α_2-antagonists can impair cognitive (working-memory) performance. (Noradrenaline's enhancement of 'posterior brain' processing is thought to be mediated via α_1 and β-noradrenergic receptors.)

Acetylcholine

Acetylcholine (ACh) is an excitatory neurotransmitter that is widely distributed within the central and peripheral nervous system. It is the product of a chemical reaction between choline and acetyl coenzyme A, catalysed by the enzyme choline acetyltransferase (ChAT). The latter is present at particularly high levels within the caudate nucleus and also the dorsal and ventral horns of the spinal cord. The rate-limiting factor during acetylcholine synthesis is the availability of choline (which is derived from the diet but also synthesized within the nervous system). Following neurotransmission, acetylcholine is catabolized by the enzyme acetylcholine esterase (AChE; Gartside & Marsden, 2006).

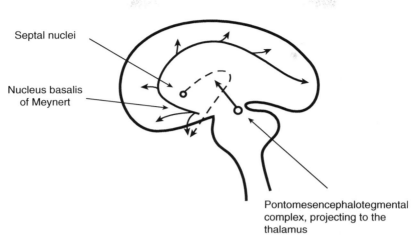

Septal nuclei

Nucleus basalis
of Meynert

Pontomesencephalotegmental
complex, projecting to the
thalamus

Fig. 62 Cartoon showing the projections of the acetylcholinergic systems within the human brain.

There are two families of cholinergic receptor: the nicotinic (i.e. the site of action of nicotine, and a site where signalling is characterized by fast excitatory neurotransmission) and the muscarinic (where neurotransmission is slower, and more sustained, as in the ganglia of the autonomic nervous system; Standring, 2005). The nicotinic system is of relevance to our concern with volition in that it is implicated in neurotransmission at the level of the midbrain (possibly impacting reward systems) and at the neuromuscular junction (in the periphery; below).

Cholinergic projections arise in the basal forebrain and pons, one key source being the nucleus basalis of Meynert, which sends important projections to the cortex (Figure 62). The lateral septum sends cholinergic projections to the hippocampus and these have been implicated in the memory impairment characteristic of Alzheimer's disease/dementia (Gartside & Marsden, 2006). There are also short cholinergic projections within many regions of the brain, especially the striatum (e.g. the cholinergic 'aspiny internuncials' that were mentioned previously; above). In Huntington's disease (chorea), the degeneration of the caudate nucleus may impact cholinergic function, as part of a complex process that eventually leads to excessive inhibition of the indirect pathway (consequent upon loss of GABA/enkephalin relays comprising its first leg) thereby leading to 'hyperkinesis', i.e. choreiform movements (see Litvan et al. 1998).

The cholinergic nuclei of the forebrain are subject to 'top-down' modulation by projections from the OFCs (and these are thought to be implicated in the recognition of rewarding stimuli in the external environment; Arnsten & Robbins, 2002).

In everyday clinical practice, it is regarded as preferable not to test cognition while patients are taking 'anticholinergic' medications (e.g. benzhexol and procyclidine), as these are likely to impact their memory and attention. That cholinergic function is relevant to memory is also implied by the use of 'anticholinesterases' – drugs that inhibit acetylcholine's catabolism (by AChE) – as putative 'cognitive enhancers' in Alzheimer's disease. However, we should acknowledge that the latter have evinced rather limited impact upon the disease's course and have also been a source of much controversy (e.g. Courtney et al. 2004).

Nevertheless, despite acetylcholine's importance to higher cognitive function (through contributions to memory and attention), from our point of view it is its contribution to volition that is crucial. Cholinergic function has the following potential impacts upon voluntary behaviour:

1. A role in striatal function is manifest through the clinical counterfactual example of anticholinergic medications reversing antipsychotic-induced parkinsonism (above);

2. Activity at nicotinic receptors in the midbrain may have a role in the 'reward' value of nicotine, and hence, in nicotine addiction (i.e. 'smoking').

3. At the level of the peripheral neuromuscular junction, acetylcholine is released at the motor endplate, causing a local potential change in the muscle fibre, which, if large enough, leads to 'propagation' (Rogers et al. 1976) and, hence, voluntary action.

So, although there is 'less to say' at the moment about cholinergic function, we can see that rather like dopamine it is capable of influencing both relatively 'low' and relatively 'high'-level voluntary behaviours. In myasthenia gravis, the problem is one of loss of (peripheral) motor function (i.e. muscle paralysis) due to the impact of the disease upon the neuromuscular junction (the 'motor endplate'; Table 4, Chapter 1). In drug-induced parkinsonism, cholinergic tone is in some way contributing to rigidity, increased muscular tone (through central, striatal mechanisms) and is counteracted through the use of anticholinergic medications. In cigarette smoking, the addict finds it hard, if not impossible, to break his 'habit'. A relatively sophisticated train of action sequences (the acquisition, smoking, and inhalation of nicotine) is attributable to the reinforcing properties (and consequences) of a cholinergic receptor's stimulation.

Glutamate

Synthesized within virtually all neurons and glia, from glutamine or from glucose via the Krebs cycle (Gartside & Marsden, 2006), glutamate is an amino acid that constitutes the major 'fast-acting' excitatory neurotransmitter within the brain. It is widely distributed; indeed, we have already encountered it in the major corticospinal and corticostriatal projections leaving the cortex, the thalamocortical projections returning there, within the basal ganglia-thalamo-cortical 'loop' systems, and also those excitatory projections leaving the sub-thalamic nuclei (above). There is also a (glutamatergic) 'perforant path' that runs between the entorrhinal cortex and the hippocampus. The pyramidal cells of the cerebral cortex (Chapter 1) and hippocampus are glutamatergic. Hence, it is clear that much of what human beings can enact, through volun-tary movement, is highly reliant upon a substrate of glutamatergic neurotrans-mission, especially that occurring within the pyramidal tracts and motor 'loops' (above).

Such neurotransmission is disrupted by the illicit substance phencyclidine (PCP or 'angel dust'). The latter antagonizes a form of glutamate receptor called the NMDA (N-methyl D-aspartate) receptor. The consequences of such antagonism include an illness that may mimic schizophrenia, also extending to a form of catatonia (when the substance user becomes mute and rigid).

More generally, NMDA receptors are thought to contribute to other vital functions, such as 'long-term potentiation' (LTP) – a process via which memo-ries may be 'laid down' (particularly relevant to hippocampal function). NMDA receptors may also be implicated in cell damage, degeneration, and death, as occurs after cerebral insult (e.g. the ischaemia that follows a 'stroke').

Gamma-aminobutyric acid (GABA)

This is the major inhibitory neurotransmitter within the nervous system and we have already encountered it within the basal ganglia-thalamo-cortical cir-cuits, and the laminae of both the cerebral cortex and the spinal cord (these being the 'homes' of numerous inhibitory interneurons). GABA neurons are widely distributed within the brain, but are particularly abundant in the basal ganglia (e.g. in the 'direct' and 'indirect' pathways; above), hypothalamus, amygdala, and other limbic regions (Gartside & Marsden, 2006).

GABA is formed from the decarboxylation of glutamate (above), a process catalysed by glutamic acid decarboxylase. Like the other neurotransmitters we have surveyed, GABA systems exhibit a range of receptor subtypes, and the $GABA_A$ receptors are particularly implicated in the actions of the benzodi-azepines (so-called 'minor' tranquillizers), barbiturates, and alcohol.

The contribution of GABA to volition will be readily inferred from its neu-roanatomical distribution (above); its involvement in the 'loop' systems, and also the spinal reflexes; however, it may also be interesting to note another line of inquiry. For, there are two curious abnormalities of motor function that are both encountered in clinical psychiatry, each of which is of rather obscure aetiology: catatonia and 'conversion' disorder (hysteria). What is interesting (here) is that both are amenable to GABAergic interventions.

In catatonia, a patient may present as mute and akinetic, they may stand in symbolic poses (for instance, as if crucified; a so-called 'mannerism'); they may also 'echo' the movements of others in their vicinity ('echopraxia'; see Chapter 2). If and when they recover, they may report: 'I knew what was happening, I just couldn't get myself to say anything … I couldn't move' (Fink & Taylor, 2003, p. 150). Catatonia can constitute a form of schizophrenia, though it may more commonly occur in depression, mania, and certain 'organic' states (e.g. following medial PMC lesions). Most of the time, it presents as a form of profound 'hypokinesia' (though 'catatonic excitement' may also occur).

In contrast, conversion disorder – otherwise known as 'hysteria' – is what Freud was describing when he saw patients (e.g. the famous 'Anna O') who could not move their limbs, even though there was no explicable 'organic' reason for their impairment (Freud & Breuer, 1991; and see Ludwig, 1972; and Spence, 1999). He posited that such a dysfunction was attributable to 'unconscious' mechanisms (we shall return to these phenomena in Chapter 7).

Now, as indicated, what is interesting about both catatonia and conversion disorder is that their respective motor impairments may be temporarily ameliorated through the administration of benzodiazepines. In their elegant monograph on catatonia, Fink and Taylor (2003) provide many such examples:

> A 42-year-old [woman] was hospitalised for depression, nihilistic ideas, motor retardation, insomnia, weight loss, and thoughts of worthlessness … A day later she was mute and stuporous. General medical, [neurological], and laboratory examinations found no abnormalities. She was given 2.5 mg lorazepam orally. Fifty minutes later, all her symptoms were reversed. She was improved and asked for discharge.
>
> (Fink and Taylor, 2003, p. 139)

Lorazepam is a benzodiazepine, used widely in 'acute' psychiatry. Patients with catatonia or conversion disorder may return to normal motor function while under the influence of such medications. Now, this does not prove that a primary disorder of GABA transmission or $GABA_A$ receptor function 'causes' such states, but it does demonstrate that motoric function is susceptible to modulation via such routes. Indeed, Fink and Taylor provide a further line of empirical evidence, in the same patient, through the one-off administration of a GABA antagonist (flumazenil):

> With her informed consent, [the patient] was given a bolus of 0.7 mg flumazenil, and almost immediately complained of dizziness, nausea, anxiety, and fears concerning accidents of family members. These fears condensed to certainty. Within two minutes, she was again mute and stuporous, and remained in this state for almost two hours.
>
> (Fink and Taylor, 2003, p. 139)

So, not only can a benzodiazepine (a GABA$_A$ receptor agonist) cause catatonia to remit, but also the subsequent administration of a GABA receptor antagonist may cause it to reappear. Furthermore, another drug that acts upon the GABA$_A$ receptor (zolpidem; not a benzodiazepine) also causes catatonia to remit (Thomas et al. 1997). So there seems to be some connection between GABAergic function, specifically GABA$_A$ receptor function, and the problem of catatonia (Fink & Taylor, 2003, p. 187).

Note also the occurrence of another possible neurochemical convergence here, manifest through the motoric consequences of glutamatergic and GABAergic receptor activity. While NMDA (glutamatergic) antagonism may render a healthy person catatonic (e.g. under the influence of PCP, above), agonism at the GABA$_A$ receptor site (in the form of benzodiazepine binding) can ameliorate spontaneous catatonia. Furthermore, in someone who has previously exhibited catatonia, a GABA$_A$ receptor antagonist (flumazenil) may precipitate relapse. Hence, it seems that both optimal glutamatergic and GABAergic function facilitate 'normal' human action.

An end to chemistry

Now, we are about to change architectures once more. However, before we do so, let us consider what we have learned from the foregoing data. We saw that neurological organization is susceptible to several different modes of description, or categorization, all of which are 'artificial' in that they are conceived of by the human mind. We seek to impose an order upon 'Nature' through different ways of 'looking at' the same complex and multifaceted system: the brain. We have 'looked at' neural projections; we have 'looked at' neurochemistry. We have pursued two architectures among many possible choices. Nevertheless, I think that we can defend our approach, not least because it yields an understanding that is credible at the (objective) level of human action, and its decomposition in certain disease states. If we saw the distinction between pyramidal and extrapyramidal (basal ganglia) systems exemplified in the pathologies of 'stroke' and Parkinson's disease (and their differing impacts upon the 'late' and 'early' components of the *Bereitschaftspotential*, respectively; in Chapter 3), then we also saw that choosing to define the systems of the brain in terms of their chemistry evoked similarly meaningful clinical distinctions: e.g. in the contrast between the inactivity of Parkinson's disease (a nigrostriatal dopamine deficiency state) and violent impulsivity (a phenomenon implicating a deficiency of serotonergic neurotransmission, particularly at the level of the OFC). Indeed, perhaps more importantly, we can now determine how 'beneficial' changes to the human condition might be instigated via therapeutic manipulations that are based upon such knowledge: replacement therapy with L-DOPA in Parkinson's disease and the use of SSRIs to combat impulsivity and 'self-defeating' habits (e.g. cutting and mutilation). Now we may proceed to yet another 'way of looking' at the brain and its 'output' (behaviour).

Cognitive architectures

The preceding sections have dealt with architectures that are very much embedded in the biology of the human organism: the patterns of projections that may be mapped out across the white matter of the cerebral hemispheres and spinal cord, the neurotransmitters which characterize certain projection fields and synapses within specified regions of the nervous system. There is a precision to such anatomy and physiology ('structure and process'; Chapter 1) that is very appealing; at times it can really 'feel' as if we are getting very close to the basis of voluntary action. However, it is important to acknowledge that we are (still) only operating at one level of understanding, while attempting to address a problem that is inherently 'multi-layered'. Anatomy and physiology concern levels of organization that the eye and the microscope may 'see' and the micro-pipette and -electrode access, but we have said hardly anything at all about sub-cellular mechanisms (what it is that happens within the neuron when an incoming signal 'arrives') and we have addressed 'higher' orders of representation merely at the level of phenomenology, e.g. when we infer that orbitofrontal lesions may precipitate 'impulsivity'. So, although it may appear something of a 'retreat' from biology, in this section, we try to understand what it is that is occurring throughout the brain when an organism (specifically 'an intelligent agent'; Shallice, 2002) behaves 'purposefully'. In order to do this we need to think computationally, combining insights from 'cognitive' and 'neuro'-psychology. In what follows, I am very indebted to the work of Tim Shallice (1988, 2002), a British neuropsychologist based for many years at the University of London.

Automation versus 'control'

Throughout this text we have expressed a recurrent interest in what it is that allows the brain to generate 'new' behaviours, to refrain from 'simply' resorting to predictable routines ('default responses'), and also what it is that allows us to 'automate' motoric procedures when setting down such 'routines'. We saw that in the animal literature reviewed by Dick Passingham, and in the human literature concerning many functional neuroimaging studies (both reviewed in Chapter 2), there was an anatomical distinction between the generation of 'novelty' and the learning of new sequences, which often implicated dorsal prefrontal systems, and the rehearsed performance of already-learned routines, which often implicated premotor and motor (i.e. 'posterior') systems. Indeed, we saw also (in Chapter 2) that there was a similar distinction between the functions of the medial PMCs (especially anterior SMA), implicated in 'internally initiated' responses, issuing forth at a time of the agent's own 'choosing', and those predictable responses – elicited by cues in the external environment – which relied for their production upon the integrity of lateral premotor systems. Furthermore, in the foregoing sections of this chapter, we have seen how an understanding of basal ganglia-thalamo-cortical 'loop' systems could inform our knowledge of such distinctions and transitions, e.g. that between new motor learning (with its reliance upon the DLPFC loop) and the later, automated, 'running of a programme' (reliant upon the 'motor/SMA' loop; see Figure 52, above). What runs throughout these distinctions is a well-known contrast between the 'controlled' and the 'routine' (i.e. automated).

Indeed, such a distinction is not only discernible in behavioural experiments. It is a well-recognized aspect of the phenomenology of everyday life.

There are daily procedures that I may carry out on some form of 'automatic pilot' and there are those that demand my immediate conscious attention. I may drive a car and ride a bike using motor routines that I have learned previously, and deployed on countless prior occasions, but there will be instances when I need to alter what I might have done 'routinely'. I may be driving along a quiet and familiar road, listening to the music in the car (Charlie Parker's *'Relaxin' at Camarillo'*) when all of a sudden a child runs out into the road and I need to brake, immediately. Alternatively, I may be driving along a familiar route, one that I take every day when I am going to work, but on a day when I am not working and when I have other, completely unrelated, errands to run. I should change my route slightly, take the second turn off and not the first, but because I am not concentrating (I am listening to Charlie Parker again!) I take the more familiar first turn (my 'default procedure'), only to discover that I am (mistakenly) heading for work.

Hence, I find myself operating at a kind of phenomenological junction: between those behaviours that I can just let 'run' (as if they were programmes) and those specific acts that require me to break my routines: those moments when 'conscious' intervention is necessary. How can one explain such vacillations?

The model that I shall describe here is the one that Tim Shallice has proposed over several decades and which has undergone sequential modifications. Essentially, it begins by stressing a distinction between routine ('unwilled') and controlled ('willed') behaviours.

Schemata and contention scheduling

Shallice (1988, pp. 328–352) posits that any voluntary task that we can perform may be described in terms of 'schemata' – automated programmes that can be 'run' on the brain, similar to computer scripts. So there might be a schema for when I 'put the kettle on', when I 'open the garage door', when I go about 'eating an apple', etc. Such schemata might be very 'simple' or they might be more complex, composed of many sub-programmes or routines. Hence, when I have a complex task to perform, such as 'collecting a friend from the railway station', one can imagine a string, or sequence, of virtual packets of behaviour – relatively simple routines that go to make up the overall act of 'collecting Nikita from the railway station'. Shallice terms such an overall plan the '*source* schema'; in contrast, the virtual string of related tasks is a sequence of '*component* schemata' (e.g. opening the garage door, opening the car, and getting inside). Not only are the component schemata relatively automated, but also the environment in which I find myself may help elicit (or 'trigger') them. Hence, if I am in the garage, and the car is also in the garage, and I have the car keys in my hand, then there is an increased likelihood that I may open the car door. While this 'makes sense' most of the time, and indeed it may be helpful when it smoothes my journey to work, it may comprise an inappropriate 'default' if I had actually entered the garage hoping to find the lawnmower! Clearly, it is most unlikely that I would make such a mistake under 'normal' conditions, but it just might happen if I am sufficiently 'pre-occupied' or 'distracted' (i.e. while my mind is 'concentrating' on 'something else').

Shallice says that such inappropriate defaults are examples of schemata being 'triggered' by cues in our external environment. They have been termed 'action lapses' or 'capture errors' (i.e. our behaviour is 'captured' by aspects of the immediate environment; p. 328). He describes his own experience:

> [T]he example … of my walking into a room I knew well and suddenly noticing that I was making a pulling movement with my arm, which I did not understand. I eventually realised what was obviously at some level 'known' – that the light switch in that room was controlled by a cord, which had got hooked up in a cupboard door. As the action was so mystifying at the time, it indicates that initiation and execution of this action was not normally controlled by a conscious intention to execute it.
>
> (Shallice, 1988, p. 328)

He goes on to mention a similar occurrence, this time affecting a monkey that has sustained a frontal lobe lesion (taken from a report by Bianchi, 1922):

> The monkey which used to jump on to the window ledge, to call out to his companion, after the operation jumps on to the ledge again, but does not call out. The sight of the window determines the reflex of the jump, but the purpose is now lacking.
>
> (Shallice, 1988, p, 329)

Hence, for both Shallice and the unfortunate monkey, the environment precipitates behaviours that seem to be without purpose. In fact, there is a 'purpose' but it is one that is unknown to the agent, and currently inappropriate, for it is based upon 'past' experience. The 'environment has changed' in Shallice's example – the cord that controls the light is lost to view ('hooked up in a cupboard door'); the 'brain has changed' in the lesioned monkey: the environment (the ledge) still elicits his jump but he no longer 'knows' what to do next. In each case, automation has been 'tricked', caught out, by a change in circumstances.

Shallice's models are aimed at providing a principled account of the computational steps or procedures that would be required to construct a purposeful behaviour *de novo*. In essence, he takes behaviour apart and then puts it back 'together' again. Hence, his earlier model introduces two concepts that are particularly useful in this regard (and they are demonstrated in Figure 63):

1. The 'routine selection' of 'routine operations' is 'decentralized' and takes place through a process called '*contention scheduling*' (in other words it is *not* reliant upon 'higher' or 'executive' resources);

2. Conversely, non-routine selection is qualitatively different and involves the contribution of a general purpose '*Supervisory Attentional System*'; the name that Shallice gives to such a higher, executive resource (Shallice, 1988, p. 332).

So, when we are engaged in routine operations, the environment assists us to a certain extent by 'triggering' low-level schemata and such schemata compete

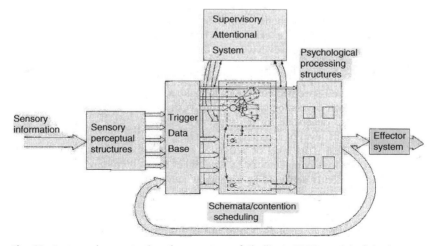

Fig. 63 Cartoon demonstrating the structure of Shallice's 1988 model of the human executive system. See text for details. Reproduced from *From Neuropsychology of Mental Structure*, Shallice T (1989), with permission from Oxford University Press.

with each other for their eventual emergence (hence, there is an evolutionary, selective, element to the model). Shallice's view is that the process of contention scheduling facilitates the emergence of the most contextually appropriate behaviour. This is brought about by a process of activation of relevant schemata with lateral 'inhibition' of those that are inappropriate. It follows that in any familiar environment there may be a set of schemata that might potentially 'work' and a smaller subset that would be optimal. Bearing in mind that a source schema is guiding the process (setting the agenda for what must occur, e.g. 'taking the car out of the garage'), one can see how an internal context is determined at the level of such (source) schemata and that contention scheduling serves to order their appropriate components (above). Hence, one can see source schemata as a means of 'biasing' the system, so that some component schemata are more likely to be selected than others because they are contextually more appropriate.

Therefore, in routine situations, much of what we do may be carried out without the need to divert 'higher', 'executive' resources to its execution. One really can move around the kitchen, 'making the breakfast', while listening to the radio or 'thinking of something else'. Furthermore, one can imagine a hierarchy of motor programmes of ascending levels of complexity – from the 'simple' schema that opens a carton of orange juice to the schema that 'lays the table' or sequences a 'full English breakfast' (but only very rarely!). The point is that lower level actions may be subsumed within meaningful action chains or sequences, and that these are nested, embedded, within the overarching purpose represented by a source schema (e.g. 'making the breakfast').

Calling in the supervisory attentional system

What happens when things get complicated? Well, in Shallice's earlier account, complications arise whenever we must 'trouble-shoot', change our plans, suppress our habits, or concentrate. Maybe we are preparing a meal we have never made before. Perhaps we are driving in an unfamiliar town or city, trying to find our way around. Perhaps we are improvising, at a keyboard, and we need to come up with something 'entirely original' (see Chapter 10). It is clear that under such conditions, 'running a programme' will not suffice. Resort to habit and automation will not be enough. So, how may we generate 'novelty'?

Shallice's solution was to invoke the concept of the supervisory attentional system (SAS). This 'higher' system acts upon the contention-scheduling mechanism, and biases ('modulates') its output. Hence, where it might be difficult to select what to do next, or to suppress what we have routinely done many times before, some aspect of the SAS allows it to specify *which* schemata are to be maximally facilitated *now*, at the level of contention scheduling. The focussing of attention upon a problem (e.g. what ingredient to add, what street sign to look out for) makes it easier to proceed. More importantly, it makes it more likely that we shall do so accurately.

However, with psychological models there is always the criticism that we may be merely replacing one kind of descriptive language with another. Instead of saying we 'made a mistake', we can now say that we were subject to an 'action error'. Are we any the wiser? Well, yes we are, up to a point. For the Shallice model allows us to begin to ascertain 'where' in the brain such processes may 'reside', and what the nature of their relationships may be.

So, for instance, on the basis of much of what we have discussed in Chapter 2, and our reference to the works of Marc Jeannerod and others, it is clear that some low-level schemata might be quite readily 'mapped' onto premotor-parietal systems. We saw that patients with some kinds of dyspraxia were unable to 'make' their hands do the tasks that they wanted them to do, even though they fully understood what it was that they needed to execute. A dyspraxic hand may be unable to execute the comparatively simple schema of 'picking up the teacup' or 'putting the letter in the mailbox'. The hand cannot adopt the shape required of it to perform such simple procedures. Of course, the hand itself is (probably) neurologically normal; it is the 'control' of the hand that is disrupted. The hand appears dyspraxic because there is a lesion of the parietal cortex or the lateral premotor region.

So, from the point of view of Shallice's model, there is a good case to be made for thinking of schemata as residing at the level of the PMCs and parietal cortices and for the basal ganglia to contribute via facilitating the sequencing of behaviours (indeed, he explicitly invokes the latter as the substrate of 'contention scheduling', 1988, p. 334).

Hence, as we have seen previously demonstrated through functional neuroimaging studies of humans, automated tasks may be carried out by more 'posterior' motor regions and these would provide suitable substrates for Shallice's component schemata and contention scheduling.

Furthermore, we may posit that the prefrontal lobes provide putative substrates for the 'higher' components of the SAS. Shallice refers to the ways in which such systems are activated when humans have to perform complex executive tasks (e.g. the WCST, above) and how those who have sustained frontal lobe lesions may be particularly impaired on these sorts of tasks (even when their intellect and other cognitive processes are relatively intact). Hence, a lesion of the cognitive SAS would predictably render certain tasks difficult – concentrating in complex situations, suppressing habitual responses (routines), which are currently inappropriate, and 'generating' new solutions to problems.

All these are clinical features of people with frontal lobe lesions but they may also be elicited empirically by the administration of the WCST and other executive tasks.

In the WCST setting, a 'frontal' patient will exhibit perseverative errors (failing to change 'rule' in the face of negative feedback; above) and they may have difficulty generating new responses.

So, the Shallice model allows us to delineate the locations and the functions of hypothetical aspects of an 'intelligent agent', an organism that may potentially 'switch' between automated procedures, 'run' in posterior motor regions, and 'controlled' behaviours, trouble-shooting, and problem solving under conditions of novelty. These latter processes, subsumed within the rubric of the SAS, may be mapped onto certain regions of the PFC.

Shallice II

However, there is still a problem with the earlier Shallice model in that it is cognitively under-specified, especially at the level of the SAS. While it is helpful to specify what it is that the SAS 'does' (e.g. 'it trouble-shoots'), it is a far more difficult proposition to conceive of how it actually does it. This is a challenge taken up by Shallice (2002) in a later iteration of his model, one that incorporates aspects of 'artificial intelligence', shared in common with so-called 'diagnostic' systems (Figure 64).

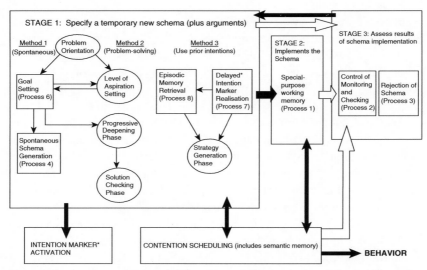

Fig. 64 Cartoon demonstrating Shallice's 2002 model of the supervisory attentional system. See text for details. With kind permission from Oxford University Press and the Royal Society of London.

Essentially, this later iteration is entirely concerned with what happens 'inside' the SAS. It specifies many sub-processes that should occur there and posits a division into three overarching sub-systems or 'stages' (Figure 64). Hence, it may be helpful to explain what it is that the SAS must do in any 'new' situation, in terms of these three stages. Shallice specifies that it must:

1. 'Specify a temporary new schema': essentially a first approximation of a response to the new problem, one that incorporates 'arguments';

2. 'Implement the new schema': essentially involving a trial run to see whether the new solution will work;

3. 'Assess results of schema implementation': in other words, form a judgement as to whether the schema is likely to 'work' as it stands or whether modification or rejection is required.

Inherent in Shallice's model is a means via which such procedures might be carried out virtually, prior to action. If consciousness can act as a kind of 'work-space' (Baars & McGovern, 1996), then the SAS may work through possible solutions without committing the organism to action. Also, inherent in the model is a certain 'level of agency' (in this context, agency is being used in a way similar to the philosophical use of the term 'intentionality'). To understand what Shallice means by agency in this regard, we need to consider a typology that he borrows from Das and colleagues (1997). Hence:

1. A 'zero-order' agent is one that responds to its environment simply on the basis of one environmental feature, in a pre-specified way (e.g. a thermostat is a zero-order agent that responds solely to room temperature; Shallice, 2002, p. 263);

2. A 'first-order' agent is one that carries an explicit model of its environment;

3. A 'second-order' agent carries more than one explicit model of its environment and may function at a higher level because it can compare these models;

4. A 'third-order' agent is a second-order agent that also possesses a 'higher'order model of its own beliefs and desires (Das et al. 1997).

Hence, a third-order agent (such as a healthy human being) is able to evaluate current schemata against an overarching aim, a kind of meta-source schema. Through such an understanding, Shallice begins to explain how the human brain (the 'intelligent agent') might hold to very long-term 'intentions', through maintaining a higher order, source schema over long periods of time (e.g. 'I want to finish writing this book'), in the face of competing contingencies (e.g. 'carry on, the chapter is nearly over', versus, 'there is a packet of chocolate biscuits in the kitchen').

Furthermore, the components of the 'new' SAS, with its stages of schema specification, implementation, and appraisal (assessment) have sub-components that we might begin to map onto prefrontal regions. Hence, Shallice postulates the following:

1. That the left DLPFC is implicated in modulating schemata at the level of contention scheduling; this is akin to the 'control' of response generation described in Jahanshahi and colleague's work (2002; reviewed in Chapter 2), and the 'sculpting of response space' referred to by Frith (2000); such a process could essentially act as a bridge between Stage 2 of Shallice's later SAS (Figure 64, above) and contention scheduling (Figure 64, below), i.e. it contributes to the 'implementation' of schemata (notice also the resemblance to the role of DLPFC envisaged in Koechlin and Hyafil's 2007 model of prefrontal function, reviewed towards the close of Chapter 2);

2. That right DLPFC is implicated in 'monitoring and checking' of behaviour according to internal criteria (a process that would be located within Stage 3 of the new model (Figure 64, right); note that the criteria would have to be 'held' or 'maintained' in some active form to facilitate such comparison;

3. That 'specification' of a required memory trace implicates right ventrolateral PFC (a region previously shown to be implicated in mnemonic retrieval; something that would occur early on, within Stage 1 of the model; Figure 64); and

4. That both the 'setting up' and the 'realization' of an 'intention' would implicate Brodmann Area10, the focus of Paul Burgess's work (outlined in Chapter 2), a process implicated in both the early and late stages of the SAS's involvement in novelty generation; i.e. 'early on' an intention is generated, 'later on' its successful implementation (or otherwise) must be checked.

Clearly, the later Shallice model is a complex volitional architecture, and one that is not fully specified in terms of its precise neuroanatomical/neurophysiological correlates. Indeed, if one looks at Figure 64, then one can see that there are still several processes awaiting such elucidation. However, one may also anticipate where this model is leading, how it might be possible to fully specify such an architecture at some point in the future.

Nevertheless, because this is a cognitive psychological model, we also have to avoid taking a retrograde step towards imagining a 'little man' (our beloved homunculus) sitting in area 10, setting out intentions, while his colleague sits in the right DLPFC 'monitoring' how things are going. We can see that there is still some way to go before we arrive at the philosopher's benchmark for a theory of human action: a factory that we might visit at night, one where we might witness all of the machines turning over without the need for a human 'supervisor' to be present. In other words, for the time being, the ghost has not yet left the machine!

Night time in the brain: Sleep architecture

It may seem strange to the reader to close this chapter, concerning 'volitional architectures', with a consideration of sleep. However, as I hope to demonstrate shortly, there is one very specific occurrence during sleep that is immensely pertinent to our pursuit of volition, the question of 'freedom', and the contribution of consciousness towards action. In this case the pertinent architecture expresses itself through time, it is a temporal architecture i.e. it is a 'process' rather than a 'structure' (Chapter 1). Hence, I hope that the reader will bear with me while I 'flesh out' what it is that we need to know about sleep. For this section, I am most indebted to an overview provided by Adam Zeman (2002).

The stages of sleep

Most adults need to spend just under a third of their lives in an altered state of 'consciousness' that seems to be essential for life, albeit arrived at via a 'mechanism of action' that is largely unknown to us. For 7–8 hours in every 24 we appear to be to all 'intents and purposes' unconscious. However, as has become increasingly apparent since its structure first attracted systematic study, sleep is actually rather more complicated than that. For, throughout an average night, a healthy sleeper oscillates between various 'stages' of sleep, of varying 'depths', each characterized by different profiles of waveform on an EEG trace. According to convention, these stages are labelled 1–4, with 1 comprising a relatively 'shallow' sleep state and 4 the 'deepest' sleep that we may attain:

1. Stage 1: During this stage the alpha rhythm (of relaxed wakefulness; above) is replaced by a mixture of high- and low-frequency oscillations. The onset of slow, rolling eye movements indicates that Stage 1 is established; it constitutes approximately 5% of one night's sleep.

2. Stage 2: The EEG reveals prominent slow-wave activity, 'theta' (4–7 Hz) and 'delta' (<4 Hz) waves, interspersed with transient features, the so-called 'sleep spindles', 'K-complexes', and 'vertex sharp waves'. The sleeper is motionless and eye movements are infrequent. Stage 2 constitutes approximately 45% of one night's sleep.

3. Stage 3: High-amplitude delta waves are present for 20–50% of the time.

4. Stage 4: High-amplitude delta waves are present for most of the time.

Stages 3 and 4 together constitute so-called 'slow-wave' sleep.

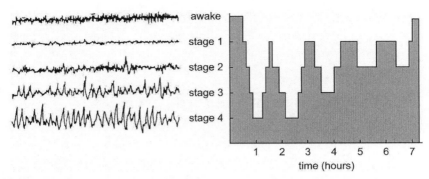

Fig. 65 Cartoon showing the stages of sleep. On the left are the EEG signals accompanying different stages of sleep while on the right is a hypothetical hypnogram. Notice that the sleeper spends longer in the deeper stages of sleep earlier in the night (stages 3 and 4) than later in the night when sleep becomes more shallow.

Now, towards the beginning of a 'good' night's sleep, we move between these four stages at characteristic intervals (as represented on a 'hypnogram'; see Figure 65). Towards the beginning of the night, we spend longer periods in deep or 'slow-wave' sleep and over the course of the night we seem to re-surface, gradually. Hence, in the second-half of a normal hypnogram it is clear that we are spending much more time in Stage 1. However, something else is also happening, for during these bouts of 'shallow' sleep we are actually entering another state: so-called 'rapid eye movement' or REM sleep, a period during which, if awoken, we may admit to having been dreaming. An adult spends approximately 20% of their night in REM sleep.

Events occurring during rapid eye movement sleep

REM sleep is characterized by the following features: an EEG pattern similar to that seen during the waking state; rapid eye movements, where the eyes move from side to side under their lids; and deep muscular relaxation, particularly of the anti-gravitational, postural muscles (note: the diaphragm is spared; we continue to breathe). In sleep studies (using EEG and EMG), the tone of the muscles of the chin and the limbs may be used as an indicator of REM relaxation.

Now, what is interesting in the context of our pursuit of volition is this 'paralysis' that occurs during REM sleep. How is it brought about? Well, it is thought that the pons initiates a hyper-polarization of the (lower motor neurons of the) anterior horns of the spinal cord via the inhibitory reticulospinal pathways (Table 3; Chapter 1). Hence, movement is 'blocked'. We become 'atonic'.

But what would happen if such a paralysis 'failed'? Well, the consequences are apparent in cats!

> Cats in whom this centre [in the pons] has been destroyed no longer show atonia during REM sleep, and as a consequence they may get up and walk around or appear to chase phantom birds, presumably reflecting their dream content. The function of this atonia centre [in the pons] may therefore be to prevent the dreaming brain from influencing the rest of the body.

> (Stradling, 2005, pp. 1409–1410)

So, our voluntary musculature (and that of the cat) is usually paralysed while we dream. One 'teleological' explanation for such a state of affairs is that it 'protects us' from 'acting out our dreams'.

This may all be stated very simply. However, consider what it actually says about evolution, action, and the role of consciousness in volition (whatever the conclusions we may now have drawn from Benjamin Libet's work and that of Patrick Haggard; in the Prologue and Chapter 3; above). It suggests:

1. That 'conscious' phenomena, or at least those forms of consciousness experienced during REM sleep, can indeed impact explicit behaviour;

2. That 'somehow' the brain evolved to 'turn off' the body's voluntary musculature 'in order to' lessen the risks of our 'acting out' our dreams;

3. That dreamt events and actions (when 'released', e.g. by pontine lesions, above) re-instate the role of (albeit altered) consciousness in action;

4. That such a relation is not confined to humans (you can 'see it' happening in cats and dogs; above); and

5. That temporal dissociations between sleep, dreaming, and paralysis may have striking consequences for human agents.

And, indeed, this is so.

In 1986, Schenck and colleagues described four men who had injured their sleeping partners or themselves as a consequence of 'dream enactments'. Prior to assessment, one man had 'attempted to strangle his wife while dreaming of fending off a mauling bear ... [H]is wife commented on his gentle nature' (Patient 4; Schenck et al. 1986, p. 298). When studied in a sleep laboratory, these men were found to have an abnormality of their REM sleep; though they entered this phase (as verified on EEG recordings) their muscles did not relax (as verified by EMG); hence, they were still able to move about (while dreaming). Recorded events included 'stereotypical hand motions, reaching and searching gestures, punches, kicks, and verified dream movements' (Schenck et al. 1986, p. 293).

Consider an example, the so-called 'Patient 1':

A 67-year-old man, with a history of more than 40 years sleep movements witnessed by his wife, began to exhibit more extreme sorts of behaviour, while asleep. He would 'punch and kick his wife, fall out of bed, stagger about the room, crash into objects, and injure himself'. His behaviours were often related to the reported content of his dreams. One recurring example consisted of his 'delivering a speech and emphasizing certain points with his right hand from which he awakened sitting up with [his] right arm outstretched and [his] fingers pointing in a manner consistent with the dream action' (Schenck et al. 1986, p. 294).

When this man was studied in the laboratory the investigators could demonstrate that during REM sleep his chin and limb EMGs each exhibited phases of activity, during which he was able to move in accordance with his dreams (see Figure 66).

In a later study of 93 consecutive patients reporting these same sorts of problems, Olson and colleagues (2000) found that the mean age of presentation to medical services was just under 65 years, a third having injured themselves during sleep and two-thirds having assaulted their spouses; dream content was altered and involved the 'defence of the sleeper against attack' in 87% of cases and the same percentage of patients responded positively if treated with clonazepam (a benzodiazepine, i.e. a GABAergic medication, above).

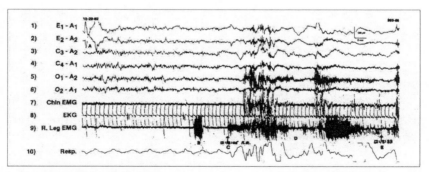

Fig. 66 EEG and EMG data taken from a patient. This patient has REM sleep behavioural disorder. During rapid eye movement sleep, when there is frequent spiking activity across the EEG, there is also associated activity within the chin leads of the EMG and within the EMG for the subject's right leg. Hence, the patient is moving while he is dreaming. There is also an increase in his respiration during these movements. Reprinted from Carlos H Schenck, Chronic Behavioural Disorders of Human REM Sleep: A New Category of Parasomnia. *Sleep* 1986; 9(2): 293–308. Permission granted through Copyright clearance centre on behalf of The American Academy of Sleep Medicine.

However, the onset of REM sleep 'behaviour disorder' (RBD), as this condition has now become known, is often a harbinger of other problems for the unfortunate patient and their spouse. Given that we know that REM paralysis relies upon activity in the pontine region, such disruptions as are seen in this condition suggest brain pathology either at this level or else impacting upon it from 'above'. Olson's data (and those of other centres) suggest a relationship with Parkinson's disease, multiple system atrophy, and dementia.

Hence, we have seen that one feature of human sleep architecture is an intermittent entry into REM sleep, a state during which we tend to dream, though we are usually protected from the consequences of our dreaming by the actions of our pons and reticulospinal tracts upon the anterior horns of our spinal cords. Though we may 'envisage' dream actions, 'Nature' prevents us from enacting them ('normally', usually). If such a system breaks down, then we may harm ourselves, and others. So, are we 'responsible'?

No! Because, to echo the words of J.F. Meister (cited in Bonkalo, 1974), *in somno voluntas non erat libera*, a sleeping person has no 'Free Will'. The men we described (above) do not consciously choose to hit their partners; they find themselves doing so. Nevertheless, we humans do seem to be 'acting' in many of our dreams. So what kinds of 'acts' are these? They seem to comprise 'virtual volitions', things that we 'might have done' in another (dreamt) environment. Yet, we are usually somewhat less than 'active' in the phenomenology of dreams. Things happen, we are engaged in 'acts', but we did not 'choose' to be there. Perhaps we are actually more akin to puppets or passengers, conveyed by the narrative of the dream and deposited into the fray. Apart from the unpleasant nature of many of those dreams reported above (by Schenck's and Olson's patients), the worst problem arises if virtual volitions are somehow allowed to proceed (i.e. if they emerge 'un-blocked' by the dreamer's pons). Whatever the 'purpose' of dreaming, its normal phenomenology seems to comprise the hallucination of action; behaviours the dreamer finds herself performing, though she is not 'really' performing them since (really) they are 'blocked' by her brain. There is still something deeply mysterious about dreaming. At the very least it serves to demonstrate that an 'un-paralysed' consciousness is capable of influencing ongoing physical action.

Indeed, what is interesting is the set of circumstances that Nature seems to have contrived 'in order to allow' competing physiological processes to coexist under normal conditions. For some 'reason' we dream. 'Voluntary' behaviours engaged in during dreams 'would' impact explicit behaviour, were it not for our state of REM paralysis. So, we are paralysed. Yet, we must continue to breathe, so our diaphragms do not undergo paralysis (only our 'voluntary' muscles' do so). Again, rather as we concluded at the close of Chapter 1, we experience a 'freedom' that is (normally) precisely modulated by natural processes. We are able to move discrete fingers as a consequence of the structure of our motor systems (e.g. the richness of the corticomotor innervation of our spinal anterior horns, synapsing at the level of the alpha lower motor neurons). We may dream about moving our fingers, but our actions will remain 'virtual' so long as our pons and our reticulospinal pathways cooperate in 'hyperpolarizing' these same anterior horns. Our 'normal' physiology protects us from our 'selves' while 'we' dream. And though we 'know', post-Libet, that consciousness does not initiate action, we find that dream consciousness will elicit veridical behaviours, movements that impact ourselves (and our sleeping partners), if we are not paralysed.

Designs for living

Each of the architectures that we have considered in the course of this chapter sheds light upon what it means to act 'voluntarily' and what it is that delineates our 'response space'. Neural 'loops' coordinate activity over distributed brain regions, they allow coherent movements to emerge; neurochemical architectures modulate neural processes, they promote volition or restraint; such systems may be conceived of cognitively, in models that we create with arrows and boxes, models that emphasize a distinction between 'routines' and 'control', the way that we structure our actions in time; and finally, our own bodies paralyse us, to 'prevent' us from 'acting' 'involuntarily', when we dream. Multiple structures and processes, all engaged in providing a coherent space for action. So it is that, in the next chapter, we consider what happens when our systems fall apart.

Chapter 5

Losing control

And if your right hand causes you to sin, cut it off and throw it away; it is better that you lose one of your members than that your whole body go into hell.[11]

Those are two very different people, the arm and I.[12]

Over the course of this book, we have gradually assembled an understanding of some of the biological conditions that must be satisfied in order for the brain to be 'able' to generate a coherent pattern of behaviour, one that on the face of it appears 'purposeful'. We followed a course of basic anatomy and physiology in Chapter 1, examined the contribution of some 'higher' brain centres (located in the frontal cortex) in Chapter 2, interrogated the timing of neural events (in cerebral motor regions) during the genesis of voluntary actions in Chapter 3, and attempted to adopt a more 'systemic' approach in Chapter 4, in order to consider some of the distributed processes (e.g. the neural 'loops' and neurochemical pathways) that seem to work in concert, in 'collaboration', during the emergence of voluntary behaviours. (Indeed, we also described a [pontine, reticulospinal] system that actually *prevents us* from moving when we are engaged in 'virtual volitions', while dreaming.)

---

[11] Matthew 5:30.

[12] The words of the very first patient described in the neurological literature as having suffered from an 'alien hand' (*avant la lettre*). The case was reported by Kurt Goldstein in 1908, and the patient was a 57 year old woman who had suffered a stroke leading to her left hand exhibiting a 'will of its own'. This citation is taken from Scepkowski and Cronin-Golomb (2003). Goldstein's (1908) original report is in German. Goldstein K. Zur Lehre der motorischen Apraxie. *Journal fur Psychologie und Neurologie* 1908; 11: 169–187. The first use of the term 'alien hand' occurred in the French literature, Brion and Jedynak coining the term *'la main etrangere'*, in 1972. Brion S, Jedynak CP. Troubles du transfert interhemispherique. A propos de trios observations de tumeurs du corps calleux. Le signe de la main etrangere. *Revue Neurologique (Paris)* 1972; 126: 257–266.

There is still much that we do not understand, but we do at least have some awareness of the brain systems that are implicated in our ability to produce what look like 'voluntary actions'.

In this chapter, we change emphasis once again. Here, we examine what can go wrong, what it is that may disrupt the 'normal' pattern of voluntary behaviour, with particular regard to those instances when human actors find that they are no longer 'in control'. Examples include limbs that 'will not do' what their owners 'wish them to do', and people who experience their movements as being controlled by 'outside' forces.

Now, it may seem strange to disrupt our narrative progression in this way, to turn from the reconstruction of 'normal' action, in order to consider what might 'go wrong' under certain pathological conditions, but I do so because I think that the lessons we may learn here serve to challenge and inform what we mean by the words 'voluntary action'. In essence, the *appearance* of 'purpose' is not enough. Here, we see that 'true purpose' requires an 'agent'. Moreover, it requires an agent who 'recognizes' herself (or himself) as such.

Hand in glove

Approximately 48 min into the film 'Dr. Strangelove' (directed by the late Stanley Kubrick), the eponymous doctor makes his appearance, portrayed by the late actor and comedian Peter Sellers (Fig. 67). This doctor is a strange cove, not least because of the antics of his 'anarchic' right hand. The latter, sheathed in a black leather glove, grasps objects tightly, 'will not' let them go, and occasionally 'performs' Nazi-style salutes. The doctor has to hit this hand in order to make it 'let go', in order to make it 'behave'. The implication is that this character, Strangelove, has a not-so-well-hidden past, a past that he cannot quite conceal because his right hand keeps 'giving him away'.

However, although it may be tempting to search for 'motive' or 'meaning' in the movements of such a limb, it seems likely that the behaviours observed are not really 'actions' in the philosophical sense of the word (Macmurray, 1991): that is, they are not 'chosen' by an agent (in this case, the fictional Dr. Strangelove). Instead, they appear to comprise a set of 'disinhibited', rather stereotypic, motor routines, which have somehow been 'released' from 'his' control (yes, we have returned to the problem of describing people in terms of their 'parts'.) So, if the Strangelove character is 'given away' by his Nazi-style salute, then it is only because such motor behaviour is so overlearnt, and hence stereotypically 'prepotent', that it emerges when his 'control' processes are compromised. (The problem is rather akin to that of a young man who stubs his toe in the presence of his censorious great-aunt: the expletive that he emits may be beyond his immediate control, in the context of his sudden experience

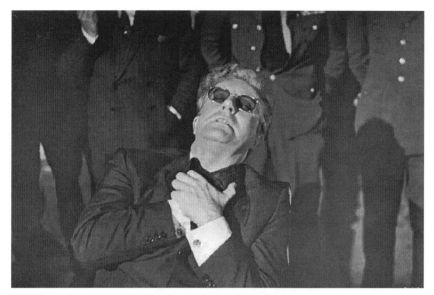

Fig. 67 A still from the film Dr. Strangelove, where the eponymous doctor (played by the actor Peter Sellers) attempts to restrain his anarchic right hand (with limited success). 'Dr Strangelove' © 1963, renewed 1991 Columbia Pictures Industries, Inc. All rights reserved, courtesy of Columbia Pictures.

of pain, but the fact that he emits it at all suggests that it forms part of his normal vocal repertoire at other times. Hence, his elderly relative has gained an unwelcome insight into his store of vocal schemata!)

Thus, if we think in terms of the cognitive model of motor control described by Tim Shallice (1988), and delineated in Chapter 4, then it is clear that Strangelove's salute emerges as a kind of rogue 'schema', a routine no longer suppressed by contention scheduling or, indeed, by the bad doctor's 'supervisory attentional system' (SAS; see Fig. 63, in that chapter). In other words, it is an 'automated routine', escaping 'his' control.

Anarchic limbs

However, as intriguing as all this may appear, why should we bother to describe and diagnose such a character, depicted in a film? Surely, he is fictional. Well, yes, Dr Strangelove may never have existed, but there are certainly human beings who *have* suffered from his (implied) pathology. There really are people who are unable to control the wayward movements of their upper limbs (and, even more rarely, their lower ones). So, consider the following examples, sourced from the neurological literature. Unless otherwise stated, all these patients were originally 'dextral' (i.e. they were right-handed).

Hands that grip and grope

1. '[A]t one point it was noted that the patient had picked up a pencil and had begun scribbling with the [affected] right hand. When her attention was directed to this activity, she reacted with dismay, immediately withdrew the pencil, and pulled the right hand to her side using the [unaffected] left hand. She then indicated that she had not . . . initiated the original action of the right arm. She often reacted with dismay and frustration at her inability to prevent these unintended movements . . . She experienced a feeling of dissociation from the actions of the right arm, stating on several occasions that "it will not do what I want it to do." '(Goldberg et al., 1981)

2. '[The patient] viewed these (autonomous) actions as unwanted, unintentional, and uncontrollable. He described the [affected] right hand as "the bad one, it has a mind of its own," and that it was "always trying to get into the act". A very specific complaint, which was chronic and persisted for a year after [his stroke], was that the patient felt that the right hand anticipated future actions and performed movements prior to the patient actually intending them. The [unaffected] left hand did not show this tendency.' (Feinberg et al., 1992)

3. 'The [affected] right hand frequently carried out complex activities that were not willed by [the patient]. These activities were clearly goal-directed and were well executed, but undesired by the patient, who used her [unaffected] left hand to try to stop them . . . [When she] had a genital itch, the right hand scratched it vigorously, in view of other people, causing considerable embarrassment to the patient, who tried to stop the right hand with her left . . . The patient considered her left hand to be the one she could trust, while the right hand, which could make motions completely without her wanting it to, was the untrustworthy one that "always does what it wants to do".' (Della Sala et al., 1991)

These are curious phenomena: right hands that do not 'obey' their mistresses and masters, right hands that seem to be 'released' from their owners' control. Indeed, this is not all that they have in common, for in each of these cases the reported behaviour occurred as a consequence of a brain lesion located in the medial premotor region of the patient's left hemisphere. This is a rare, but characteristic, sequence of events. In a right-handed patient, a brain lesion (often a stroke involving the anterior cerebral artery; Scepkowski and Cronin-Golomb, 2003) impacts the dominant (left) hemisphere's medial premotor system and then the previously dominant (right) hand exhibits dysfunctional behaviours: disinhibited gripping and grasping movements (rather similar to those exhibited by the fictional Dr. Strangelove). The patient is then reduced to trying to control the hand in abnormal ways: by holding it, hitting it, putting it in a pocket or in a glove, tying it to the body, or even sitting on it. Such a limb is often said to have a 'mind of its own'.

The first recorded description of such pathology was provided by Goldstein in 1908, and is found in the German-language literature. The same phenomenon later acquired the diagnostic label of the 'alien hand', following its description in the French literature by Brion and Jedynak in 1972. More recently, Della Sala and his colleagues (1991) have called such hands 'anarchic' because they do not do what their owners wish them to do. (We seem never to be too far from invoking hierarchical structures in neurology: we have 'release' signs following frontal pathology [Chapter 1], a counter-revolutionary neurotransmitter in the form of serotonin [Chapter 4], and now we encounter anarchic limbs that rebel against their owners' supervisory control!)

From our perspective, there are several key points that are of interest here:

1. The affected hand makes movements (i.e. it is not 'still' or, neurologically, 'silent'); this suggests that it is 'released', to move.

2. Those movements are targeted on stimuli in the environment (or within the body); in other words, they seem to be reactive movements, contingent upon sensory stimulation.

3. There seems to be a kind of 'purpose' or 'goal-directedness' to such movements.

4. Though the authors publishing these clinical descriptions often term the anarchic movements 'actions', it is clear that they are not voluntary actions, chosen by an agent (i.e. the patients deny 'authorship' of such movements.)

5. The subject, the patient, cannot 'control' the hand directly (she or he has to resort to physical force or other unusual tactics).

6. Generally speaking, it is the right hand that behaves in this way (following a left medial premotor cortical lesion, though this is not exclusively the case).

7. Usually, the patient still regards the hand as being 'hers' or 'his' (i.e. 'belonging' to her or him) albeit possessing a 'mind of its own'.

How do we account for such strange occurrences? One early explanation was provided by Denny-Brown (1958), who suggested that such dysfunction (which he termed 'magnetic apraxia') was attributable to a failure of the anterior regions of the left hemisphere to inhibit the posterior regions, notably the left parietal lobe. Hence, if the parietal lobe remained intact (after a frontal lesion), then the programmes necessary to enact grasping movements would persist, while the inhibitory control of these (potential) movements, instantiated in frontal regions, was lacking (as a consequence of the frontal lesion). Hence, it would appear as if the contralateral (right) hand was 'magnetically' drawn towards objects in the environment as a result of motor disinhibition (at the level of the cortex).

A more recent theory posits a similar mechanistic formulation (albeit in terms of medial and lateral, as opposed to anterior and posterior, frontal lobes): Goldberg and Bloom (1990) attribute anarchic behaviours to the disturbance of a hypothetical balance normally pertaining between the medial and lateral premotor systems. According to their 'dual premotor system theory' (Goldberg and Bloom, 1990), the situation is that the medial and lateral premotor systems, though both involved in the programming of motor acts (as elucidated in Chapters 2 and 3), usually hold each other in some kind of balance or mutual inhibition. Hence, while the medial premotor system (especially the SMA) is implicated in 'internally initiated' actions, the lateral premotor system is implicated in responses to cues in the external environment (a distinction that we also encountered in Dick Passingham's [1993] analysis of the non-human primate literature; see Chapter 2). Thus, it is hypothesized that there is a neurological balance (at the level of the premotor cortices) between acting according to our 'internal' goals and those that are cued by the (immediate) external environment.

One may now see how a number of different literatures seem to converge upon a single understanding of how motor system 'errors' might arise. We saw that Tim Shallice (1988) described 'action lapses' or 'capture errors' as occurring when an agent acted upon their environment without willing or wishing to do so (as when Shallice himself performed a habitual movement out of context, inappropriately). In Shallice's model(s), such errors reflected the failure of the contention scheduling system to adequately order component schemata (i.e. the components of a corresponding 'source schema'). Furthermore, if the SAS was itself compromised, then there might be no neural means via which such errors could be 'corrected' (by overseeing structures, within the motor hierarchy). So it is that in the 'dual premotor system theory' such motoric errors, such episodes of 'capture' by the environment (of a vulnerable motor schema, which is 'triggered' by sensory cues, as occurs when the patient grasps and scribbles with a pencil [see the first case in this subsection]), are attributable to the (still-functioning) lateral premotor system. Furthermore, this schema emerges because there is some corresponding failure by the medial premotor system to set an agenda or to 'choose' appropriate actions at that moment (perhaps because the agent is distracted or not 'attending' to their behaviours, their movements).

So, following a medial premotor cortical lesion, this may be what happens: the medial system is lesioned, the lateral system preserved. Perhaps, the impact of such a lesion on the medial system is that it 'releases' the lateral premotor system to 'act' on the environment. Therefore, what emerges is the lateral system's best approximation of an appropriate behaviour, given the objects or cues available within that environment. Hence, 'it' scribbles with a pen (or scratches the patient's genitals).

However, notice also that by providing such a reading of the evidence, we are implicitly affirming some form of motor hierarchy. For, we seem to be preferentially endowing medial premotor systems with some element of 'responsibility' for our more 'purposeful' activities, while suggesting that a 'disinhibited' ('released' or at least 'preserved') lateral premotor system 'doing its best' is not good enough; it is volitionally inadequate. Losing the influence of the medial premotor system renders the patient's movements quasi-purposeful but unhelpful, self-defeating even. Indeed, in the cases described earlier in this chapter, we see that the patients, in order to control their errant right hand, often have to deploy the unaffected left. They have to 'correct' their behaviours.

However, as fascinating as all this is, it is still rather speculative, phenomeno-logically and descriptively. So, is there any way in which we might 'tighten up' our understanding of what the errant hand and its 'controller' are up to? Well, fortunately, there is, for in an elegant study of such an affected patient (named 'JC') by Giovannetti and colleagues (2005), the authors made some progress towards delineating the conditions that facilitate such an affected hand's misbehaviour (and the unfortunate agent's lack of control).

> JC was a 56-year-old right-handed man who had suffered a stroke involving the left medial frontal region of his brain, extending into his corpus callosum (that white matter bundle connecting the left and right cerebral hemispheres; Giovannetti et al., 2005; Fig. 68). After some weeks, it was noted that JC's right hand would (uncontrollably) reach for, grasp, and use objects in his environment. JC and his wife reported that the hand 'reached for light switches (echoes of Shallice [1988] here; see Chapter 4), repeatedly pressed buttons on the television remote control, and groped for his left hand or face during sleep' (p. 77). JC stated, 'The hand does what it wants to do'; 'it has a mind of its own.'

Now, what is especially interesting about their report is that Giovannetti and colleagues actually went on to test JC in a series of settings, to see what it was that his (affected) right hand did wrong. They tested him to see whether the hand might be 'distracted' by objects that were close to it (spatially) or that resembled the 'correct' (i.e. contextually appropriate) object in some meaningful ('semantic') way. In other words, in a crowded environment,

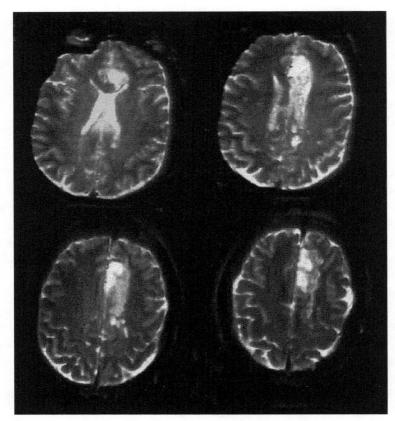

Fig. 68 Structural magnetic resonance imaging scan showing transverse planes through the brain of the patient JC described by Giovanetti and colleagues. The patient has a lesion in his left medial frontal lobe (on the right of the images shown). The lesion extends to the anterior cingulate cortex and also the corpus callosum. Reprinted from *Neuropsychologia* 43/1, Reduced endogenous control in alien hand syndrome: evidence from naturalistic action, Giovanetti T, Buxbaum LJ, Biran I and Chatterjee A (2005) with permission from Elsevier Ltd.

would the anarchic hand make mistakes that were governed by the proximity of a distracting object or by an object's semantic relationship to the object for which the affected hand 'should' have reached? So, if there were pencils, pens, and test tubes on a table, would 'it' pick up the nearby test tube instead of the (required) pen (because the former lay closer to the real 'target') or might it pick up a pencil because the latter resembles a pen in function (i.e. they are semantically related)? In their experiments, Giovannetti and colleagues found that the former was the case: that is, the errant hand was 'tricked' by spatial proximity rather than by semantics. In other words, it grasped at what was 'close to hand' at the time.

Furthermore, in another experiment, they tested whether giving JC other demanding tasks to do (simultaneously) would impact his impaired ability to try to control the errant right hand. While he 'dual-tasked', would the anarchic behaviour get better or worse? They found that it became worse. Compared with the errors that he made with his relatively 'good' hand, and with behaviours exhibited by a healthy control group, JC made disproportionately more errors with his (affected) right hand when his attention was distracted (i.e. when he had to undertake other tasks at the same time). The authors concluded that this showed that JC was (usually, 'normally') deploying his executive resources in an attempt to control his anarchic right hand. Hence, control decreased and performance deteriorated when those executive resources were expended on some other (simultaneous) task (Giovannetti et al., 2005).

The authors also used their findings to offer some simple therapeutic interventions to assist JC in managing his errant hand: he should try to 'keep his environment stark and free of distractor objects' (so that there was nothing nearby to 'attract' the right hand; we return, here, to the phenomenology of 'magnetism' invoked by Denny-Brown [1958]), and he should avoid 'working on more than one task at a time' (so that his 'executive' would not be compromised, overextended; p. 86).

So, taking these observations and experimental data together, JC's plight suggests that in his and similar cases, schemata are 'released' following a medial premotor lesion. Such schemata may be 'triggered' by objects in the external world, objects that are in close *spatial proximity* to the affected hand. Furthermore, it seems to be the case that 'higher' supervisory systems are habitually engaged in attempting to 'control' the affected limb, albeit rather unsuccessfully, because when the executive is further 'loaded' with additional tasks to perform the limb's behaviour is rendered even worse.

Therefore, if we now return to our consideration of the 1988 Shallice model (Fig. 63), we might posit that the left medial premotor lesion sustained by JC has interfered with the ability of his 'contention scheduling' system to select the most appropriate schema for his current environment. Instead, the current environment elicits ('triggers') schemata (from the lateral premotor system) and the resources of the SAS are then diverted towards trying to inhibit or 'correct' such 'capture errors'.

Indeed, this hypothesized propensity towards movements being 'triggered' by sensory stimuli is borne out in a further case report provided by Yamaguchi and colleagues (2006). They described a woman with a problem very similar to JC's: she had a right hand that behaved anarchically as a consequence of a medial premotor lesion in the left hemisphere (involving the left supplementary motor area [SMA] and anterior cingulate cortex [ACC] but not extending as far as the corpus callosum). However, what Yamaguchi and colleagues did which is interesting is that they tested the responsivity of this woman's brain to tactile sensory stimulation. In other words, they stimulated her right and left median nerves (at the wrists) and measured 'somatosensory-evoked potentials' (SEPs) across her scalp (these are electroencephalographic signals denoting sensory processing). They found that stimulation of the right hand, as opposed to the left (and in contrast to a group of control subjects), elicited heightened activity over the left frontal and parietal regions. Such activity occurred at more than 30 ms after the initial stimulus, suggesting that the substrate of such exaggerated response potentials was not peripheral (i.e. not to do with the incoming, afferent nerve supply) but located relatively 'late' or 'high up' within the cerebral sensory processing systems. Yamaguchi and colleagues explain their findings in terms of their patient's SMA lesion having led to a failure of inhibition of somatosensory responses to objects in her environment. Hence, objects might be hypothesized to elicit (or 'trigger') anarchic movements more easily (see Figs. 69 and 70).

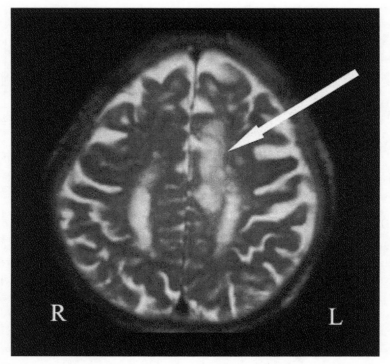

Fig. 69 A magnetic resonance imaging scan showing a left-sided medial frontal lesion. Reprinted from *Journal of Clinical Neuroscience* 13/2, 279–282, Somatosensory disinhibition and frontal alien hand signs following medial frontal damage, Yamaguchi S et al (2006) with permission from Elsevier Ltd.

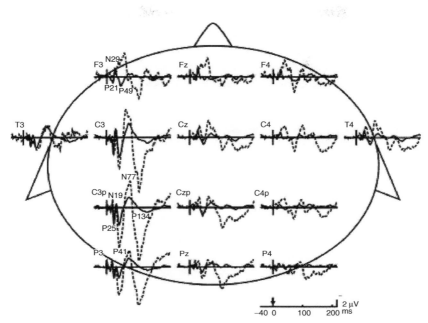

Fig. 70 A figure showing evoked potentials in the brain of the patient described by Yamaguchi and colleagues in 2006. The potentials (SEPs) are evoked in response to stimulation of the median nerve of the right upper limb. Notice that sensory evoked potentials are greater over the left side of the brain, corresponding to the position of the left frontal lesion. The implication is that the lesion leads to disinhibited sensory processing of incoming stimuli. Reprinted from *Journal of Clinical Neuroscience* 13/2 279–282, Somatosensory disinhibition and frontal alien hand signs following medial frontal damage, Yamaguchi S et al (2006) with permission from Elsevier Ltd.

Notice also that, once again, it is the medial premotor system that (through its counterfactual absence) is revealed as being pivotal to the emergence of 'internally initiated', that is, (truly) 'goal-directed', actions. For, although an anarchic limb might appear to express a pseudo-purpose, implying a defective goal, the agent (the subject) relies for their (authentic) internally initiated behaviours upon the medial premotor system being intact. Hence, this literature converges with that describing the effects of much larger lesions of the medial premotor and prefrontal regions (described in Chapter 2), where a subject may be rendered akinetic and mute, where they may cease to have the 'will' to generate new behaviours. Cases such as JC's are not 'as bad as that'; however, they too lack the ability to 'control' their own emergent behaviours so that they end up witnessing (with some distress) the behaviour of an errant, anarchic hand (as was the case with the lady whose genital itch led to such embarrassment; Della Sala et al., 1991).

Hence, there seems to be something central about the role of the medial premotor and prefrontal systems in the control of action that is revealed (counterfactually) by the effects of medial frontal lesions on motor behaviour, in much the same way as this region was implicated in 'internally initiated' acts through the electroencephalographic and functional magnetic resonance imaging (fMRI) studies of healthy volunteers described in the work of Libet (Prologue), Haggard, Cunnington, and others (Chapter 3).

Hands that fight each other

Anarchic limbs generate other sorts of problems for their 'owners'. One of the most peculiar is the emergence of 'intermanual conflict'. Consider these cases, again sourced from the neurological literature:

1. 'Astonishment and frustration were expressed [by the patient] regarding her inability to voluntarily release her grasp of objects in the [affected] left hand. She would attempt to restrain the unwanted movements . . . by keeping her hands folded together or by gripping an object in [her] left hand. The left hand would perform activities with objects around her in a compulsive way that was not associated with a feeling of voluntary control . . . [It] was noted to wander around in the 'alien mode' when not restrained . . . [However] [a]nother incident occurred when the [unaffected] right hand picked up a bowl of hot soup and the left hand threw it to the ground. On another occasion, her left hand began to remove a cigarette from her mouth as she was about to light it with the right hand. She stated that the left hand "was trying to keep me from smoking".' (Goldberg and Bloom, 1990)

2. 'She often spoke to her own [affected] left hand, asking it to perform some movement, but the hand "did only what it wanted to". In bimanual tasks (e.g. lighting a match) she tried to use only her [unaffected] right hand but was regularly impeded by her left hand's groping. At that time she experienced the lack of ownership of her left hand and could not indicate her own among others' hands . . .' (Trojano et al., 1993)

3. 'Sometimes the [affected] left hand would pick up a cup and move it into the path of the [unaffected] right hand so as to interfere with eating. While playing checkers on one occasion, the left hand made a move that [the patient] did not wish to make, and he corrected the move with the right hand; however, the left hand, to the patient's frustration, repeated the false move. On other occasions, he turned the pages of a book with one hand while the other tried to close it; he shaved with the right hand while the left one unzipped his jacket; he tried to soap a washcloth while the left hand kept putting the soap back in the dish; and he tried to open a closet with the right hand while the left one closed it.' (Banks et al., 1989)

Such cases add another level of complexity to the problem of the anarchic hand, for here we have two hands 'belonging' to the same agent but seemingly 'engaging' in some form of combat. How might this be possible?

One answer may reside in some of the data that we have already described in Chapter 3 concerning the immediate antecedents of voluntary movement under 'normal' conditions and also the (pathological) re-emergence of so-called 'mirror movements' in adult life (Farmer, 2005). Recall that it was revealed through both forms of literature that the dominant (usually left) hemisphere's motor centres make a contribution to the control of movements initiated by the motor centres of the non-dominant (usually right) hemisphere. Hence, if the pathways running between such motor centres were interrupted (e.g. by pathology), then it became possible for the non-dominant hemisphere to elude the 'normal' influence of its ('dominant') neighbour, so that unusual movements might emerge. Hence, we saw how mirror movements might arise in a resting left hand when a ('normal') right hand moved (because the left hemisphere's motor control centres no longer inhibited those of the right hemisphere). The right hemisphere 'escaped' inhibition by the left; hence, the left hand moved, as a 'mirror' to the (normal movement of the) right.

Thus, it is interesting to note that in those cases of anarchic limbs where the affected limb interferes with the normal functions of the unaffected limb, it is often the case that the lesion affects the corpus callosum and that the 'affected' hand is (again) on the left and the 'unaffected' (i.e. 'normal') hand on the right. Hence, once again, we have gained an insight into the functional hierarchies pertaining to the dextral cerebral motor system, an insight that is provided by the impact of a lesion (sometimes a resection of the corpus callosum for the treatment of intractable epilepsy, sometimes the consequence of a stroke or a tumour). When this hierarchy 'fails', the right hemisphere's motor systems are 'released' and the contralateral, left, hand behaves abnormally.

Again, from our perspective, it is interesting to note that

1. The affected hand makes *movements* (i.e. it is not 'still'); hence, it appears to be 'released'.

2. Those movements are *targeted* on objects in the environment or the actions of the 'unaffected' hand; in other words, they are stimulus-driven (i.e. reactive).

3. There seems to be a 'purpose' or 'goal-directedness' to such movements (albeit a rather 'mischievous' one).

4. This purpose often seems to be at 'cross-purposes' with those of the 'unaffected' hand (obviously, any authentic 'purposes' are those of the agent, the subject, but nevertheless are *expressed* via the actions of the 'unaffected' hand).

5. Therefore, the 'purpose' of the anarchic hand seems to be *contingent upon* that of the unaffected hand.

6. The subject, the patient, cannot 'control' the hand directly (but has to resort to physical force or 'talking to' the limb).

7. Generally speaking, it is the left hand that behaves (is affected) in this way (e.g. following a callosal lesion; though this is not always the case).

8. The patient sometimes says that the hand has a 'mind of its own'.

9. The patient sometimes misidentifies the hand as belonging to 'someone else'.

10. Overall, the phenomenology suggests that, in the dextral brain, the left hemisphere is hierarchically superior to the right hemisphere in terms of motor control because, when the communication pathway between the hemispheres is severed, it is most often the left hand (i.e. the 'effector' of the right hemisphere motor system) that 'misbehaves'.

Hence, once again, we seem to be learning things about the 'normal' state of neurological affairs through the consequences of their disturbance by cerebral disease. If we consider the 'normal' motor system to comprise an ascending hierarchy of schemata, component schemata nested within evermore sophisticated source schemata (i.e. action programmes, from flipping a coin to writing a letter to travelling the world), then we may posit that (deep enough) fault lines within such a hierarchy, akin to the cracks forming within an ancient pyramid, may reveal subcomponents that are potentially separable from their hierarchically 'superior' control processes. Such subcomponents may be elicited (i.e. 'triggered') by events and cues within the organism's immediate external environment, whereupon quasi-purposeful behaviours emerge. However, these behaviours are only ever 'quasi-purposeful': they may 'look like' actions, when witnessed by an external observer, but they are not authentic voluntary acts. The agent did not choose them, and the hierarchy did not 'select' them. Indeed, they were 'released' as a consequence of its fragmentation.

So, when the female patient scratches her genitals, or the man in the checkers game appears to move twice (first when the affected left hand moves, second when the right hand corrects that behaviour), it may be embarrassing and confusing. The agent has a limb that is literally 'beyond her control'. She has an intention that is 'truly' hers and some emergent behaviour, which contradicts that intention. It literally opposes 'her' Will. Hence, some of her behaviours are authentic whereas others represent the output of rogue schemata.

Furthermore, these scenarios demonstrate something that is rather similar, in principle, to the problem of rapid eye movement (REM) sleep behavioural disorder, which we described at the close of Chapter 4: most of the time, we humans are spared the fractionation of our voluntary motor processes by neural mechanisms that maintain some form of 'order', some form of coherence, hierarchies pertaining to 'medial trumps lateral' in the premotor system and 'left trumps right' in the (dextral) cerebral motor system. We do not respond to or grasp every object in our immediate vicinity because there are 'built-in' controls within our nervous systems that seem to suppress such automatic responses. We do not act out the content of our dreams because the hyperpolarization of our spinal cords' anterior horns prevents us from doing so. However, if control processes fail, then we may grasp at what 'we' do not 'want' and strike out at those with whom we sleep when 'we' did not 'mean to' do so. Furthermore, we (as a community) seem to equate 'responsibility' with precisely such a 'meaning to' do something. We do not hold the patient responsible for the behaviours of her errant (anarchic) hand; we do not blame the man who strikes out in his dreams, because his spinal cord is no longer hyperpolarized (during REM sleep). Hence, a very simple view of responsibility seems to be that we require some form of symmetry between desire and behaviour, between 'intentions to act' and those behaviours that emerge. If intentions fail (to control an errant limb) or behaviours emerge unintended (as in a dream state), then we, as a community, seem to suspend moral judgement. This is something that we shall return to later in this book.

Putting it all together

Finally, knowing what we now know, it is interesting to consider a further case taken from the neurological literature, in order to recognize that each characteristic of this (new) patient's story, despite being rather bizarre, now seems to 'make sense'. The patient concerned had probably suffered a right-sided cerebrovascular accident (a 'stroke') though a computed tomography (CT) scan of her brain was reported as 'normal'.

> Voluntary movements of her [affected] left hand required visual control. Voluntary movements of her [unaffected] right hand were accompanied by mirror movements of the left hand. During physical examination, the left hand involuntarily grasped a pair of scissors. The patient reported loss of control of the left arm when it pulled her clothes and grasped persons and objects. The left arm constantly moved under the blankets at night, thus impairing sleep . . . Interestingly, the patient was neither afraid of, nor annoyed by, her hand and, in describing it, used the metaphor of a child who could not be trusted.

> (Kikkert et al., 2006)

Notice how, in this case, the left hand is disinhibited: it not only grasps objects unbidden (by the subject) but also becomes active (it exhibits mirror movements) when the 'good' hand is in action. The patient tries to monitor the anarchic limb's performance, by keeping it under visual control, but the limb evades such 'supervision'. It seems as if neither contention scheduling nor the SAS can bring the limb to task. In light of the data that we have already considered, we can now see how each of these disparate features might arise, and how they are 'understandable', given the structure of the human cerebral motor system.

Losing agency: somatoparaphrenia

A feature of both the foregoing forms of the anarchic limb is that, by and large, the subject (agent) maintains a metaphorical distance from the behaviour of their errant member. It is 'as if' the limb has a 'mind of its own'; it is 'as if' it is a 'child' who 'cannot be trusted'. Indeed, we have seen more than once how patients describe a breakdown in trust, a failure of reliance upon this part of their body. Yet, they usually seem to 'know' that the limb is still 'theirs'. Despite the very abnormal situations in which they find themselves, they retain an awareness that the problem is inherently physical, to do with their body (and their brain). They do not invoke delusional explanations. They do not claim to be 'possessed'.

However, it would be premature to conclude that this is never the case. As we have seen, in the clinical example provided by Trojano and colleagues (1993), when we move from the medial aspect of the frontal lobe back towards the corpus callosum and further posterior towards the sensory brain (especially the parietal lobe), there may be times when a patient sustaining such a lesion fails to recognize their upper limb's movements as 'belonging to them'. Indeed, if we travel even further, we shall find that there are two ways in which owner-ship, or possession, breaks down among such 'alien limbs' (here, we have returned to Brion and Jedynak's [1972] memorable term la main etrangere):

1. A limb, recognized as being integral to the subject, may come to seem as if it is under someone else's *control*; or,

2. A limb may not be *recognized* as being (physically) integral to its owner at all (i.e. it no longer 'belongs' to them).

So it is that with some right-sided and more posterior cortical (and subcortical) lesions, the subject's sense of agency over her body may be radically altered. In one case, it seems to be the movements of her limb that have become 'alienat-ed' ('1' in the preceding list); in the other, it seems to be the limb itself, its physical integrity, that is no longer recognized (i.e. it has become 'other'; '2'). Hence, in the following case, the patient clearly experiences her agency as having been ceded to 'someone else'.

> She said: 'Suddenly I had a strange feeling on my left side; later I could not recognize the left arm as my own; I felt it belonged to someone else and wanted to hurt me because it moved towards me; I saw it quite big and distorted like a monster; I was terrified.' During the third episode[,] which was witnessed by one of the authors[,]

she said: 'Look, it's coming; please help me.' (The patient was a 50-year-old right-handed woman who had previously sustained a right parietal haematoma secondary to a ruptured arteriovenous malformation).

[Leiguarda et al., 1993]

There appear to be at least two things happening in this case: the disinhibition of the affected limb, so that motor control is lost, and a concomitant failure to recognize the limb as the subject's own. Hence, there seems to be an inherently sensory component to the disturbance (accompanying the motoric disinhibition).

In such cases, the phenomenology of the anarchic or alien limb blends with that of another condition mentioned in classical neurological texts. Critchley (1953) described what he called 'somatoparaphrenia', an ailment affecting subjects who, following right-sided parietal lobe lesions, perceive the left sides of their bodies as being 'possessed' or 'controlled' by outside ('alien') entities. This really does begin to appear 'psychotic' in severity, with the person actually believing that they are 'inhabited' by another, that someone else is moving within the left side of their body. Modern accounts continue to appear (e.g. Nightingale, 1982). Indeed, the suggestion that such experiences are dependent upon the state of the right parietal cortex has gained some empirical support through more recent investigations demonstrating that a procedure known to change parietal activity may terminate such perceptual abnormalities. That procedure is called 'vestibular stimulation' and involves injecting cold water into the outer ear on the left side of the body (an intervention that demonstrably impacts neural activity in the right parietal cortex and surrounding regions; see Bottini et al., 2001).

Bisiach and colleagues (1991) have elegantly demonstrated temporary reversal of somatoparaphrenic delusions following such vestibular stimulation. Here, an investigator is examining an affected patient's left arm:

Examiner: Whose arm is this?
AR [the patient]: It's not mine.
Examiner: Whose is it?
AR: It's my mother's.
Examiner: How on earth does it happen to be here?
AR: I don't know. I found it in my bed.
Examiner: How long has it been there?
AR: Since the first day . . .

Immediately after vestibular stimulation, the examiner asks the patient to show her the patient's left [affected] arm.

AR: (Points to her own left arm.) Here it is.
Examiner: (Raises the patient's left arm.) Is this arm yours?
AR: Why, yes . . .

On the following morning . . . the examiner asks AR again whose is AR's left arm while pointing to it.

> AR: It's my mother's . . .

(abridged from Bisiach et al., 1991)

As noted, Bottini and colleagues (2001) have shown that left-sided vestibular stimulation modulates activity in right parietal lobe-related areas, among others. So, we seem to have a case of (rather familial!) 'possession' that is apparently 'cured' (albeit temporarily) through the use of cold water. Nevertheless, later on, the abnormal experience returns.

Hence, although a return to phrenology is to be avoided, it would appear that the right parietal cortex does have a particular relevance to disturbances of subjective agency and that manipulation of parietal activity (albeit indirectly and in conjunction with effects on related brain regions) may substantially alter subjective experience of the body. Moreover, we now have a possible means of understanding some of the very strange experiences reported in the context of schizophrenia, when people may come to believe, quite literally, that their thoughts and actions 'belong' to someone else.

Agency lost: 'alien control'

So, all of the above leads us to an (even more) extreme situation, one in which a human subject comes to believe that their thoughts and actions are directed, at a distance, by some external force or person. Here, control is not 'merely' lost but is also externalized: something or someone else is moving the patient. Now, such is the apparent illogicality of this claim that it may assist the reader if I provide some 'flavour' of what it is that the person, the patient, is claiming, reporting. The following is a selection of examples, drawn from medical and philosophical publications:

1. 'A former patient of the Heidelberg clinic, a well-educated individual who a little later became acutely ill with schizophrenia, wrote an account of these . . . phenomena: "On the following morning I was put into a most peculiar mood by this machine or whatever it is . . . All the night through I was fully sensible and quite clear . . . [T]he machine . . . was fixed in such a way that every word I spoke was put into me electronically and I could of course not avoid expressing the thoughts in this peculiar mood . . . At times I was given back my natural way of thinking . . . I feel the machine is getting me down mentally more and more and I have several times asked for the current to be turned off and my natural thinking returned to me . . . I want to make another point . . . when one reads all this it seems the greatest nonsense ever written but I cannot say anything else except that I have really felt all this,

though unfortunately I have never understood it.'"(abridged from Jaspers, 1963, pp. 579–580)

2. 'A patient said: "I never shouted, it was the vocal cords that shouted out of me . . . The hands turn this way and that, I do not guide them nor can I stop them."'(Jaspers, 1963, p. 23)

3. 'A 29-year-old shorthand typist described her actions as follows: "When I reach my hand for the comb it is my hand and arm which move, and my fingers pick up the pen, but I don't control them . . . I sit there watching them move, and they are quite independent, what they do is nothing to do with me . . . I am just a puppet who is manipulated by cosmic strings. When the strings are pulled my body moves and I cannot prevent it." '(Mellor, 1970, pp. 17–18)

4. 'A 26–year-old engineer emptied the contents of a urine bottle over the ward's dinner trolley. He said, "The sudden impulse came over me that I must do it. It was not my feeling[;] it came into me from the X-ray department, that was why I was sent there for implants yesterday. It was nothing to do with me[;] they wanted it done. So I picked up the bottle and poured it in. It seemed all I could do." '(Mellor, 1970, p. 17)

5. 'A 29-year-old housewife said, "I look out of the window and I think the garden looks nice and the grass looks cool, but the thoughts of Eamonn Andrews [a TV personality of the time] come into my mind. There are no other thoughts there, only his . . . He treats my mind like a screen and flashes his thoughts onto it like you flash a picture." '(Mellor, 1970, p. 17)

6. 'At one point, [the patient] can hardly speak and his protruding tongue seems to trip him up as his words falter. The interviewer makes a remark about the difficulty that he is having [speaking]. The patient answers that the Devil is trying to prevent him from speaking. Over the course of some minutes he is unsure whether the interviewer might be possessed and doing these things to him. At one point, he storms out of the room. Two or three minutes later, he is back to apologize. He has concluded that God is in the interviewer as well.' (Spence, 2002, p. 164)

7. 'On the same ward, there is a young woman who has schizophrenia and whose symptoms are centred on eyes. She stares closely at people but asks that they do not look back at her. If they do, she seems to . . . experience others' thoughts as entering her head. She asks repeatedly for reassurance: "Can this kind of thing really happen?" '(Spence, 2002, p. 164)

8. 'A man opened the door. He was young, thin, and dishevelled, with beads of sweat on his forehead, and matted hair . . . He let us in. There was no carpet

and very little furniture . . . Why [had he been] screaming? He did it to stop the thought interference. It was the only way. Thoughts came into his head, all the time, from outside. The screaming seemed to clear his mind, helped him regain control, but then he'd need to scream again.' (Spence, 1999, p. 489)

As the reader may have gathered, there is a great deal of variation among such accounts. Some people are describing interference with their thoughts, others interference with their actions. Some make specific claims about individual acts, others about a sequence of experiences, sometimes extending over days. Some describe their impulses, even their moods, as being imposed upon them. So, we have to acknowledge that psychotic illnesses rarely present us with the stereotypic symptoms that we might expect of a purely somatic, 'physical disorder' (e.g. right-sided abdominal pain localizing to the 'iliac fossa' and associated with 'rebound tenderness' 'equals' appendicitis). The phenomena that we encounter in psychiatry are often aberrant 'signals' emerging from within a highly idiosyncratic personal and social situation; one has to listen to people ('patients') carefully, and often at length, to 'hear' what it is that they are saying. Indeed, such aberrant phenomena may be very difficult for anyone to describe, to 'put into words'. Nevertheless, we might posit that there are emergent commonalities, central features that arise and cohere across such accounts. So it is that, in general, these patients (in the preceding examples) are describing a sense of separation, alienation, from their most intimate agentic experiences: their thoughts are being interfered with; their impulses are not their own; their actions are specified by external agents, machines, or people at a distance (Spence, 2001). The common theme is one of a loss of 'agency'. The person is no longer the author of their own thoughts and deeds. Someone, something else, is implicated; there is 'interference'.

Now, such phenomena have attracted the description 'alien control', not because the malign force described is necessarily believed to be extraterrestrial in nature but because it lies outside of (i.e. it is 'alien to') the person who describes it. Furthermore, as implied, alien control is often (though not always) a symptom of schizophrenia.

A note, on schizophrenia

What is schizophrenia? Well, it is a phenomenologically heterogeneous condition that tends to present in early adulthood, just as a young person is beginning to establish an independent life. The symptoms are indeed highly variable but can be characterized by the occurrence of abnormal beliefs (often delusions), experiences (commonly auditory verbal hallucinations, i.e. 'hearing voices'), abnormalities of behaviour (e.g. disorganized speech and movement), and in relative contrast, so-called 'negative symptoms' (lack of speech, lack of volition, lack of emotional experience and expression, etc., which we shall consider in Chapter 6). In general, the negative symptoms of schizophrenia are more difficult to treat; they tend to be less responsive to pharmacological and other therapies (Mortimer and Spence, 2001).

Schizophrenia affects approximately 1% of the population, impacting equal proportions of men and women (during early adulthood), although the clinical manifestations tend to be more severe among young men (as is the case with several other disorders of neurological development). Although 10% of those affected may be relatively fortunate in that they may make a complete recovery following their first illness episode, most will not be so lucky; many patients follow either a 'relapsing or remitting' course, that is, a life punctuated by recurrent 'breakdowns', or else suffer a gradual functional decline, perhaps steepest over the first 5 years of the illness, before reaching a plateau-like period of relative symptomatic stability. Therefore, as schizophrenia can be a chronic illness, there are many adults who will remain on antipsychotic medications for very long periods of time (and some of the adverse effects of such medications on voluntary motor systems were rehearsed in Chapter 4).

Violating personal space

Now, if we return to the more florid ('positive') symptoms of schizophrenia (e.g. abnormal thoughts and experiences), then central to our (historical) understanding of the disorder has been a hypothesized disturbance of so-called 'ego boundaries', reflected in the hypothesized inability of the patient to differentiate internal events (e.g. thoughts) from external occurrences, and vice versa. Hence, a thought may sound like an external 'voice', and a gesture exhibited by a stranger in the external environment may impact the patient's mind (as was reported by Patient 7, in the preceding case reports). Such boundary violations are enshrined in the so-called first rank symptoms (FRSs) of schizophrenia, described by the German psychiatrist Kurt Schneider (1974; Table 11). Among such symptoms are those of alien control, as we have just described them, alternatively labelled as 'passivity phenomena', 'made' thoughts, and 'made' movements, terms denoting (again) that patients experience their autonomy as being usurped by alien, outside forces (see Mullins and Spence, 2003).

Is this solely a disorder of the motor system?

Now, when one talks to people who experience these sorts of phenomena (symptoms), one of the notable features of their reports is that they can be remarkably specific. A 'spirit' or persecutor controls *certain* movements, not just any movement. Someone might report that a computer programmes

Table 11 First rank symptoms of schizophrenia (of Schneider)

First rank symptom	Comments
Delusion	
Delusional percept or 'primary' delusion	A delusion (a firmly held, false belief, based on false premises, that is incorrigible and out of keeping with sociocultural background) that suddenly appears fully formed in the mind, from 'out of the blue', and is unrelated to the current mood or social context.
Auditory hallucination	
Audible thoughts (thought echo)	Literally hearing one's own thoughts echoed as 'speech' (*echo de la pensee*).
Voices arguing or discussing	Voices talking about the patient (in the third person).
Voices commenting on the patient's actions	So-called 'running commentary' (where a voice or voices continually comment on what the patient is doing).
Passivity of thought	
Thought withdrawal	Thoughts are 'taken out' of the subject's mind.
Thought insertion	Thoughts are 'inserted into' the patient's mind.
Thought broadcasting (diffusion of thought)	Thoughts are 'broadcast' to others, at a distance.
Passivity experiences; delusions of control	
Passivity of affect ('made feelings')	Emotions are influenced by outside forces.
Passivity of impulse ('made drives')	Impulses are influenced by outside forces.
Passivity of volition ('made volitional acts')	Actions are influenced by outside forces.
Somatic passivity (influence playing on the body)	Delusions of alien penetration.

certain of his limb movements while he is walking; he 'knows' this because these (specific) movements feel 'kind of spongy'. However, there are other movements that he experiences as entirely 'normal'. Someone else reports that thoughts are being 'put into his head'. Not all thoughts, just some thoughts. The affected thoughts can 'feel' electric. He may even be able to point to their site of entry. Indeed, often, patients evince a very physical, so-called 'concrete' way of talking about psychological phenomena that are usually ('normally') experienced as rather diffuse (non-localizable) mental events: a patient reports that he can 'feel' a thought, it is 'electric', and it is 'felt' to be in one part of his head; there may be a machine, a 'chip', allegedly inserted there. Something 'must' have been done, while he was asleep; something happened 'during the night'.

So, if we take such accounts at face value, then it seems to be the case that the 'experience' of thinking and moving, of volition itself, is sometimes radically disturbed in these people, and that such disturbance is at least partially *sensory* in nature. In other words, *it has to do with the experience of one's own volition, one's own 'agency'.*

Furthermore, although such a patient's (actual, veridical) movements usually appear (grossly) normal, they may evince subtle abnormalities when they are studied under experimental conditions. Hence, there are several accounts of (alien control or passivity) patients failing to correct fine errors in their motor performances when they are denied direct visual feedback of their movements (e.g. Frith and Done, 1989). It is as if they do not quite know 'where' their limbs are, in terms of egocentric space. Indeed, it has long been proposed that proprioception (afferent sensation) may be subtly deficient in such people (Angyal, 1936).

If one accepts the (phenomenological) data that the patients themselves have provided, then it seems possible that such impairments are actually action-specific: it is almost as if certain component 'schemata' (to borrow from Shallice's 1988 model; Fig. 63) are 'faulty' in some way, and crucially, rather than giving rise to grossly abnormal action performances, they give rise to grossly abnormal *experiences* of action performance. There is something wrong with the way that certain (and sometimes quite specific) thoughts and movements are 'experienced'.

Now, from which brain systems might such bizarre symptoms arise? Well, the neurological cases that we have already considered in the foregoing sections (e.g. somatoparaphrenia) would suggest that damage to the parietal lobes could be a suitable candidate for investigation. Nevertheless, how could such an abnormality be, computationally, implemented neurobiologically? What is the 'nature' of the deficit? As was alluded to previously, one theoretical account of alien control or passivity attributes it to a failure of 'monitoring' of ongoing action, and more specifically, to a failure by the brain's motor programming systems to *predict* the future (sensory) consequences of emergent acts. Normally, through a hypothesized process called 'forward modelling', the brain predicts its own outcome states following future acts. So, if I were to suddenly lift my arm, then my brain would have already computed the sensory stimuli arising from such an act. Indeed, a deviation from such predictions should alert the brain to potential errors and the possible need for motoric corrections. Furthermore, were there to be a fault within the system, then my action might *feel* as if it had come from 'nowhere', as if an outside force were responsible for its production. Indeed, bearing in mind what we have already learnt from the specificity of some patients' reports, it might even be the case that 'forward modelling' is deficient for certain acts and not others (hence, some steps are experienced as 'spongy', others are not; some thoughts feel 'electric' whereas others do not.)

Alien control, in the brain scanner

Now, one benefit to have been derived from the recent emergence of functional neuroimaging techniques is that they have allowed investigators to examine the cerebral motor system directly and to locate functional abnormalities *in vivo*, in life. In one such study, conducted with colleagues at the Hammersmith Hospital in London in the 1990s, I was able to use positron-emission tomography (PET) scanning to examine the cerebral activity associated with moving a joystick, held in the right hand, in freely chosen directions and in stereotypic patterns among people with schizophrenia experiencing alien control ('passivity', 'made' thoughts, and 'made' actions), other patients experiencing schizophrenia but in the absence of alien control or passivity phenomena, and a group of healthy 'controls'. In each case, the subjects moved the joystick in time with a pacing tone (at 0.33 Hz). They were also scanned while 'at rest', as they listened to the same pacing tone but remained still (Spence et al., 1997).

During the scan sessions, some alien control or passivity patients experienced acute symptoms, consistent with ongoing sensory disturbance. Here are some of their verbatim accounts:

> 'I felt like an automaton, guided by a female spirit who had entered me during it [the movement of the joystick].'
> 'I thought you [the experimenter] were varying the movements with your thoughts.'
> 'I could feel God guiding me [during a joystick movement].'

So, what did we find? We found that, compared with the other groups, the 'alien control or passivity patients' exhibited relative hyperactivation of their right inferior parietal cortices (Brodmann area [BA] 40, an area implicated in spatial awareness and programming) and left SMA (BA 6, a region implicated in the programming of action; Fig. 71) while they engaged in 'voluntary' movements. Indeed, we also found that this pattern of abnormal activity remitted as the symptoms went away (all subjects being scanned on a second occasion some weeks later).

Hence, our findings are consistent with the view that those systems engaged in the programming of action in egocentric space (i.e. the premotor and parietal cortices) are disturbed among those patients who experience alien control

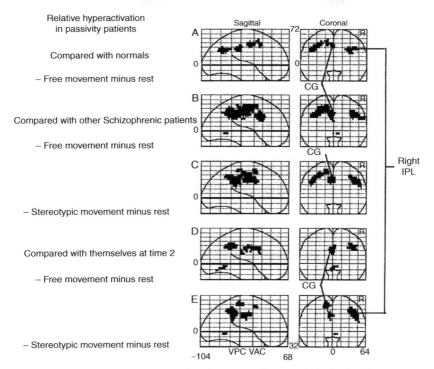

Fig. 71 Statistical parametric maps showing areas of increased activation in the brains of patients with schizophrenia, suffering from passivity phenomena (delusions of alien control), while they move their right upper limbs. Each comparison with a control data set reveals relatively increased activity in the right inferior parietal lobule (IPL) and also the cingulate gyrus (CG). (From Spence et al., *Brain* 1997; 120: 1997–2011). With permission from Oxford University Press.

or passivity phenomena (Spence et al., 1997). It really does seem as if there is a 'logic' to the abnormalities such patients describe, although we are obviously some distance from providing what might be called an 'exhaustive' account of their phenomenology. For instance, although we may now have clues about the commonalities that underpin such strange phenomena ('alienation' implicating motor programming systems), we have no 'biological' explanation for why one patient invokes the role of a female spirit during their movements and another God.

There is also a further, subtle finding, which deserves mention. For, the abnormality of right-sided parietal systems, revealed among the patients experiencing alien control or passivity, was not solely apparent when these subjects *chose* the direction of their joystick movements. Parietal (and SMA) hyperactivation also occurred during movements that were entirely (externally) specified by the experimenters. So, when subjects moved the joystick in a simple sequence of clockwise movements, one movement at a time, the aberrant pattern of cortical activity was also detectable. Again, this was in marked contrast to both the comparator groups (i.e. the 'other' schizophrenia patients and the healthy controls), and the alien control or passivity patients themselves when they had recovered (Fig. 72).

So, if we think back once more to the Shallice 1988 model of the SAS and contention scheduling system (Fig. 63; Chapter 4), it seems likely that parietal dysfunction in the presence of 'alien control or passivity' symptoms implies an abnormality at the level of schemata, as the dysfunction may be visualized (using PET scanning) during both 'internally chosen' and 'externally specified' actions. It is *not* specific to those behaviours that are 'chosen' by the agent (which, hence, implicate the SAS). The problem is located 'below' the SAS. Why do I say this? Because, the movements that elicit parietal lobe abnormality are not solely those that demand a decision from the subject's 'higher' centres. The movements concerned can be entirely externally specified. Thus, the abnormality central to alien control or passivity phenomena seems to reside at that level of the model that is 'common' to both automated (routine) and controlled ('willed') movements, and that level is located relatively 'low' down, within contention scheduling.

Subsequent studies have replicated the finding of parietal abnormality in the presence of such symptoms, with one recent study doing so while patients performed self-paced finger movements in an MRI scanner (Fig. 73). Ganesan and colleagues (2005) demonstrated that abnormal parietal activity (seen in those with FRSs of schizophrenia) follows action-related activation of the motor cortex (i.e. at a temporal delay), a finding that would be consistent with alien control or passivity phenomena arising from abnormal sensory awareness, post-action initiation.

More recently, another group has shown that schizophrenia patients reporting motor alien control or passivity phenomena (e.g. 'made' movements) exhibit reductions in right parietal and left prefrontal cortical grey matter, relative to other schizophrenia patients (Maruff et al., 2005). A study of students with high 'schizotypy' scores (thought to be related to schizophrenia) revealed that those who feared 'losing control of their thoughts' exhibited reduced SMA grey matter volume (Matsui et al., 2002).

Taken together, the developing literature on alien control or passivity phenomena suggests that the disturbed sense of agency described in schizophrenia implicates the parietal cortices (concerned with spatial and bodily

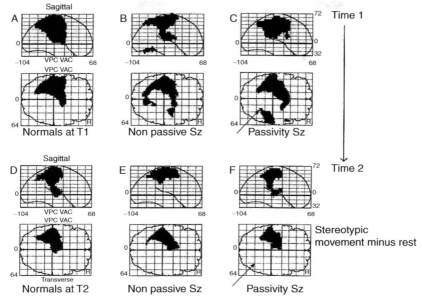

Fig. 72 Statistical parametric maps, showing areas of increased activity when subjects move their right arms in order to move a joy stick in a stereotypic, pre-specified, sequence of movements. At time 1, healthy controls and non-passive schizophrenic patients do not activate their right parietal cortex. However, at time 1, patients experiencing passivity phenomena do activate their right parietal cortex during the performance of stereotypic sequences. The arrow in the upper figure shows the area of the right parietal cortex activated. At time 2 (~ 6 weeks later), none of the groups exhibit right parietal activity during the performance of stereotypic movement sequences (see lower row of figures). (From Spence et al., *Brain* 1997; 120: 1997–2001), with permission from Oxford University Press.

awareness) and possibly key planning and programming areas within the frontal lobes (i.e. the left dorsolateral prefrontal cortex [DLPFC] and SMA, respectively).

Some tentative conclusions

Throughout this chapter, we have focused very much upon abnormalities of volitional experience: the plights of those who have (verifiably, objectively) lost control of their limb movements and those people who experience a disordered 'sense' of control, albeit in the presence of relatively preserved movement (at least in terms of its objective appearance). We have seen that human subjects, agents, may be deprived of both their motoric control and their sense of agency (their 'authorship' of action). Relatively complex behaviours may arise unbidden (via 'anarchic hands') or under the 'influence' of 'external

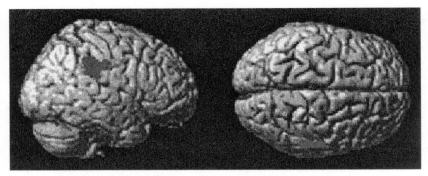

Fig. 73 Images of a magnetic resonance imaging scan showing areas of increased activation in patients with schizophrenia while moving their right index finger 'spontaneously'. The area of activation lies in the right parietal cortex. Activity is greater in those patients who experience the first rank symptoms (FRSs) of schizophrenia (including alien control). (From Ganesan et al., American Journal of Psychiatry 2005; 162(8):1545). (See colour plate section).

forces', as when a patient with schizophrenia moves her hand but *feels* as if she is subject to the play of 'cosmic strings'.

What may we conclude? Well, at the very least, we might conclude that no account of human action (and, therefore, human moral responsibility) is ever complete in the absence of a subjective report, a 'view from within', provided by the agent. Just because behaviours may 'appear' purposeful does not mean that they are. Some quite complex behaviours can emerge without their conduit's 'consent'. So, when we wish to apportion responsibility, we are not merely identifying an organism, a set of bones and joints, muscles and nerves that 'conveyed' the pattern of movement to the environment; we are saying something important about 'its' underlying volitional processes: the symmetry pertaining between desires and deeds, intentions and actions.

Anarchic and alien motor phenomena of the kinds that we have described seem to arise from structural or functional abnormalities located in several distributed, but no less specific, brain regions, and seem to constitute impairments of agency, mediated via at least two mechanisms:

1. A disinhibition of 'lower' motor centres giving rise to relatively stereotypic and contextually inappropriate motor routines (as occurs following medial frontal and callosal lesions); in other words, the kinds of movements that might have 'given Dr. Strangelove away';

2. A disturbance in the perception of voluntary movement, so that control of movement (agency) is attributed to an alien entity (phenomena associated

with right parietal lobe lesions and epilepsy, and focal hyperactivity in the context of schizophrenia).

A full understanding of this second perturbation of agency will require considerable empirical ingenuity. It seems (at least to me) to be far more complex than the earlier category of perturbation ('1'). Current models of alien control invoke deficits in proprioception and putative motoric 'feed-forward' mechanisms. Yet, there is little current understanding of why one mode of thought or action should be affected, and not another, and why one patient invokes the power of X-rays to control them and another a 'female spirit'.

Chapter 6

Failing to act

Avolition manifests itself as a characteristic lack of energy and drive. Subjects are unable to mobilize themselves to initiate or persist in completing many different kinds of tasks. Unlike the diminished energy or interest of depression, the avolitional symptom complex in schizophrenia is usually not accompanied by saddened or depressed affect. The avolitional symptom complex often leads to severe social and economic impairment.[13]

Apathy is defined as lack of motivation not attributable to diminished level of consciousness, cognitive impairment, or emotional distress.[14]

In this chapter, we attempt to address one of the most severe and persistent forms of volitional disturbance observable in human beings, namely, the apparent *absence* of voluntary behaviours: actions and ideas. Such 'avolition' may occur as part of a 'symptom complex', really an assemblage of *observable* deficits or 'signs' constituting a 'negative' syndrome, a perceived absence of behaviour. Indeed, it is the *lack* of movement, speech, emotion, and (from what one may gather, 'externally') 'inner speech' or thought that comprises such a syndrome's essential unity.

What is more, the problem of 'avolition' also serves to provide an example of a phenomenon to which different practitioners and indeed different branches of medicine have applied different descriptors in order to express rather similar concepts. Hence, whereas a psychiatrist may describe a slowed, predominantly

---

[13] The definition of 'avolition' taken from Nancy Andreasen's (1983) Scale for the assessment of negative symptoms (the SANS). [Andreasen NC. Scale for the assessment of negative symptoms. Iowa City: Iowa, 1983.]

[14] Taken from Marin RS, Biedrzycki RC, Firinciogullari S. Reliability and validity of the Apathy Evaluation Scale. Psychiatry Research 1991; 38: 143–162.

silent, and grossly dishevelled patient as 'avolitional' (exhibiting 'psychomotor poverty', if they believe the 'underlying' diagnosis to be one of schizophrenia or 'psychomotor retardation' if they believe the underlying diagnosis to be one of depression), a neurologist may use the word 'apathetic' to describe an apparently similar patient, manifesting a hypothesized lack of motivation, or 'abulic', when they describe an observed absence of (an, as yet, hypothesized) 'Will' (Chapter 2). (Notice that the psychiatric terms used tend to describe an observation whereas the neurological terms tend to imply a proposed causal mechanism.)

Now, admittedly, it is likely that psychiatrists and neurologists most often encounter different kinds of clinical situations: traditionally, psychiatrists have seen patients with 'functional' disturbances of the nervous system (at various times hypothesized as being 'psychological' or 'neurochemical' in causation, 'aetiology', and potentially reversible in outcome), whereas neurologists have tended to see those with 'organic' or 'structural' abnormalities of the nervous system (often regarded as untreatable). However, with advances in biomedical investigational techniques and applied therapeutics, these received distinctions now seem markedly deficient: psychiatric disorders may well have pronounced organic components and, nowadays, neurological diseases are often (at least partially) treatable.

Nevertheless, there is an extent to which psychiatrists may often be assessing patients who demonstrate a marked *narrowing* of response repertoires (manifest through repetitive patterns of limited behavioural diversity: e.g. self-defeating or self-harming behaviours), and neurologists may often be seeing those who have lost all (or most) of their voluntary behaviours (as is the case with the sequelae of massive 'strokes', especially the akinetic mutism consequent upon medial prefrontal or anterior cingulate cortical lesions; the 'off-state' of Parkinson's disease; and the 'organic' causes of apathy).

Thus, there may be a great many possible causes of an 'avolitional' or 'apathetic' syndrome (see Table 12, for a selection) and the specific words deployed by doctors to describe these phenomena, scattered throughout different medical literatures, serve to provide us with an insight into their diagnostic deliberations. (Indeed, in the next chapter, we shall examine what has become a rather divisive example of this same problem of [apparently] impaired volition, a clinical state that attracts various descriptors, across disciplines, each loaded with radically different assumptions: 'hysteria', 'conversion disorder', 'medically unexplained' symptomatology, 'functional disorder', and so on; Chapter 7; see also Spence, 2006a, 2006b.)

Table 12 Some causes of avolitional presentations

Syndrome
'Gross' structural pathology (i.e. tumours, 'strokes')
Cortical: prefrontal, medial frontal, anterior cingulate, or supplementary motor areas (SMAs)
Subcortical: striatal, basal ganglia, thalamic nuclei
Small-vessel vascular impairment (e.g. brainstem 'stroke')
Degenerative processes (e.g. frontotemporal dementias)
External to the brain: meningioma (over the frontal lobes)
Functional/neurochemical disturbance
Parkinson's disease and related syndromes (Parkinson's 'plus')
Catatonia (may be related to mood disorders, delirium, schizophrenia)
Schizophrenia: severe psychomotor poverty ('negative') syndrome
Depression: severe psychomotor retardation
Manic stupor
Epilepsy
Complex partial status (a protracted seizure arising from a localized source in the brain, which does not 'generalize'; hence, the patient does not exhibit tonic-clonic movements but is still in an altered state of consciousness.)
Exogenous
Infections: classically, the frontal lobe syndrome of end-stage syphilis ('General Paralysis of the Insane': GPI)
Substance misuse: PCP ('Angel dust') overdose
Head injuries: concussion
Environmental: long-term institutionalization, repeated trauma
Dissociation
'Shock'
'Hysteria'
Dissimulation
Munchausen's syndrome (the pursuit of medical care for intangible gains: e.g. repeated medical investigations)
Malingering (the pursuit of medical care for tangible gains: e.g. to avoid legal processes)
'Instrumental psychosis' (feigned psychosis in someone who has 'really' suffered from it in the past; the current episode is posited to avoid situational difficulties: e.g. a court appearance.)

Reflecting upon the contents of Table 12, it is also clear that the apparent absence of behaviour may present great diagnostic challenges to the treating clinician. Some of the possible causes of such impairment may constitute very serious illnesses indeed, such as frontal lobe tumours, 'strokes', or dementias, whereas others may pose very real problems for interpersonal, therapeutic relationships (e.g. 'Is this patient deliberately feigning the impairment in order to avoid court proceedings?'). Even the most sophisticated clinical investigations may provide only part of the solution. Clinicians and their colleagues may have to give prolonged, careful attention to acquiring (unobtrusive) clinical observations: watching the patient's behaviour in different contexts, in different companies. (This is something that we shall return to in Chapter 7.)

However, for the remainder of the present chapter, I shall focus on providing a selective review of some of the possible mechanisms via which a human actor may be deprived of their 'volitions', essentially their ability to generate spontaneous activities, 'in the world'. I shall not reprise those disorders that we have mentioned elsewhere (e.g. the consequences of a 'stroke' for limb movement or speech production [Chapters 1 and 2], or of Parkinson's disease for 'internally initiated' action [Chapters 2–4]). Instead, I shall focus on a specific exemplar of the psychiatric paradigm, as manifest in the symptom and/or sign of 'avolition' observed in schizophrenia, and an example of a very similar neurological syndrome that may be precipitated by lesions of many potential sites within the central nervous system, each impacting a final common pathway and resulting in the appearance of 'apathy'. Essentially, we shall proceed from a frontal, 'cortical' account of volitional impairment to a more systemic analysis, one in which we invoke the multiple hierarchical levels discernible throughout one of the basal ganglia–thalamocortical loop systems (delineated in Chapter 4; i.e. involving the anterior cingulate cortex [ACC]).

So, to reiterate, the point of this chapter is to characterize how a human being might be deprived of their spontaneity, their behavioural flexibility—a varied response repertoire.

Avolition in schizophrenia

In order to convey an insight into how the 'negative' symptoms of schizophrenia may impact a person, I offer the following example, abridged from an earlier published account (Spence and Parry, 2006). In this case, our patient was a young man who we had found living 'rough', on the streets:

> At the age of seventeen [the patient] was discharged from local authority care and spent the next 20 years roofless on the streets. He never claimed state benefits and lived

off the food he found in rubbish bins. He moved from city to city, recognized by police but not subject to assessment until he came to the notice of a psychiatric team treating the homeless. After following [the man] around the city and attempting to engage with him, they detained [him] for assessment under the United Kingdom's *Mental Health Act.*

When seen in the ward . . . [initially, this young man's] . . . ethnicity could not be determined because he was so unkempt, his long hair matted into dreadlocks. His clothes and shoes needed to be cut from him. It emerged that he is Caucasian. [He] said little but when he spoke he reported voices commenting upon his behaviour. He had lived without social contact for most of his adult life and his only desire was to 'keep walking'. He did not use or understand denominations of money. He was edentulous, his gums lined with dental abscesses. Blood tests revealed low serum folate (consistent with malnutrition).

[The patient] exhibited marked executive deficits on formal neuropsychological assessment. His verbal fluency was particularly reduced . . . While waiting ([for] over a year) for a rehabilitation placement [to become available; he had not responded to a series of trials of medications] he continued to exhibit avolition [lack of volition] and alogia [lack of speech], needing to be reminded to change his clothes and wash his hair. He displayed a stereotypic pattern of behaviour. He always sat in the same place in the television room (among others though not speaking to them). He rocked to and fro on his chair. Over a year many chairs were replaced as he broke them through rocking . . . When taken to see the rehabilitation unit, he walked back four miles rather than stay. He wanted to live on the acute ward.

In recollecting this man, I recall several features that we did not include in our initial account. Indeed, I should mention that he was not *totally* apathetic, for he exhibited two sorts of behaviour that suggested that he might be capable of 'enjoying himself'. On occasions, he could be seen riding on laundry trolleys (i.e. he pushed them along the ward corridors and then stood on their rails, 'riding' them until they came to a halt); on other occasions, he would go to the ward's videotape library to seek out a specific film, in order to play it on the ward's video player (John Travolta enthusiasts may be heartened to learn that the single film our patient watched, over and over again, was 'Saturday Night Fever'.) Furthermore, this man was not devoid of what we might construe to be *moral* behaviours: he would approach the nursing staff if he found money on the floor, handing it over to them; he would also go to them if he saw another patient in distress. He would not say very much but would point.

So, although it is clear that this man exhibited markedly *restricted* behavioural repertoires, and clearly suffered from a debilitating mental illness, he remained a human subject, an agent, still capable of performing some very specific ('goal-directed') acts when 'necessary'. Nevertheless, his range of acts was very limited.

In the language of psychiatry, our patient reported a 'positive' symptom of schizophrenia in that he 'heard voices' commenting on what he was doing (see Table 11, Chapter 5). He also exhibited marked 'negative' symptomatology:

1. 'Avolition': He performed relatively few purposeful acts, and exhibited a limited range of behaviours, mainly comprising stereotypic motor routines (e.g. rocking to and fro in his chair, walking up and down the corridor); he also evinced poor self-care and hygiene.

2. 'Alogia': He exhibited little spontaneous speech and markedly reduced verbal fluency when tested under formal conditions (i.e. he might typically generate only two or three 'words beginning with the letter S' in one minute).

3. 'Asociality': Though he sat in the 'day room', among others, he did not interact with them; generally, he chose not to interact.

4. As hinted earlier, we were only able to *infer* this man's capacity for enjoyment (indirectly), from specific samples of his observable behaviour: the riding about on laundry baskets and the repeated watching of a single film. Otherwise, from an external perspective, it would have been quite easy to conclude that our patient was 'anhedonic' (i.e. that he lacked the capacity for pleasure).

5. 'Affective blunting': His 'affect', that is, the observable range of expressed emotions conveyed to others via facial expression, intonation of voice, or expressive hand gestures, was markedly 'blunted' or 'flattened' (i.e. restricted). Indeed, it was largely absent.

Hence, our patient exhibited a 'full house' of the negative symptoms of schizophrenia, those symptoms (more accurately termed 'signs') that denote the absence of specific 'higher' functions: volition, speech, social interaction, the experience of pleasure, and the expression of emotion. What neural processes do we think might be implicated in the generation of such a clinical profile?

Well, if the concept of 'volition' attempts to capture the performance of 'purposeful' behaviours, undertaken by humans, then of course 'avolition' describes an absence, particularly a failure, on the part of the subject (agent) to *initiate* spontaneous, 'goal-directed' acts. Such a failure of initiation is incorporated into Andreasen's (1983) definition of avolition (see the beginning of this chapter). It is also readily apparent in our patient's very limited behavioural repertoire. Though he might occasionally carry out goal-directed activities (as he did when he left the rehabilitation unit and walked back to our ward, and when he repeatedly sought out the same videotape, of 'Saturday Night Fever'), his self-care was generally stymied by a failure to act. Hence, he was dishevelled and generally 'stuck', most of the time performing repetitive, purposeless routines (i.e. 'stereotypies'), such as rocking to and fro on his chair. For a young man, he is greatly impaired compared with his peers.

Therefore, in the light of what we have gleaned from preceding chapters of this book, we might posit that although our patient does not seem to *perform* behaviours in an abnormal way (e.g. his hand movements are not 'dyskinetic' as he inserts the videotape into the video player; he is capable of pushing, holding onto, and balancing on rather precariously loaded laundry trolleys), he *initiates* few 'cognitively demanding' modes of behaviour: conversations do not arise, he does not cook or wash, he does not read or write, he does not draw or craft objects. Indeed, apart from walking up and down or rocking to and fro (both, essentially, repetitive activities), his motor acts lack 'goals'; he largely operates according to routine.

Hence, it would be fair to say that the brain regions engaged in *generating* behavioural diversity might be functionally (and/or structurally) deficient in this man: the dorsolateral prefrontal cortex (DLPFC; anterior to Broca's area; hence the absence of spontaneous speech acts), the ACC (any 'drive' towards behaviour is only fitfully apparent: e.g. seeking out the John Travolta videotape), and also, possibly, Brodmann area (BA) 10 (at the frontal poles; Chapter 2; the only evidence of our patient 'planning' for the future or experiencing 'prospective memories' or 'delayed intentions' is again provided by his pursuit of the Travolta film). So, is there any empirical evidence that is consistent with these hypotheses? Well, although we do not have the relevant organic data relating to our patient (he consistently declined most forms of investigation, and indeed, all modes of brain scanning), there are studies that speak to this issue.

Avolition in the brain

In a positron-emission tomography (PET) study of 30 patients with chronic schizophrenia, scanned while they were 'at rest' (i.e. lying with their eyes closed, 'doing nothing' in the scanner), Liddle and colleagues (1992) utilized a within-group correlational design to examine the relationship between subsyndromes of schizophrenic symptomatology and resting state brain activity. With regard to the psychomotor poverty subsyndrome (i.e. the 'negative' syndrome that we described earlier, which incorporates the symptoms of avolition and alogia), they demonstrated an inverse correlation between the severity of such symptoms and prefrontal regional cerebral blood flow (rCBF, an index of neuronal activity; Fig. 74). Hence, the worse a patient's psychomotor poverty (avolition, alogia, etc.), the lower their prefrontal cortical activity when at 'rest'.

Fig. 74 Data from a positron-emission tomography study of people with chronic schizophrenia, scanned in the resting state. There is an association between reduced resting state prefrontal activity (as indicated in the image) and increased severity of the psychomotor poverty syndrome, characterized by avolition and alogia. Reprinted from the *British Journal of Psychiatry*. Patterns of cerebral blood flow in schizophrenia, Liddle PF et al, 1992, 160 pp 179–186 with permission from The Royal College of Psychiatrists.

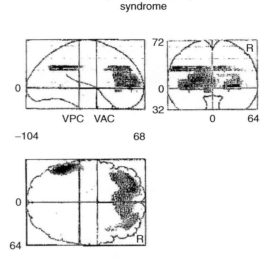

Psychomotor poverty syndrome

Negative correlations

The implication of such a finding is that reduced frontal lobe activity is associated with reduced behavioural expression (in the forms of purposeful behaviours and speech acts). Hence, these data are congruent with the pre-frontal cortex's implied role in the emergence of spontaneous behaviours (Chapter 2); however, in this case, the inference is drawn from an association between a relative *absence* of cortical activity and an *absence* of action. So, in essence, we gain the impression that frontal lobe activity may be a necessary condition for humans to be able to generate spontaneous acts (at least in the context of schizophrenia). Furthermore, since Liddle's work was published (in 1992), other studies of the (schizophrenic) negative syndrome have yielded congruent findings (e.g. Heckers et al., 1999).

So, if the frontal lobes are the focus of abnormal function in people with schizophrenia who exhibit markedly reduced volition, is the problem solely one of 'function' (i.e. 'activity') or could it also be related to underlying brain 'structure'? Such a question has important ramifications: for instance, if the nature of the deficit was purely 'functional', then one might posit that it would be more easily 'reversed' (e.g. through the use of suitable medication) than an underlying structural deficit (how might one ever 'restore' structure in a living human brain?).

Well, Chua and colleagues (1997) studied a small group of patients with schizophrenia, again utilizing a within-group correlational design, to examine the relationship between cortical *grey matter volume* and symptom severity.

This study is conceptually very similar to that of Liddle and colleagues (1992), which examined the *functional* correlates of the psychomotor poverty syndrome. Indeed, in the later study, Chua and colleagues found that worse psychomotor poverty syndrome was associated with reduced prefrontal grey matter volume (particularly in the left hemisphere; Fig. 75). Hence, reduced spontaneous behaviour (among people with schizophrenia) not only exhibits a correlation with reduced *activity* in the prefrontal cortex (Liddle et al., 1992) but also may indicate an underlying reduction in local (left prefrontal) grey matter volume (Chua et al., 1997).

Now, admittedly, Chua's was a very small study (assaying only 12 people); however, its findings are congruent with those of other studies that have reported a relationship between prefrontal structure and severity of 'negative'

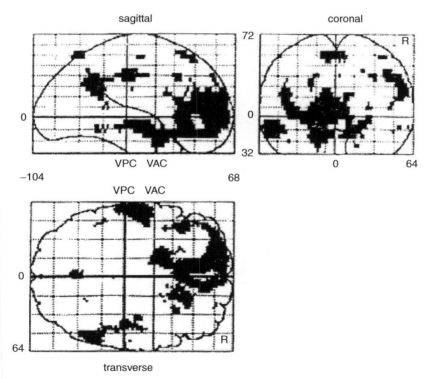

Fig. 75 A statistical parametric map relating to structural magnetic resonance imaging data derived from people with schizophrenia showing that increased severity of the psychomotor poverty syndrome is associated with reduced grey matter density, particularly within the left prefrontal lobe and also within the left temporal lobe. Reprinted from the *British Journal of Psychiatry*. Grey matter correlates of syndromes in Schizophrenia, Chua SE et al, 1997, 170 pp 406–410, with permission from The Royal College of Psychiatrists.

schizophrenic symptomatology (e.g. Gur et al., 1998; Sallet et al., 2003; Wible et al., 2001; Wolkin et al., 2003). Prefrontal structural abnormality and reduced behavioural repertoire do seem to be correlated, in people with schizophrenia. Furthermore, in a recent study at our own laboratory, Tom Farrow and I examined the relationship between 'unconstrained motor activity' in people with chronic schizophrenia (i.e. the extent to which they 'moved around' over 20 h spent in a research ward, as measured using a wrist-worn 'Actiwatch' device) and the volume of key prefrontal regions in their brains (namely, the DLPFC and the ACC), as measured using magnetic resonance imaging (MRI). We found a positive correlation between the amount of freely occurring ambulatory activity and the volume of the left ACC (Farrow et al., 2005; Fig. 76).

Now, this is of interest in that the ACC is an area where large lesions may render the subject 'akinetic', immobile (Chapter 2). So, our data suggest that (in people with schizophrenia) the *volume* of this area may also impact a measure of *mobility*. Hence, although this study did not elucidate the 'complexity' of such motor behaviour (it merely assayed its volume), it does suggest that specific 'executive' structures may constrain freely undertaken behaviour (at least in the context of schizophrenia). Therefore, if they are correct (i.e. replicated by other labs), these and similar findings (e.g. Chua et al., 1997) may be a cause for some concern: they seem to suggest that those who exhibit

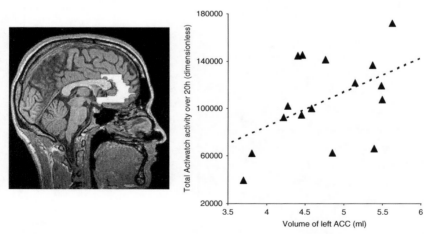

Fig. 76 Data from a magnetic resonance imaging (MRI) study showing that in people with chronic schizophrenia the volume of daytime activity is positively correlated with the volume of their left anterior cingulate cortex (ACC). Reprinted from the *British Journal of Psychiatry*. Structural brain correlates of unconstrained motor activity in people with schizophrenia, Farrow T, F et al, 2005, 187 pp 481–482, with permission from The Royal College of Psychiatrists. (See colour plate section).

avolition may do so as a consequence of the *structure, and the function,* of their brains (admittedly, causation cannot be inferred from statistical association, but nevertheless such a link becomes plausible.) Also of concern would be other studies that find a progressive element to prefrontal volume reduction in schizophrenia (e.g. Gur et al., 1998; Madsen et al., 1999; Salokangas et al., 2002). So, although pharmacological interventions might be able to modulate the hypoactivity of the prefrontal cortex in this disorder (e.g. Honey et al. 1999; Hunter et al., 2006; Spence et al., 1998; Spence et al., 2005), it is less clear how such therapies might be able to ameliorate the effects of gross morphological (i.e. structural) disturbance.

Genetic constraints

Now, if the prospect of a (brain) structural contribution to the emergence of avolition is a cause for some concern (in view of its possible contribution to *constraining* potential functional recovery), then another potential constraint is also becoming increasingly well characterized in current neuroscientific research: that of a subject's genotype, their genetic endowment. Therefore, although the limitations of space preclude our reviewing the genetics of schizophrenia at any length, it is appropriate to say a little about this important issue here and now.

In general, it is widely accepted that 'schizophrenia' is a highly 'heritable' syndrome: relatives of affected patients are themselves at increased risk of developing the disorder, in accordance with their genetic proximity to an index (affected) patient. Hence, although the prevalence of schizophrenia in most communities is on the order of 1%, the lifetime risk of developing the disorder in one who is a full sibling of an affected patient is approximately 10% (and 5% if one is a 'second-degree' relative, such as a half sibling). The identical twin of an affected patient has a 50% lifetime risk of developing the disorder (Note that although markedly heritable, the condition is not *entirely* genetically mediated—i.e. the 'congruence' exhibited by identical twins is not 100%.)

Nevertheless, although there is clearly a genetic component to the emergence of schizophrenia (borne out by twin and adoption studies), a big problem for the field continues to be the relative paucity of (well-replicated findings of) single genes conveying a large risk. What seems to be the case is that what we call 'schizophrenia' is a heterogeneous syndrome transmitted via a polygenic mechanism, that is, by multiple genes, each of small effect. Hence, the search for contributory genes and causal pathways requires very large studies (of thousands of subjects, in order for each of them to have sufficient statistical power) and may, even then, yield information that is of very limited practical application. In other words, it is unlikely to be 'simply' a question of screening out one or two 'disease' genes from affected families; it is far more likely to be the case that many genes of small effect will be found to be widely distributed among the 'normal' population and also that such genes may well have 'normal' functions, perhaps only conveying 'risk' as such when they are present in certain noxious combinations with other 'risk' genes. So, really, there might not even be such a thing as a single 'gene for schizophrenia'.

Therefore, if we come to considering the genetic pathways via which 'avolition' might become manifest in human subjects, it is again likely that genes of small effect may be relevant, and that multiple genetic substrates may be implicated. Hence, in the following subsections, I shall consider just two genetic contributions to the putative 'deficit' state observed in schizophrenia, one of which we have touched upon previously (in Chapter 4). I should also state that in both of these cases the effect wrought by the gene upon cognitive and/or symptomatic function in schizophrenia is also discernible among 'healthy' subjects. Thus, it is not so much that patients suffer a unique 'genetic hit', but more that they have a particularly 'bad case' of something that is also discernible across the wider community or population.

Genes impacting cognition

As we established, at some length, in Chapter 4, dopamine is a neurotransmitter that is pivotal to the physiology of volition. Indeed, deficits in dopaminergic neurotransmission are most obviously implicated in Parkinson's disease. However, they are also believed to contribute to the pathophysiology of 'negative' symptoms in schizophrenia (Mortimer and Spence, 2001). Hence, it has been postulated that although the positive symptoms of the disorder (such as delusions and hallucinations; Table 11) implicate subcortical and limbic system dopaminergic excess, negative symptoms (such as avolition) reflect a cortical hypodopaminergic state (Abi-Dargham, 2003). Therefore, the problem of schizophrenia is a pernicious one for pharmacological therapists, for in seeking to reduce dopaminergic neurotransmission (at the level of the striatum and limbic system), in order to control 'positive' symptoms, they risk making the 'negative' symptoms of the disorder worse (through reducing cortical dopaminergic function).

Now, as was outlined in Chapter 4, pertinent to the levels of dopamine in the prefrontal cortex are the specific conditions of its metabolism. In the prefrontal cortex, dopamine elimination is crucially dependent upon its catabolism by the enzyme catechol-O-methyltransferase (COMT; this may be contrasted with the conditions pertaining subcortically, where there are additional means of dopamine elimination from the synaptic cleft). Hence, factors that reduce the efficacy of COMT in metabolizing dopamine may be expected to lead to a relative enhancement in the latter's cortical activity (i.e. dopamine will persist longer in the synaptic cleft, thereby becoming more 'efficient'), whereas factors leading to more rapid dopamine elimination from the synaptic cleft will render the neurotransmitter less efficient (Chapter 4). So it is that in so-called 'knockout mice', lacking the gene that encodes COMT, cognitive performance is actually enhanced (because cortical dopamine remains unmetabolized for longer).

Now, as stated previously (in Chapter 4), in humans, the gene encoding COMT contains a common functional polymorphism (Val108/158Met) that has been found to influence cognitive performance in healthy people and those with schizophrenia (Egan et al., 2001). Indeed, the *COMT* genotype is related, in an allele dosage manner, to performance exhibited on the Wisconsin Card Sorting Test, explaining 4.1% of the variance in the frequency of perseverative errors (perseveration, in this context, denoting the continued performance of behaviours that are no longer contextually appropriate). As the 'Met' allele is associated with slower metabolism of dopamine, homozygotes for this allele make less perseverative errors than homozygotes for the 'Val' allele, with heterozygotes performing at intermediate levels (Egan et al., 2001). Hence, if we regard perseverative patterns of behaviour as being indicative of avolition (as they were in the case of our homeless man [Spence and Parry, 2006]), then we may posit that the *COMT* gene provides one example of a gene that may contribute to the clinical picture of avolition—reduced behavioural diversity. However, the effect is likely to be a small one. There may well be a great many genetic contributions to such a complex phenotype as 'avolition'.

Genes impacting symptoms

Indeed, the recent literature has provided another clear example of such a genetic contribution. This one takes the form of a gene that has been considered a 'risk gene' for schizophrenia, albeit of small effect size. The gene concerned codes for dysbindin, a protein, present in the brain, which binds α- and β-dystrophin (components of the 'dystrophin–glycoprotein complex', which is itself implicated in influencing glutamatergic neurotransmission in the brain). The gene coding for dysbindin has been implicated in conveying risk for schizophrenia because its region of the genome (located on chromosome 6p22) has been found to be 'linked' to the occurrence of schizophrenia is some familial pedigrees. Indeed, one form of this gene, the 6-locus 'CTCTAC' haplotype, is significantly over-represented among Caucasians with schizophrenia (see DeRosse et al., 2006).

So, if a gene is implicated in causing schizophrenia, might it be implicated in causing certain, specific symptoms of the disorder? This is the line of reasoning adopted by DeRosse and colleagues (2006) who examined the dysbindin genotypes of 181 people with schizophrenia and compared these with their (lifetime) exhibition of avolition, alogia, and affective 'flattening' (all negative symptoms of the disorder). Although the dysbindin genotype did not seem to be related to other aspects of the syndrome (gender, age of onset, length of illness, etc.), it was related to the lifetime severity of negative symptomatology (Fig. 77). Hence, in those patients who possessed one or two copies of the CTCTAC haplotype (for the dysbindin gene), each of the negative symptoms was significantly over-represented across the course of their illnesses. This finding provides direct evidence for the biological impact of a genotype (impacting neural function) upon the clinical severity of avolition (and alogia and affective flattening) in schizophrenia. Again, such an effect is likely to constitute only a small contribution to the total avolition discernible among people with schizophrenia (indeed, only 26 of the 181 patients in DeRosse's sample carried the index haplotype), but nevertheless it gives us another insight into the multiple pathways via which the brain may be rendered 'avolitional'.

A putative model of avolition

Therefore, if we attempt to synthesize the findings that we have just rehearsed regarding the putative neurobiology of the 'negative', 'psychomotor poverty',

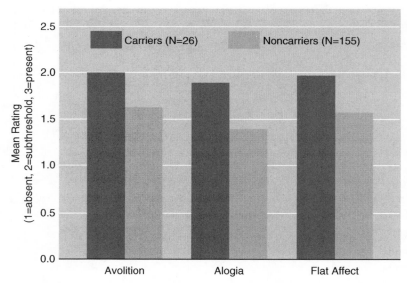

Fig. 77 Graph showing that carriers of the index dysbindin genotype exhibit more severe negative symptoms of schizophrenia than those patients who do not carry the index genotype. (From DeRosse et al., *American Journal of Psychiatry* 2006; 163: 532–534). (See colour plate section).

or avolitional syndrome encountered in schizophrenia, then we may be able to distil a small number of reasonably definitive statements, propositions that might form the basis of a preliminary model of avolition (and its associated deficits), about this disorder:

1. Avolition and alogia are characterized by deficits in responsivity, both in terms of the spontaneity with which responses to the environment are generated and also their relative novelty or complexity. Those who are 'avolitional' exhibit limited behavioural repertoires: they execute fewer actions and those actions that they do execute are of less variety (than is the case in 'health')—that is, they tend to be stereotypic. Now, if we were to view such symptoms as predictive 'neurological markers' of putative pathology, then we should have predicted that they might implicate the prefrontal cortices: avolition *resembles* the consequences of prefrontal and anterior cingulate or medial premotor cortical pathology, seen in 'neurological' cases; alogia *resembles* the syndrome of 'dynamic' or 'transcortical motor' aphasia, which itself implicates regions of the frontal lobe anterior to Broca's area (see Dolan et al., 1993, for confirmation of this 'prediction'.)

2. When contemporary neuroimaging techniques are applied to groups of patients satisfying the diagnostic criteria for the syndrome of schizophrenia, and when such patients are compared with each other by using within-group correlational designs, then those who exhibit a more severe psychomotor poverty subsyndrome (incorporating avolition and alogia) also exhibit greater prefrontal lobe deficits, whether in terms of 'function' or 'structure' (e.g. Chua et al., 1997; Liddle et al., 1992).

3. The beginnings of the 'genetics of avolition' are currently discernible within the literature concerning the genetics of schizophrenia itself. Although it is unlikely that there will be single ('avolitional') genes of large effect, it is likely that several or many genes may serve to contribute small effects to such a clinical profile, each impacting the biology of those systems that underlie the ability of the organism to generate behavioural diversity. In the case of a complex phenotype, such as 'voluntary action' or 'behavioural diversity', it is quite likely that there may be very many candidate systems wherein genetic variation might act to influence 'higher' orders of emergent behaviour, via multiple mediating pathways. Indeed, so far, a reasonable case may be made for 'normal' variants of the *COMT* and dysbindin genes impacting such processes. It is also of note that each of these variants impacts a major neurotransmitter system: the dopaminergic and glutamatergic systems, respectively, systems that we know to be implicated in the genesis of volition (Chapter 4). Hence, one may hypothesize that avolition 'should' be more

pronounced in those patients who carry both the Val/Val functional polymorphism of the *COMT* gene (at the 158, Val108/158Met, codon, on chromosome 22: 22q11.1-q11.2) and the CTCTAC haplotype of the dysbindin gene (at 6p22).

If we were to synthesize these, admittedly disparate, data, then we might arrive at a model such as that depicted in Fig. 78. In this cartoon, we move from a representation of 'developmental' factors on the left, towards 'current anatomy' in the middle, and emergent 'behaviours' on the right. Hence, a number of early influences, exemplified here by the *COMT* and dysbindin genotypes, might contribute to the development of an organism and persist in exerting an influence on its current anatomy and physiology (centre). Moreover, the current anatomical and/or functional status of the individual forms the underlying matrix of a system in which 'higher' neurological centres are 'able' to modulate 'lower' centres (in a way clearly derived from Shallice's 1988 model; see Chapter 4), and where adequate functioning of such higher centres (in the prefrontal and medial premotor cortices) *should* facilitate the emergence

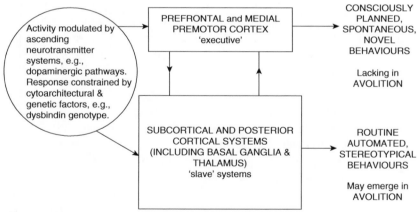

Fig. 78 Cartoon demonstrating the basis of avolition as seen in schizophrenia. At the centre of the figure, the normal components of the human motor system are represented, divided between an executive (above) and subordinate slave systems (below). The executive is required for the performance of spontaneous or novel behaviours. The subordinate slave systems are sufficient to perform routine, automated or stereotypical behaviours. In avolition, there appears to be a relative deficit in the function (and also the structure) of the executive system, as exemplified in studies by Liddle, Chua, and others. Hence, avolition may be associated with a deficit in the functioning of the prefrontal executive. The cause of such deficits may include genetic factors such as the dysbindin and other genotypes (see left of figure).

of novel, complex, or attention-demanding actions (represented on the upper right of the cartoon).

However, should the organism fail to modulate 'lower' centres, then complex behaviours will become more difficult to generate and stereotypic responses (mediated via those 'released' lower centres) will predominate. So it is in the avolitional brain where we may posit that a failure of 'higher centres' to adequately modulate 'lower' systems leads to the emergence of repetitive stereotypic behavioural sequences. In such a system, incremental impairments of higher centres, for example, as a consequence of multiple genetic influences (and adverse environmental events), would be expected to contribute incremental impairments of behaviour diversity. Hence, it follows that restoration of prefrontal and/or medial premotor cortical function 'should' restore behavioural diversity (and our group has begun to publish evidence of such an effect, consequent upon the administration of a so-called 'smart drug' [Hunter et al., 2006; Spence et al., 2005; and also Farrow et al., 2006]; see Chapter 10). So, although we have not yet 'solved' the problem of avolition, it does at least appear to be increasingly tractable. We know where some of the problems lie and we have an 'idea' of what a solution 'should' look like: it should comprise the restoration of behavioural diversity (Chapter 10).

Is there any difference between avolition and apathy?

As promised, we now prepare to 'step sideways' from the psychiatric to the neurological clinical literature. For, as was alluded to at the very beginning of this chapter, the phenomenon that a psychiatrist would describe as 'avolition' bears a resemblance to what a neurologist would call 'apathy'. Indeed, the definitions of these conditions (as offered at the head of the chapter [Andreasen, 1983; Marin et al., 1991]) seem very similar. Furthermore, if there are differences, then these often seem to comprise matters of perspective: psychiatric definitions often stress an *observation* (because psychiatric aetiologies may be complex and/or currently unknown) whereas neurological terms often imply an *aetiology* (or cause); in other words, whereas 'avolition' describes the absence of observed voluntary behaviours, 'apathy' implies that such an absence is attributable to a lack of motivation or drive (on the part of the patient).

However, if the phenomena so described were, in essence, actually rather similar, then we might expect to find that they exhibit similar biological correlates; and, to an extent, this is true. So, in the following section, I shall describe the neural correlates of apathy, beginning with its cortical correlates (which are again predominantly frontal in location) before moving on to consider specific case reports demonstrating the underlying importance of one of the basal ganglia–thalamocortical loop systems to motivation (drive) and its impairment (apathy).

Apathy in the brain

The symptom of apathy has attracted increasing interest in recent years, following the publication of a seminal paper by Marin (1991), which set out the features of this condition and the syndromes with which it is most often associated. Hence, although apathy may accompany a great many neurological syndromes, there is a certain regularity to the locations of maximal pathology identified within each of these disparate disease states (Table 13). Indeed, as a 'rule of thumb', apathy is particularly likely to be encountered in the presence of *medial* frontal lobe lesions, disorders of the basal ganglia that are associated with *hypokinesia* (i.e. reduced movement) and reduced excitatory neurotransmission to the medial frontal cortex, and lesions 'lower' down the central nervous system, which may be posited to interfere with ascending neurotransmitter systems. Indeed, as we shall demonstrate shortly, a case can be made for lesions at multiple levels of the anterior cingulate ('limbic') loop system precipitating apathy in previously healthy subjects.

So, if the medial frontal lobes make important contributions to the physiology of 'motivation' and 'drive' (Chapter 2), then one might posit that any

Table 13 Neurological conditions associated with apathy

Causes of apathy
Conditions impacting the frontal lobe, including schizophrenia and frontal lobe injuries and dementias
Lesions of the right hemisphere
Lesions close to the midline of the brain, especially anterior cingulate cortices, supplementary motor areas (SMAs)
Vascular lesions of the basal ganglia and thalamus
Lesions after carbon monoxide and manganese poisoning
Movement disorders associated with hypokinesia rather than hyperkinesias; hence, Parkinson's disease and Progressive Supranuclear more than Huntington's chorea
Disorders impacting the anterior cingulate ('limbic') and orbitofrontal 'loop' systems Amphetamine and cocaine withdrawal 'Apathetic' hyperthyroidism Long-term institutionalization

Source: Derived from Cummings (1993), Litvan et al. (1998), and Marin et al. (1991).

neurological condition that impacts these regions could potentially precipitate apathy; and, there is evidence in favour of this view:

1. In a study of two samples of people affected by schizophrenia, one exhibiting apathy and the other not, and a healthy control group, Roth et al. (2004) found that those schizophrenia patients who were apathetic exhibited smaller volumes of both frontal lobes, compared with both comparator groups.

2. In a study of 148 patients with varied (presumed) causes of dementia (these were necessarily provisional diagnoses as the patients were alive when scanned), Rosen et al. (2005) found a particular association between apathy and frontotemporal dementia and, within this syndrome, between apathy and reduced volume of the ventromedial superior frontal gyrus (an area lying in the medial prefrontal cortex; Fig. 79).

Hence, it would seem that despite very different proposed aetiologies, conditions that impact the frontal cortex (especially the medial frontal cortex) are more likely to render patients apathetic.

Thus, once again, we have a putative 'cortical' account of apathy (as we had for avolition), one tending to implicate that region of the frontal cortex most

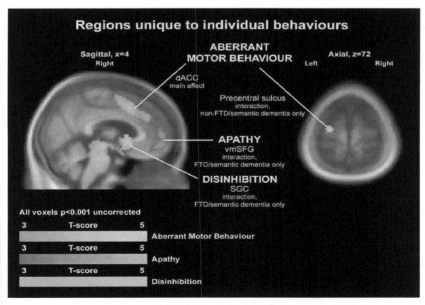

Fig. 79 Image showing the structural brain correlates of abnormal behaviours in people with different forms of dementia. Note that apathy is associated with grey matter deficits within the ventromedial superior frontal gyrus, as indicated in blue. (Rosen et al, *Brain* 2005; 128: 2612–2625) with permission from Oxford University Press. (See colour plate section).

obviously involved in the emergence of motivation, or drive, towards action. However, if this is the case, and if the basal ganglia–thalamocortical loop systems (that we discussed in Chapter 4) are as central to voluntary behaviour as we have implied, then is it not possible that apathy might be precipitated by pathology residing within the 'underlying' levels of such a loop system? And if we specify the successive levels located within the anterior cingulate ('limbic') loop (i.e. the caudate nucleus at the level of the striatum, followed by the ventral pallidum, followed by the output nuclei of the thalamus; Fig. 80), might we not discover evidence of apathy being precipitated by lesions at each of these levels? Well, for the most part, this is the case:

1. Grunsfeld and Login (2006) describe the case of a 57-year-old woman who was rendered apathetic ('abulic') when an endoscopic procedure targeting her sinuses went wrong; the endoscope pierced her brain, impacting her right caudate nucleus (Fig. 81): 'Prior to the surgery she had worked full

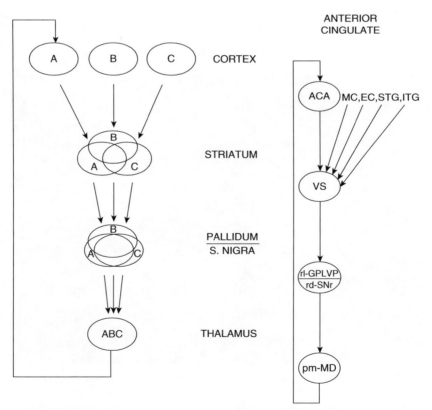

Fig. 80 Schematic of the generic structure of the basal ganglia–thalamocortical loops (left) and the specific structure of the anterior cingulate loop (right).

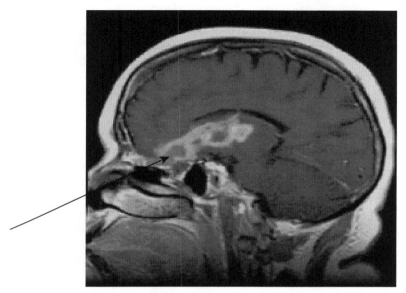

Fig. 81 Structural magnetic resonance imaging MRI scan seen in the sagittal plane showing the brain of a patient who experienced apathy after an endoscope perforated her skull and impacted upon her right caudate nucleus. The arrow indicates the course of its trajectory. (From Grunsfeld and Login, *BMC Neurology* 2006; 6: 4). With permission from Biomed Central.

time as an aide in a centre for learning disabled children plus an additional 20 h weekly as an aide in a home health agency. She also was involved extensively with her church and community activities. After recovering from the surgery, she was unable to return to work. She would sit at home and do nothing. She did not even wish to drive her car any longer.'

2. Endelborghs and colleagues (2000) describe the case of a 58-year-old man who developed a 'stroke' while undergoing coronary artery angiography; he was to remain apathetic over 18 months; the 'stroke' involved both his thalami (Figs. 82 and 83): 'The patient's behaviour had dramatically changed. Instead of the active man he used to be, he had become an apathetic, passive, and indifferent person who seemed to have lost all emotional concern and initiative. His affect was clearly blunted. The patient remained indifferent to visitors or when he received gifts. He did not show any concern for his relatives or his illness and manifested no desire, no complaint, and no concern about the future. The patient, who used to be a successful travelling salesman, had entirely lost concern about his business. There was a striking absence of thoughts and spontaneous mental activity. He rarely spoke spontaneously and took no verbal initiative. When asked about the content of his

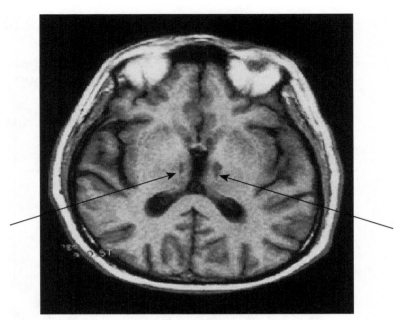

Fig. 82 Structural magnetic resonance imaging scan seen in the transverse plane showing the brain of a patient demonstrating bilateral infarctions of the thalamic nuclei. (From Endelborghs et al., *Stroke* 2000; 31: 1762–1765).

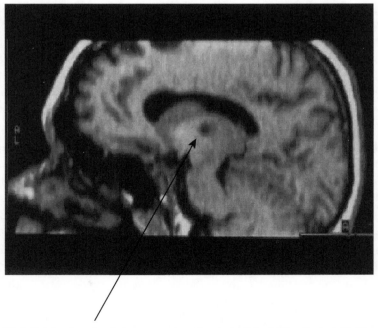

Fig. 83 A structural magnetic resonance imaging scan of the brain, displayed in the sagittal plane, showing an area of thalamic infarction. (From Endelborghs et al., *Stroke* 2000; 31: 1762–1765). (See colour plate section).

thoughts, the patient claimed he had none, suggesting a state of mental emptiness.' As may be seen in the man's published single photon-emission computed tomography (SPECT) image, the disturbance of his functional brain activity is not restricted to the sites of his structural lesions (i.e. his thalami); instead, it extends superiorly to affect his caudate nuclei and medial frontal cortices (an example of 'diaschesis'; Chapter 2).

3. Van der Werf and colleagues (1999) describe the case of a 44-year-old man who suffered a similar 'stroke' during the course of a spinal operation; he was also rendered apathetic, investigations revealing the site of the stroke to be the intralaminar nuclei of the right thalamus (Fig. 84): 'At the time of surgery, he owned a flourishing company selling flower bulbs, and occupied

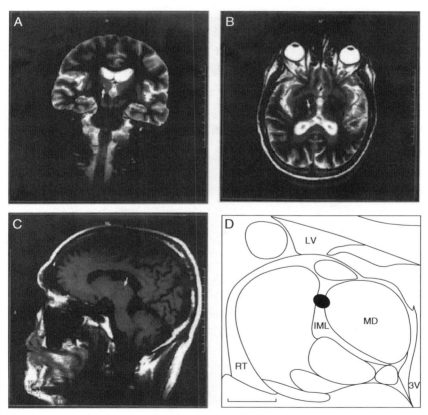

Fig. 84 Images showing the position of an intrathalamic lesion in a patient rendered apathetic. In each case, the arrows point to the position of the lesion. Reprinted from the *Journal of Neurology, Neurosurgery and Psychiatry* 1996; 66: 36–42. Neuropsychological correlates of a right unilateral lacunar thalamic infarction. Van Der Werf YD, Weerts JGE, Jolles J et al, 1999, 66/1 with permission from the BMJ publishing Group Ltd.

many board positions in his field of work, but was unable to keep up these activities after the operation. He is currently doing odd jobs at his company[,] which is now run by his wife . . . When left to himself, he will tend not to initiate any activity. Having been a lively and creative character, involved in sports and described as a great family man, he had become apathetic and lethargic. His wife describes how he can be found sitting in his bedroom on his own, when his family is downstairs on social evenings. This behaviour seems not to arise from discontent or anger but from disinterest. He shows a remarkable lack of facial and verbal expressiveness and initiative but is perfectly compliant.'

It is hard to escape the conclusion that such patients have been robbed of something that was essential to them, as people. It is almost as if they provide modern accounts to parallel that of Phineas Gage (Chapter 2). How might the person described as 'remaining' in each of these accounts 'measure up' to the person who entered hospital for each of these fateful procedures? It is hard to avoid the conclusion that they are 'no longer' the people they once were. Just as Phineas Gage was 'no longer Gage'.

Conclusion

The purpose of this chapter has been to examine some of the dysfunctional processes via which a human agent may be deprived of their ability to act. We have seen that there is a wide range of terms deployed, across medical disciplines, in order to describe such phenomena and that often the same brain systems are implicated in their emergence: the frontal lobes, especially the medial prefrontal and premotor cortices, and the components of the anterior cingulate ('limbic') loop system, that is, specific, related subcortical nuclei. What is most striking is the impact on a formerly 'normal' human being of such apparently focal, discrete disturbances: actions cease, emotions are no longer discernible, and thoughts are apparently absent. These are devastating conditions, impacting not solely the patient but also their families, the people with whom they had enjoyed their premorbid 'relationships'. For, under such conditions, relationships are radically perturbed: the patient does not communicate, he does not act; he does not seem to 'care'. However, the situation is not entirely hopeless. In Chapter 10, we shall review one of the methods that clinicians have deployed to restore such actions, to counteract avolition and apathy.

Chapter 7

Hysterical agents

['Anna O'] was sitting at [her father's] bedside with her right arm over the back of her chair. She fell into a waking dream and saw a black snake coming towards the sick man from the wall to bite him . . . She tried to keep the snake off, but it was as though she was paralyzed. Her right arm, over the back of the chair, had gone to sleep and had become anaesthetic and paretic . . . Next day, in the course of a game . . . a bent branch revived her hallucination of the snake, and simultaneously, her right arm became rigidly extended . . . [15]

[I]t is not the muscles which refuse to obey the will, but the will itself which has ceased to work.[16]

In the foregoing chapters (Chapters 5 and 6), we examined a variety of volitional disturbances that might be broadly identified as falling into two categories or sets:

1. Patients who experience their own sense of *agency* as being radically perturbed, either as a consequence of an objective 'misbehaviour' exhibited by one or more of their limbs or as a consequence of grossly disturbed sensation (i.e. the 'feeling' that something or someone, alien to themselves, is 'in control' of their thoughts and movements; Chapter 5). Where organic abnormality can be demonstrated, it often implicates the medial premotor cortices, corpus callosum, or parietal cortex (especially on the right).

2. Patients who exhibit pathologically restricted behavioural repertoires (e.g. 'avolition', 'apathy', etc.), so that both the volume of their purposeful

---

[15] The seminal case of 'Anna O', one of the first hysterical patients reported (by Breuer) in Freud & Breuer (1991, pp.93-94). [Freud S, Breuer J. *Studies on hysteria*. London: Penguin, 1991. Translation by James and Alix Strachey, first published in *The Standard Edition of the Complete Psychological Works of Sigmund Freud*, Volume II, by the Hogarth Press and the Institute of Psycho-Analysis, London, 1955.]

[16] Brodie, 1837, cited in Merskey, 1995, p. 16. [Merskey H. *The analysis of hysteria. Understanding conversion and dissociation.* London: Gaskell, 1995.]

activity and its relative complexity are much reduced (Chapter 6). The latter constitutes an objective disorder of *action* (actually profound 'inaction'). Where organic abnormality can be demonstrated, it often implicates the frontal lobes and specific subcortical nuclei (see Table 13).

Now, in this chapter, we consider a further mode of volitional disorder, one that shares certain of its features with each of the above (at times), although it also appears rather different. Hence, in so-called 'hysteria' or 'conversion disorder'

1. Patients exhibit objectively unusual motor behaviours (that may be exaggerated or diminished in volume), which are apparently without any organic ('biological') cause, yet they (the patients) deny authorship of these behaviours (in other words, they deny *agency*).

2. Nevertheless, careful observation of these same behaviours leads to the (admittedly, uncomfortable) conclusion that they resemble purposeful *acts* (i.e. patients must 'attend' to their performances, in order for their 'symptoms' to persist; distraction or sedation leads to a 'normalization' of motoric behaviour, in marked contrast to most forms of 'organic' movement disorder; and, some pivotal neurological investigations suggest that such patients' aberrant behaviours are 'controlled' by 'higher centres', centres that are themselves involved in voluntary behaviour.)

3. Hence, while 'hysterical' patients report a disturbance of agency, their doctors witness unusual action performances (Spence, 1999).

Moreover, there is often a further problem that intrudes upon the evaluation of such patients, one that is borne of the circumstances under which they may present to medical services. In the following paragraph, I revisit the description of a fictional case, one that exemplifies many of the issues that arise in 'real-life' practice. This sketch is adapted from Spence (2006a):

> A middle-aged man, who worked as a schoolteacher, was found in possession of child pornography and then developed difficulty speaking. He mumbled replies through tightly closed lips. However, he was able to cough and swallow normally. He denied any knowledge of the material found. He was tearful and appeared depressed. His wife reported that he had manifested similar symptoms when money had gone missing from their bank account some years before. Physical examination was largely normal, apart from hypertension. The patient's wife also noted that he still spoke 'normally' in his sleep.

Now, though fictitious, this case exhibits several features that we shall return to, again and again, in the course of this chapter:

1. The motor symptoms exhibited by the patient may be construed as having arisen at a 'convenient' moment in his life.

2. His motor impairments were inconsistent over time (i.e. they 'came and went').

3. The circumstances of his presentation were such that there were reasons why the patient may not have been 'liked' by others (including investigating health-care professionals).

4. There is often an association between hysteria or conversion and concurrent depression (and personality disorder).

5. Doctors may be especially wary of 'missing' rare disorders, unusual disease presentations, so they may investigate the patient extensively.

6. However, they may also be wary of being 'duped'; such a case provokes suspicion.

The 'meaning' of hysteria

From a strictly 'Freudian' point of view, such a case arises because of a conflict located within the individual (the 'patient') concerned. Such a conflict is hard to resolve. Hence, some temporary respite ('a primary gain') may be achieved by 'converting' the conflict into a 'symptom' (one that often seems to bear a symbolic significance; hence, in the [preceding] example that I have invented, one might imagine that there is something 'unspeakable', which the patient cannot admit to or avow—e.g. perhaps he is a paedophile; see Fingarette [1969] for more on the theme of 'disavowal'). Crucially, such a 'conversion' takes place outside of awareness: that is, it is *unconsciously* mediated. In essence, the patient's unconscious spares the patient's conscious mind any further suffering. Hence, the 'primary gain' essentially comprises a reduction of conflict-related anxiety. Moreover, once his symptoms have emerged, there is the possibility that the patient may accrue further benefits: in adopting the so-called 'sick-role', he may be cared for by others, released from his normal obligation to work, and even excused legal accountability, and so on. Such benefits constitute the so-called 'secondary gain'.

Nevertheless, by now, the reader may well have recognized that there are also profound problems with the concept of hysteria: there are no objective features that adequately distinguish it from malingering; everything depends upon the credence attributed to the patient's account; and, there is the necessary, albeit problematic, invocation of a Freudian 'unconscious' (something that is terribly unfashionable in contemporary psychology!).

So it is that in this chapter, we repeatedly encounter a rather strange array of unusual motor performances, one that appears 'volitional' in its phenomenology, even though the 'sufferer' (the patient) denies their 'authorship' or 'agency' of these behaviours. In medical practice, such scenarios commonly attract the diagnostic labels 'hysteria' or 'conversion disorder' (concepts which therefore seek to explain the seemingly inexplicable in terms of the Freudian 'unconscious'), or 'functional' or 'psychogenic' disorder (which may be regarded as less theoretically driven, though they nevertheless imply that the problem is 'all in the mind'; Spence, 2006a). Indeed, as we shall see, a great deal has been written concerning the putative causes of such phenomena and their possible 'meanings' for their hosts (the patients).

The limits of observation

However, before we proceed any further, it is worth pausing to note (once again) that any adequate characterization of a person's (an agent's) volitions, their 'purposeful' behaviours and, indeed, their 'intentions', rests on (our hypothetical) ability to access their conscious states of mind. Nevertheless, it is in precisely these sorts of clinical situations that we are confronted with the essential *imperceptibility* of another's conscious states. Much depends upon what a patient *tells* us about their perceptions of their motor system's 'inner' functioning (i.e. their 'first-person' account). A 'third-person' observer or interviewer simply does not 'know' what his (first-person) interlocutor is thinking. Hence, everything rests on what we *imagine* the 'other' to be thinking and intending (and we could so easily be wrong).

Furthermore, it is not enough to imagine that we can merely fall back on objective observation to augment our information, in order to completely 'solve the problem'. This simply won't do: although we hold out the existence of conscious and unconscious aetiologies underpinning such movement dis-orders, we cannot discern, merely by looking at the patient, which aetiology is currently in play; again, we cannot 'tell what they are thinking'.

So, although current diagnostic systems seem to posit a psychic physician(!), one who can tell what their patients are thinking and intending (if you don't believe me, see Table 14), it would seem advisable to retain a sense of our own fallibility (a fallibility that becomes even more obvious when we come to consider the literature concerning human deception, in Chapter 8).

Therefore, as we have rehearsed in previous chapters (especially in Chapter 5), we are confronted with the difficulty of trying to establish whether a form of 'symmetry' exists between another person's intentions and their actions, thoughts, and deeds. In the present case, an abnormal behaviour appears purposeful, yet the patient denies purpose. Nevertheless, we have 'only' their word for their 'ignorance' of its causation. Hence, there is either an asymmetry pertaining between their 'intentions' and their 'actions'—that is, their 'will' is impeded (in some sense)—or there is no such asymmetry—that is, their intentions and actions are actually aligned, and the (invisible) intention of the agent is actually to deceive us.

What is hysteria?

Well, as we have stated already, in hysteria, it is posited that a physical symptom or sign is produced by a psychological mechanism, one that is triggered by a conflict within the patient. Crucially, there is no explanatory physical cause that can be demonstrated.

Hence, the fundamental problem in hysteria is this: *How can a motor or sensory symptom be produced in the absence of a physical cause?* The man or woman so afflicted reports that they cannot raise their arm, cannot speak out, or see; yet, physical investigations prove negative and, when sedated or observed unobtrusively over time, symptomatic inconsistencies arise.

> One ['paraplegic'] patient was observed skipping in the physiotherapy department. One, with an ostensible triparesis, assisted the doctor taking blood with her allegedly paralyzed arm. Another got herself back normally into a wheelchair having fallen out of it.
>
> (Baker and Silver, 1987)

However, despite these inconsistencies, the diagnostic systems applied (e.g. the *Diagnostic and Statistical Manual*, 4th edition [DSM IV; American Psychiatric Association, 1994]) are quite specific that the patient experiencing and exhibiting such symptoms and signs is *not responsible* for their production: that is, they are not 'feigning' (Table 14). Hence, the physician is called upon to judge what the patient is thinking and not doing, that is, to perceive that they are *really* trying to move, speak, or see and are not 'merely' pretending to be impaired. This is a complex task and, as we shall see (in the following), the use of terminology in this area suggests considerable uncertainty among physicians as to what it is that they are diagnosing.

Table 14 Selected criteria for the diagnosis of Conversion Disorder (300.11) in the Diagnostic and Statistical Manual, 4th edition (DSM IV)

DSM IV criteria A–D for conversion disorder
One or more symptoms or deficits affecting voluntary motor or sensory function that suggest a neurological or other general medical condition.
Psychological factors are judged to be associated with the symptom or deficit because the initiation or exacerbation of the symptom or deficit is preceded by conflicts or other stressors.
The symptom or deficit is not intentionally produced or feigned.
The symptom or deficit cannot, after appropriate investigation, be fully explained by a general medical condition, or by the effects of a substance, or as a culturally sanctioned behaviour or experience.

Source: From the American Psychiatric Association (1994).

Terminological ambiguity

Consider the following comments from the published neurological literature:

1. 'I have said to the patient 'I know from experience that your pretended [symptom] is the result of some intolerable emotional situation. If you will tell me the whole story I promise absolutely to respect your confidence, will give you all the help I can and will say to your doctor and relatives that I have cured you by hypnotism.' (Sir Charles Symonds [1970], cited in Merskey [1995])

2. 'Organic tremor is aggravated by taking the attention away from the area involved and usually improves when attention is directed towards the involved limb . . . Functional or psychogenic tremor disappears when attention is withdrawn from the limb or area involved. I will give $25.00 to the first [doctor] who can prove me wrong.' (Campbell, 1979)

3. 'The abductor sign is a useful test to detect non-organic paresis, because (1) it is difficult for a hysterical patient to deceive the examiner . . .' (Sanoo, 2004)

From these statements, one might conclude that although the neurologists concerned are ostensibly commenting on 'hysterical', 'conversion', 'functional', or 'psychogenic' disorders (terms that have been used interchangeably within the literature for some time), at some level they are acknowledging an element of deception on the part of those whom they diagnose. Hence, the apparent levity at the close of example 2; it is difficult to think of another medical condition where such a challenge might have achieved publication. There is, perhaps, something almost unique about this diagnosis (hysteria), in terms of the difficulties that it produces for patients and doctors alike. Does the doctor *really* believe in the Freudian mechanisms instantiated within the diagnostic systems? Is the doctor acting in good faith if they suspect that the patient is actually feigning? Is there even any such condition as 'hysteria' or is it merely a pragmatic label that serves to postpone confrontation? What are the feelings provoked within physicians when they examine and investigate such patients? Some of these difficulties are summarized in Table 15.

The problem with hysteria as a diagnosis is that it immediately sets up certain dualisms, dichotomies which may prove to be both inaccurate and unhelpful: Is it a disorder of body (or brain) or mind, one that is organic or 'psychogenic', or conscious (i.e. feigned) or unconscious (the product of hysterical conversion)? Is there a deceiver and their deceived (and which is which), and is there a villain and a victim (and who are they)?

Table 15 Some difficulties for patients and doctors when the diagnosis is hysteria

From the patient's perspective	From the doctor's perspective
Obscure terminology and 'diagnoses'.	Various terms are applied. (It is not always clear whether illness or malingering is being diagnosed.)
The cause is unknown.	Aetiology is unknown.
There are no pathognomonic signs (hence, there is no final 'proof' of illness).	There are no pathognomonic signs (hence, no 'closure', the diagnosis is never 'made', but remains conditional).
The risks of elaboration (to 'prove' that one is 'really' ill).	The fear of missing organicity.
The question of veracity (knowing one may not be 'believed').	The question of veracity (not wanting to be 'fooled').
The stigma of the psychiatric (the final referral after negative findings).	The risk of overinvestigation (and repeatedly chasing rare disorders).
The implications of litigation, such as following a traumatic precipitant (the patient may be understandably ambivalent, wanting to prove harm was done while also wishing to recover.)	The implications of litigation (symptoms may not resolve until legal matters have been settled; hence, the risk of inferred deception, also therapeutic nihilism.)
The risk of being 'difficult', diagnostically or personally.	'Malignant alienation' (failing to help those whom one does not like).

Source: Adapted from Spence (2008).

A phenomenological approach to hysteria

Perhaps, one way through this apparent quagmire is to concentrate, for the time being, on the objective 'signs' rather than the theories and abstractions that accrue around this disorder. What happens in the clinical encounter? Well, the phenomenology of hysteria has been widely described and revisited recently (see Halligan et al., 2001; Merksey, 1995; and Hallett et al., 2006). In the following, I shall focus very much on the *motor* symptoms and signs, largely because these are objectively verifiable and their analysis yields some important clues as to what is going on in this disorder (Table 16).

The central finding in the case of motor hysteria is that a movement disorder, either a deficit or an excess of motoric activity, is found to be without demonstrable organic basis. However, in addition, the physical findings on clinical examination do not 'behave' as they should. Hence, the patient may exhibit paralysis in one context but not in another. A tremor may come and go but not in the ways associated with organic disease. Through distraction or sedation, the physician may reveal preservation of normal function when the patient's attention is directed elsewhere.

Table 16 The phenomenology of motor hysteria and/or conversion

Phenomenological characteristics
Relatively acute onset, classically following an emotional precipitant.
Biologically implausible (behaves as if 'anatomy did not exist' [Freud]).
Variable manifestation (symptomatic inconsistency).
Normal movement emerges with distraction (e.g. on the Hoover test) or with sedation (e.g. with benzodiazepines).
If the symptom is a tremor, it reduces during the performance of rhythmic tapping with the contralateral limb.
If the symptom is an abnormality of gait, it appears uneconomic: it is more energy demanding than alternate forms of locomotion, given the implied deficit.
Co-morbid diagnoses are frequent, commonly depression and/or personality disorder.

Distraction

> Ask a patient to press [the] heel [of their hysterically 'paralyzed' leg] down on the bed while lying supine. When the patient finds that he or she cannot do it, the [physician's] hand is placed under that heel and the patient is asked to lift the opposing ['normal'] limb. The synergistic response of the 'paralyzed' leg produces pressing down of the heel while the 'good' leg is lifted.
>
> (Merskey, 1995, p. 203)

This procedure is known as the Hoover test and it is a means of eliciting neurological inconsistency from a 'hysterical' patient (i.e. our 'hysterical agent'). When performing this test, the physician is examining a patient who is apparently unable to extend their affected leg: that is, they cannot press it down, onto the couch or bed, when asked to do so. Yet, when they are asked to flex their contralateral, 'unaffected' leg, raising it up in the air, the affected limb extends: now it can press into the surface of the bed. So, why did it extend under one condition and not the other? The circumstances of the test suggest that while the patient was primarily attending to their 'abnormal' limb, normal actions were impeded. However, when their attention was diverted to their 'normal' limb, normal movement returned in the 'affected limb'. Hence, there is some connection between the patient's attention to action and their performance of abnormal acts.

In a patient presenting with a unilateral tremor, an organic tremor would persist during the performance of rhythmic activity carried out by the contralateral, unaffected limb, yet in hysteria the outcome is different (O'Suilleabhain and Matsumato, 1998). In the hysterical patient, their tremor reduces when they must attend to their 'good' limb. They cannot 'maintain' their abnormal movement. Hence, once again, it seems as if their attention to action is pivotal in maintaining abnormal motoric performance.

The implication (as in Campbell, 1979) is that the patient's motoric function is most likely to be normal when they are *not attending* to their affected limb, and that when they do attend, their attending itself somehow interferes with movement: that is, it makes it more likely that the emergent movement will be abnormal.

Sedation

Similar conclusions may be deduced from the consequences of using benzodiazepines, barbiturates, or general anaesthetics in hysteria:

> [I]n the stage of excitement the patient will struggle, cry out . . . He will often regain consciousness whilst he is in the act of moving the arm which was formerly paralyzed or using the voice which was formerly dumb.

> (Adrian and Yealland, 1917)

Hence, whether by distraction or sedation, when the physician interrupts the patient's attentional processes, they can reveal the preservation of normal action (in the previously affected domain). This phenomenology has been elaborated upon at length elsewhere (Spence, 1999, 2001, 2006a, 2006b). For the present, its principle implications are the following:

a) While the patient with hysteria is presenting with manifest physical signs of motoric abnormality, there are, latent within him or her, the necessary processes required to carry out physical actions normally.

b) The maintenance of the hysterical sign appears to be dependent on the patient's ability to attend to its production.

c) Distraction or sedation reveals the emergence of normal action.

d) Hence, attention is central to the patient's performance of the abnormal act.

A cognitive architecture

Therefore, the foregoing discussion demonstrates that hysterical phenomena in the motor domain behave like purposeful acts: the patient must attend in order to produce them; distraction or sedation impairs their performance. So, knowing this, can we specify the cognitive neurobiological substrate for such acts?

Well, as we know from the descriptions offered in Chapters 2 and 4, there is a longstanding, computational distinction that may be drawn between those motor behaviours that organisms perform 'automatically' and those that require conscious attention to action. Such a distinction separates those behaviours that have become routine or automated from those that are difficult, complex, or newly acquired. Furthermore, if we borrow the model developed by Tim Shallice and his colleagues (e.g. Shallice, 1988; Shallice and

Burgess, 1996; Chapter 4), then we can identify the putative roles of specific brain regions contributing to the performance of such different modes of behaviour:

1. Although the engagement of 'lower' brain systems, exemplified by the lateral premotor and primary motor cortices, and subcortical foci such as the basal ganglia and cerebellum, may be sufficient to enable the performance of routine tasks,

2. 'Higher' ('executive', 'supervisory attentional system') centres, coterminous with the prefrontal and medial premotor cortices, are implicated in the performance of more novel or complex behaviours.

3. In addition, such higher, executive centres may become involved once more when an already automated task becomes the focus of renewed attention (see Passingham, 1996).

As we know, such a theoretically driven distinction (between the novel and the automated) has its basis in biology. Hence, there is the example of transcortical motor or dynamic aphasia, wherein a patient (often suffering from the effects of a left-sided prefrontal lesion) is unable to generate spontaneous, new speech, though they can repeat the speech of others (see Chapter 2). Similarly, in many functional neuroimaging experiments involving healthy subjects, patterns of frontal activation elicited by novel behaviours and routines have been shown to differ, for example, during verbal fluency (when the subject's free selection of words beginning with a given letter elicits greater prefrontal, executive activation than the passive repetition of other people's words [Frith et al., 1991a and b; Spence et al., 2000]) or during motor skill acquisition (when initial prefrontal activation gives way to posterior and inferior brain activation as the new task becomes automated [Jenkins et al., 1992]). Indeed, in Chapter 4, we examined the relevance of successive basal ganglia–thalamocortical loop systems to such a progression during 'learning'.

The underlying principle in each of these scenarios is that prefrontal, executive systems appear to be selectively engaged whenever a task demands attention or the generation of novelty, whereas posterior and inferior systems suffice when that task has become routine or automated.

Hence, turning once more to hysteria, as we have already seen, the generation of hysterical motor phenomena seems to require the patient's attention to action: while the physician examines the dysfunctional limb or domain, the symptom is present, but if the patient is distracted or sedated, then the symptom remits. Normal motoric function is more likely to re-emerge under these latter conditions. Therefore, from a cognitive perspective, the latent, preserved, 'normal' behaviour resembles a motor routine that can be performed by subordinate brain systems without the intervention of the prefrontal executive (indeed, it re-emerges when the latter is impacted by distraction or sedation). In contrast, hysterical motor phenomena appear to be products of that executive, and seem to require its engagement (see Figs. 85 and 86).

Evidence of the executive

If the above hypothesis (that executive systems are implicated in the genesis and maintenance of hysterical phenomena) is correct, then this should be demonstrable within the domain of pathophysiology. Is there any evidence derived from cognitive neuroscience that the executive is implicated in the cognitive neurobiology of hysteria? Well, a number of studies of hysterical movement disorders shed some light on this question.

An electromyographic study of patients exhibiting tremors, performed by O'Suilleabhain and Matsumoto (1998), is informative. They studied patients with Parkinson's disease, essential (i.e. 'benign') tremor, and psychogenic tremor. They found that the latter group differed from the former groups in two important ways. First, the tremors exhibited by patients of the first two groups oscillated at *different* frequencies across their affected limbs (within the same subject); however, those in psychogenic disorders did not (i.e. in a given patient exhibiting psychogenic tremors, all affected limbs oscillated at the *same* frequency). Second, whereas the former tremors continued to oscillate when the organic (Parkinson's disease and essential tremor) patients

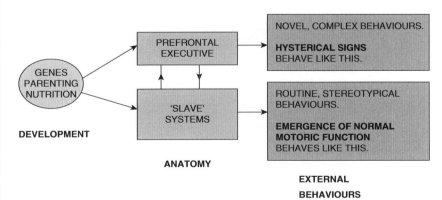

Fig. 85 Schematic demonstrating the basis of hysterical motor phenomena with respect to the organization of the human executive motor system. Hysterical movements behave like intentional actions and hence implicate the prefrontal executive. When physical examination elicits normal motor function, this emerges as a product of intact lower motor systems.

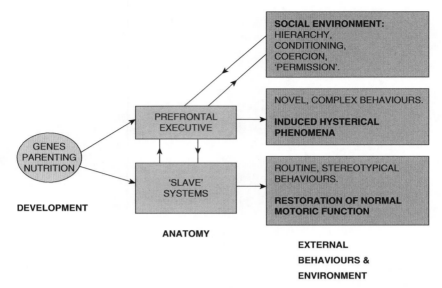

Fig. 86 Schematic demonstrating the influence of social environments on the function of the prefrontal executive. Hysterical phenomena may come and go in response to the social milieu of the patient. Certain environments encourage the exhibition of hysterical motor signs (as was the case in Charcot's Salpêtrière Hospital) whereas other environments serve to reverse such behaviours. The impact of social environments on prefrontal function is underspecified.

were required to tap out rhythms with their contralateral limbs, those due to psychogenic factors were interrupted. The authors concluded that whereas multiple 'oscillator systems' within the central nervous system generated Parkinsonian and essential tremors, psychogenic tremors seemed to rely on *single* oscillators. This means that psychogenic tremors behaved more like voluntary behaviours:

> In psychogenic tremor . . . we propose that the motor system per se is intact, and that rhythmic contractions are mediated by top-down synchronization involving a common oscillator system, perhaps at a higher cerebral level. The tendency of psychogenic trem-or to attenuate when patients are distracted could be explained by a requirement for such high-level involvement.

(O'Suilleabhain and Matsumoto, 1998)

A somewhat similar conclusion emerges from an electroencephalographic study of patients exhibiting psychogenic myoclonus (muscle spasms). As we know from the work of Benjamin Libet, Patrick Haggard, and others (reviewed in the Prologue and Chapter 3), under normal conditions, a spontaneous voluntary act is preceded by an electroencephalographic signal over the vertex, termed the readiness potential or *Bereitschaftspotential*, a signal that is thought to emerge from the medial premotor cortex (supplementary motor area [SMA]). Terada and colleagues (1995) found that such potentials also occurred in five of the six patients with psychogenic myoclonus whom they studied. 'Therefore, it is most likely that the jerks in these patients were generated through the mechanisms common to those underlying voluntary movement' (Terada et al., 1995).

Turning to abnormalities of gait and posture, the available behavioural data suggest that something similar may be happening (i.e. these behaviours are not 'routine': they seem to require *executive* control). The postures adopted in the hysterical realm are not those that would be adopted through purely physical expediencies because they are ergonomically 'uneconomic': that is, they require more energy for their maintenance than alternative modes of locomotion, which subjects would normally be expected to adopt if physically ill (Lempert et al., 1991). Furthermore, hysterical postures are also improved by distraction.

Now, there is a small literature, mostly comprising case reports and small case series, reporting the application of functional neuroimaging techniques (e.g. positron-emission tomography [PET] or functional magnetic resonance imaging [fMRI]) to hysterical disorders. However, it should be noted that frequently there are confounding factors at play (Table 17). So far, most cases described have exhibited co-morbid disorders (such as depression and/or personality disorder) and most have emerged from tertiary treatment centres, so that the patients described may not be typical of hysterical patients in general. However, if there is a common theme that emerges, then it tends to be that where there are sensory deficits (e.g. hysterical anaesthesia or blindness) there is associated hypoactivation of the relevant sensory cortices and evidence of disturbed function in 'higher' frontal regions (Mailis-Gagnon et al., 2003; Tiihonen et al., 1995; Vuillemeumier et al., 2001; Werring et al., 2004; Yazici and Kostakoglu, 1998). However, when the presenting dysfunction is one of motor disturbance, then there is evidence of either excessive activation of inhibitory prefrontal (orbitofrontal) cortices (Marshall et al., 1997) or a suppression of activity in prefrontal (dorsolateral) cortices involved in action generation (Spence et al., 2000). A common view has emerged: lower centres are somehow inhibited or suppressed by 'higher' centres.

Nevertheless, it should be noted that the specificity of these findings is currently uncertain: there is considerable overlap between the functional neuroimaging findings described in these (hysterical) disorders and those emerging in other literatures describing such conditions as chronic fatigue syndrome, somatization disorder, dysmorphophobia, and other anomalies of bodily experience (see Spence, 2006c, for a recent overview). Furthermore, whether a functional neuroimaging approach might ever be capable of distinguishing 'hysteria' from 'feigning' has only been put to the test on one occasion (so far): we reported distinct prefrontal correlates of attempted

Table 17 Problems for neuroimagers wishing to study hysteria

The problems
A scarcity of cases
Scarcity of control groups in reported studies
Symptomatic heterogeneity (thereby making the recruitment of patient groups difficult, and complicating comparison across studies)
Frequent co-morbidity (especially depression and personality disorder)
Difficulty in identifying and assembling suitable control groups (e.g. 'depressed' and 'personality disordered' groups in addition to 'healthy controls')
Studies tend to emerge from tertiary centres (thus, cases are likely to be atypical.)
May be confounded by reporting bias (those with coherent positive findings more likely to be written up and accepted for publication than negative findings.)
Establishing a suitable protocol for the scanner (whether to choose a task that the patient can perform, and hence risk problems with interpretation, or choose a task they find difficult and risk non-adherence or performance as a confounding variable)
Most studies have not addressed the issue of 'intent' (i.e. how do investigators establish whether or not patients are 'trying' to perform the task?)

movements during performance of a motor task by patients with hysterical motor weakness, people performing the task normally, and a small group of subjects who we had taught to 'fake' limb weakness (Spence et al., 2000). The results are displayed in Fig. 87. One preliminary conclusion may be that, for all their phenomenological and electrophysiological similarities, hysterical motor phenomena and feigning or malingering are not necessarily the 'same', neurobiologically.

The place of the social

From the foregoing review, with its emphasis on both the behaviours and the brains of individual patients, it is possible to overlook the fact that all hysterical phenomena arise within social milieus, and that this applies whether one considers their initial appearance 'in the community' or their manipulation in therapeutic encounters (Spence, 1999; and see Wenegrat, 2001). Indeed, if this were not the case, then the presence or absence of staff would not have its (noted) effect in the modern setting and unobtrusive observation of patients would not yield evidence of 'symptomatic inconsistency' in the way that it does at present (see Baker and Silver, 1987).

However, the influence of the social is all the more apparent if one considers the specific social conditions that spawned the emergence of the modern literature on hysteria. At the end of the nineteenth and the beginning of the twentieth centuries, there were three settings in which reported case material was

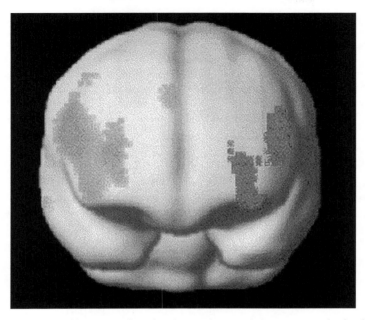

Fig. 87 A smoothed brain template showing positron-emission tomography (PET) data obtained from patients with hysteria, healthy controls feigning motor abnormality, and healthy controls performing motor tasks normally. Patients exhibiting hysterical motor phenomena had reduced prefrontal activation in the left dorsolateral and ventrolateral prefrontal regions (red). In contrast, healthy subjects who are asked to deliberately feign motor impairment had reduced activity in the right prefrontal regions (green). Reprinted from *The Lancet* 355/9211. Discrete neuropsychological correlates in prefrontal cortex during hysterical and feigned disorder of movement. Spence SA et al (2000) with permission from Elsevier Ltd. (See colour plate section).

particularly abundant and influential: Charcot's practice at the Salpêtrière Hospital in Paris, Freud's private practice in Vienna, and the battlefront of the First World War. When reading such historical accounts, one is often struck by the possible contribution of particular personal and social factors to the emergence of some of the more bizarre phenomena described. For instance, consider the impact of Charcot's personality and his milieu on other people's behaviour.

The production of signs

> Strange things were said about [Charcot's] hold on the Salpetriere's hysterical young women and about happenings there . . . [D]uring a patient's ball . . . a gong was inadvertently sounded, whereupon many hysterical women instantaneously fell into catalepsy and kept [the] plastic poses in which they found themselves when the gong was sounded.

> (Ellenberger, 1994)

The resolution of signs

There was . . . a young lady who had been paralyzed for years. Charcot bade her stand up and walk, which she did under the astounded eyes of her parents and of the Mother Superior of the convent in which she had been staying. Another . . . was brought to Charcot with a paralysis of both legs. [He] found no organic lesions; the consultation was not yet over when the patient stood up and walked back to the door where the cabman, who was waiting for her, took off his hat in amazement and crossed himself.

(Ellenberger, 1994)

What is occurring beneath the surface of such spectacular enactments and miraculous recoveries? Well, we seem to witness the manifestation of the force of Charcot's personality and the belief that others had in him, both in his manipulation of their behaviour and the elicitation of their recovery. According to Brant Wenegrat (2001), these sorts of concentrations of diagnosis and cure, occurring within very specific clinical settings and involving powerful medical figures, should make us question the veracity of the disease model being propounded. Wenegrat has studied many of our own culture's more florid contemporary neurotic and subcultural afflictions (including possession, multiple personality disorder, and alien abduction) and concluded that they involve role enactments, arising under the influence (conscious or otherwise) of powerful people (often, medical doctors). We should be particularly cautious when a new diagnosis or disorder, lacking demonstrable organic pathology, exhibits incidence rates that fluctuate widely, where certain clinicians diagnose many, most, or all of the cases (and others do not) and where prestige accrues (to either doctor or patient) through the accordance of 'special' status.

Such considerations are especially relevant when we consider the emergence of hysteria, under particular conditions of inequality and disempowerment. It has been argued that Charcot's patients came from rural poverty and faced uncertain futures (including a life of prostitution) if they did not 'perform' in his clinical setting (for a most graphic demonstration of this thesis, see Didi-Huberman, 2003). Similarly, we can see in the early psychotherapeutic work of Freud an emphasis on the plights of women drawn from the bourgeoisie, who were subject to the inalienable power and control of men. Then, later, among the soldiers who exhibited unusual movements in the First World War, we see the explicit application of power, through rank and social class structures, under conditions of very real danger (where the consequences of both failing to fight and recovering in order to fight could be death, by firing squad or enemy fire, respectively):

'[T]he patient must be convinced that the physician understands his case and is able to cure him . . . [T]he best attitude to adopt is one of mild boredom bred of perfect familiarity with the patient's disorder . . .'

(Adrian and Yealland, 1917)

'[Hysterical paralyses respond to] a little plain speaking accompanied by a strong faradic current.'

(Adrian and Yealland, 1917)

'Without any further discussion the motor areas of the cortex were mapped out roughly [on the patient's skull], the measurements being repeated aloud to impress and mystify the patient. He was told [that] as soon as the shoulder area of the cortex was stimulated by faradism he would be able to raise his shoulder and that the rest of the arm would recover in the same way . . . He [moved] at once [after electricity], and in a few minutes the whole of the paralysis had disappeared and he could raise 30 pounds.'

(Adrian and Yealland, 1917)

It is important to recognize what is being described here, events that occurred in wartime England. You have just read accounts of how medical doctors administered electricity to soldiers, men who had already risked their lives for their country under the most inhumane of conditions. The 'goal' appears to have been their subsequent return to the Front. That there may have been a gulf in understanding, reaching out between the 'physicians' and the 'men', is indicated (I believe) in this following account, reported by May (1998):

I found him staring into the fire. He had not shaved and his trousers were half open. I could get nothing out of him . . . He did not appear to be ill. We agreed to let him rest, to let him stay in his billet till the battalion came out of the trenches. But next day when everyone had gone up the line he blew his head off. I thought little of it at the time; it seemed a silly thing to do.

Hence, I hope that the reader may accept that any comprehensive account of hysterical motor phenomena must reserve a place for the 'social', for 'con-specific' influences, for the role of the interpersonal, influences exchanged between human actors. One hypothesis might be that the presence of 'superiors' in the prevailing social hierarchy impacts the executive system of the hysterical patient, such that the emergence of further hysterical motor signs is either facilitated or prevented (as in the Charcot examples recounted earlier), through either an inhibition of the executive (allowing the emergence, we might even say the 'escape', of 'normal' motor routines) or its facilitation, through coercion or the 'permission' granted to generate new, perhaps even extravagant, motor behaviours (as when the gong sounded during the dance at the Salpêtrière).

The nearest our modern, cognitive literature has come to exploring this feature of hysteria (the putative role of powerful 'others') is in the modelling of symptoms using hypnosis, where susceptible subjects are influenced to produce physical signs resembling those of hysteria (indeed, it is of interest that one such study in the literature reported functional brain images very similar to those of a hysterical patient studied by the same group.) There is clearly a need for further work in this area.

'Others' and others: a note on Zizek

From this account, we may conclude that the motor behaviours exhibited by people with hysteria behave rather like purposeful actions, although patients deny awareness of their causation. Indeed, our diagnostic systems contain both the stipulation that such motor phenomena be (potentially) subject to voluntary control and the criterion that we conclude that the patient is not consciously producing them (i.e. that they are not feigning; Table 14). Instead, we must believe that hysterical phenomena are generated from within the patient's psyche, while not reflecting their sense of agency (their conscious awareness of their own volition).

Hence, it might be concluded that although the cognitive neurobiological approach taken in this chapter can predict the brain systems that 'should' be involved in the generation of the behaviours described (Fig. 85), and that this is consistent with what we know of the empirical literature to date (explained in the preceding), nevertheless, in a sense, we are no nearer to discovering the nature of the underlying pathophysiology itself and its relation to the contents of consciousness. How do we answer the fundamental question that we set ourselves at the very beginning of this chapter?

How can a motor or sensory symptom be produced in the absence of a physical cause?

Or, to put things in another way: Have we really made any advance beyond Sigmund Freud, and his invocation of the role of the psychodynamic unconscious? My response is that 'yes, we have', for we have demonstrated that consciousness and, more specifically, *attention* are required for the production of hysterical motor phenomena. It is the diversion of attention away from such symptoms and signs that leads to their resolution. It is the dimming of conscious awareness through sedation or anaesthesia that renders activity normal again. Hence, we may state quite explicitly that attention, *not the dynamic unconscious*, is what maintains hysterical signs. Thus, some progress has been made, though no firmer conclusions may be drawn at present.

Nevertheless, there is a strand of contemporary psychodynamic thought that may be of relevance when considering the 'content' of hysterical symptoms. By content we mean the particular manifestation of hysteria exhibited, such as a weakness of the right hand, or a speech impediment. How might we understand these phenomena without recourse to speculative interpretation (e.g. 'the patient cannot move her arm because, unconsciously, she wishes to hit her father')?

In the following, we offer one view that may inform any future attempts to reconcile psychodynamic understandings of hysteria with those derived from cognitive neuroscience. However, in order to do this, we need to consider the work of Jacques Lacan (1901–1981) and its extension in the current writings of Slavoj Zizek (see Myers, 2003, for an accessible overview). We must also introduce some Lacanian terms that will be pivotal to describing hysteria.

The Real and the Symbolic

Stated simply, Lacan described a distinction between the nature of reality itself, the Real, which is the true nature of the world, beyond our language and ultimate comprehension, and the Symbolic, the common language system that we use to describe what may be put into words. We may not have any choice over the nature of the Symbolic universe that we inhabit, for we are brought up to speak a given language by our parents, and when we use words we are usually borrowing them, their meanings having been determined by others before us (Chapter 2). Hence, we can be said to inhabit the Symbolic, and we have only partial awareness of the Real (that which is underpinning our existence and is beyond words).

Now, Zizek's contribution to this field has been to extend the Lacanian account into politics and the arts in quite engaging and exciting ways. For instance, he has written much about the films of Alfred Hitchcock and the manifestations of paternal authority and power in the work of the modern film director David Lynch (Zizek, 1991, 2000). He has also described how the Real may rupture the Symbolic order, in circumstances where words will not suffice, such as in the immediate emergence of violence, or trauma, or even of the obscene. For, if a film comprises a conventional 'Hollywood' narrative, then Zizek argues that it cannot withstand the inclusion of truly obscene, explicit material, for this constitutes the intrusion of the Real, and so the narrative, the Symbolic order, is ruptured. Therefore, a conventional Hitchcock narrative would be ruptured if the auteur showed the audience explicit sexual material, rather than resorting to conventional Hollywood 'signifiers': the lights are dimmed, a saxophone plays romantically in the distance, and night becomes morning. Now, for our current purposes, it is interesting to consider this tension between the Symbolic and the Real and to see what relevance each might have to the clinical case of hysteria.

We have noted earlier (in Table 16) Freud's remark that hysteria behaves as if 'anatomy did not exist', referring to the symptomatic inconsistency apparent on physical examination and observation. The symptoms and signs of hysteria do not reflect neurological reality; instead, they reflect the patient's idea or understanding of neurology. To borrow the Lacanian terms just described, the

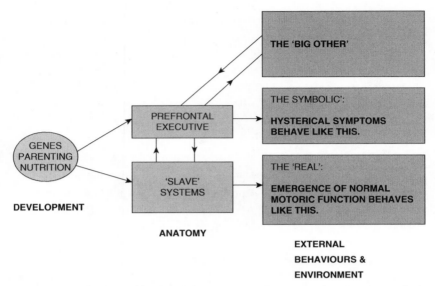

Fig. 88 Schematic showing how contemporary Lacanian terminology may be applied to the phenomenology of hysteria. In this case, the social milieu is represented by the 'Big Other'. Hysterical symptoms represent the symbolic order whereas the emergence of normal motor function reflects what Lacan would call the 'real'.

patient's symptoms and signs comprise expressions of the Symbolic order (i.e. the lay cultural view of what a given neurological syndrome comprises) not the Real (i.e. the 'true' biology constituting our nervous systems). Hence, in hysteria, the Symbolic attempts to obscure the Real.

However, what happens in the clinical examination, if we combine the Lacanian account with a rehearsal of the Hoover test, is that the patient begins by performing the Symbolic (in the apparent inability to extend the 'affected' leg) but, when distracted, evinces the Real (a non-linguistic sign, which comprises solely the physical): the 'affected' limb extends normally, pushing into the bed when the contralateral 'good' leg undergoes flexion. Hence, we may begin to substitute the Lacanian terms for those deployed in our cognitive neurobiological account of hysteria (moving from Figs. 85–88). The symptom expresses the Symbolic; the restored, normal function evinces the Real.

But that is not all. For the Zizekian account of artistic works also places especial emphasis upon male power, the dominance of the social order beyond the family (the so-called Big Other). Such power may be perverse and arbitrary; the 'subject' is literally subject to its will. Indeed, we see this power in action in tyrannical states and abusive homes; those who hold the power may literally do 'whatever they like' to those who are without it, the powerless.

So, this provides another perspective from which to view the conditions prevailing at the outset of modern accounts of hysteria, where the power discrepancy between doctors and their patients was most pronounced and where the consequences for those patients seen and assessed (particularly at the Salpêtrière and at the Front) could be most severe indeed.

Hence, to summarize: we may combine our recognition that the cognitive executive is pivotal to the maintenance of hysterical phenomena with an acknowledgement that their symptomatic content reflects the cultural understanding of a disease (i.e. it reflects the Symbolic order). When the symptom remits, through distraction, sedation, or the influence of the physician, the Real emerges, the normal, motor routine, which is procedural and beyond words. The influence of specific, sometimes powerful, human beings and of human culture is itself manifest both in the symptom and in the timing of its relapse and resolution. The Big Other (culture) and 'others' (our conspecifics) affect the way human beings behave. Any final cognitive neurobiological account of hysteria must find a way of acknowledging and investigating these elements of the Real.

Chapter 8

Deceivers all

Defenceless villages are bombarded from the air, the inhabitants driven out into the countryside, the cattle machine-gunned, the huts set on fire with incendiary bullets: this is called *pacification*. Millions of peasants are robbed of their farms and sent trudging along the roads with no more than they can carry: this is called *transfer of population* or *rectification of frontiers*. People are imprisoned for years without trial, or shot in the back of the neck or sent to die of scurvy in Arctic lumber camps: this is called *elimination of unreliable elements*. Such phraseology is needed if one wants to name things without calling up mental pictures of them.[17]

The honest man must be a perpetual renegade.[18]

There are two problems that acquire increasing salience as we make our journey through this book. First, if we really wish to approach an understanding of human volition, that is, *intentional* voluntary behaviour, then it is clear that there are more pressing behaviours in want of such elucidation, than the mere movement of a joystick in circles or the generation of individual words beginning with the letter 'S' (while lying in a brain scanner; Chapter 2). For, much of what really matters in human affairs is altogether more complex than these highly artificial behavioural 'abstractions' and often rife with conflicting ethical imperatives. Second, the more that we wish to understand what humans actually do in 'real life' (and how they go about doing it), the greater is the

---

[17] George Orwell. An extract from 'Politics and the English language', cited in Bromwich D, Euphemism and American violence, *New York Review of Books*, April 3rd 2008, 28–30 (citation is from p. 28).

[18] From the French writer Charles Peguy.

relevance of *other* people, other actors. For, although the human brain is an organ encased in bones, it is also an organ situated within a community of other brains. Others may facilitate or set the boundaries of our acts. Eventually, we all impact upon the 'interpersonal' (and see Chapter 7).

So it is that in this chapter we address what is currently known about the cognitive neurobiological basis of an inherently interpersonal behaviour—that is, deception, deceit, or lying—by which we mean the deliberate attempt to mislead another person by creating a false belief in their mind. Indeed, although the literature concerning the neurobiology of lying is altogether 'younger' than those assayed in earlier chapters of this book, it is one that has already witnessed tremendous advances within the space of less than 10 years. Furthermore (and as has been exemplified by the content of the preceding chapter, concerning 'hysteria'), there are many situations in human life where we must either take the intentions of another agent on trust (i.e. 'at face value') or else accept that we cannot 'know' what another person is thinking, and hence persist in attempting to manage our consequent uncertainty.

There is a very real limit, a phenomenological boundary, to the extent to which we may 'read' others' minds and we would do well to remember this, especially when the consequences of failure are severe (for 'us' or 'them'). However, notwithstanding this problem, there is the prospect that we might eventually understand ourselves rather better if we could study deceit under controlled conditions and learn what it is about our brains (and, ultimately, our genetic endowment) that enables 'us' (as a species) to behave in this way. Furthermore, should we discover that 'higher' brain centres are necessarily implicated in deceit, then might that not tell us something interesting about the 'responsibilities' of a deceiver? *A deceiver is*, by definition, *necessarily aware of what they are doing.* I shall say more about these issues in due course.

Telling lies and influencing people

> *Lie: a false statement made with the intention of deceiving.*
>
> (*Chambers Concise Dictionary*, 1991)

Despite injunctions to the contrary, human beings engage in lies and deceit on a fairly regular basis, although not necessarily always in order to 'dupe' others. While children may be told that lying is bad, they might also be told not to be rude, not to hurt others' feelings or appear insensitive. Hence, there is an implied limit to 'reasonable' disclosure. Indeed, in later life, a totally frank exchange of views may leave both parties feeling rather bruised and it is commonly conceded that a certain amount of 'tact and diplomacy' or 'information management' is necessary when navigating one's path among one's neighbours (see Vrij [2000] for an accessible overview). Hence,

> '[O]ne must know best how to colour one's actions and to be a great liar and deceiver.'
> (Niccol Machiavelli, 1999, p. 57)

In formal social psychological research, two findings are highly replicated: first, lies are very common (daily events), especially those that are told to life partners and parents, and second, humans are poor at detecting when they are being deceived (Vrij, 2000). So, although many subjects might believe that they are astute detectors of deception, the empirical data suggest that most of us are operating at, or a little above, the level of chance. Hence, in one seminal study, Ekman and O'Sullivan (1991) reported the following levels of deception detection among various professional groups (where 50% would have equated to 'chance' or random levels of accuracy):

U.S. Secret Service agents: 64%
Federal polygraphers: 56%
Robbery investigators: 56%
Judges: 57%
Psychiatrists: 58%
College students: 53%

Furthermore, in an enormous meta-analysis of more than 200 studies describing the combined responses of 24 483 subjects, Bond and DePaulo (2006) found that the average deception detection rate lay in the region of 54% (i.e. little better than chance).

Hence, although some Secret Service personnel, and indeed some convicted offenders, may detect deceit at 'better-than-chance' levels (Ekman and O'Sullivan, 1991; Granhag and Stromwall, 2004), we humans generally share a 'truth bias': that is, we tend to assume that others are speaking truthfully (even when they are not). Moreover, there may be sound (admittedly teleological) reasons for such a bias: not to believe others would eventually render one 'paranoid' (in the lay sense of the word); all information would require independent verification and cross-checking; life would be lived most inefficiently. Indeed, as demonstrated by recent economic scares, and widespread political disengagement, a lack of trust greatly impedes social intercourse; it is mutually disadvantageous (Galbraith, 2004; Oborne, 2006). Also, a breakdown of trust may be associated with other signs of social pathology: in recent studies, the magnitude of economic polarization (inequality) has been implicated in the increasing mistrust, depression, and violence seen in some Western democracies (Layard, 2005; Wilkinson, 2005). So, although trusting others might seem 'naive' at times, it also appears to constitute a healthier way of life.

Nevertheless, in the struggle for survival, even an evolved process may leave us with vulnerabilities when we enter the 'wrong' environment, and it has been posited (by game theorists) that the truth bias detectable in human interactions leaves open the way for a small number of 'freeloaders', 'cheats', or psychopaths to prosper (Mealey, 1995). The theory is that while most subjects adopt a trusting policy, a small number of cheats might 'get away' with cheating, so long as they are diffusely distributed among the population. Hence, they can always move on and away from those they have cheated once they have conned them. If, however, a subject becomes recognized as a cheat, then their survival depends upon their adopting either a rapid change of location or a radical change of policy! Notice, also, that a society largely composed of cheats and misanthropes would be very likely to stall (who would enter into any kind of binding agreement if they assumed their interlocutors to be liars?). Therefore, in a mutually paranoid society, life would be constrained to immediate, short-term contingencies; there could be no long-term planning, and no lasting agreements or alliances.

Conversely, the attempt to deceive another also tells us something rather interesting about the mind of the putative deceiver. It suggests that he understands, implicitly or explicitly, that different people may hold different perspectives on the same subject, simultaneously; in other words, agents experience different thoughts (O'Connell, 1998). Hence, at some level, the deceiver possesses a 'theory of mind' and this would appear to be a prerequisite for his assumption that what he says or does (i.e. his intended deceit) is not immediately detectable by his interlocutor. The deceiver requires such a theory of mind in order for him to believe that he might actually be able to create a false belief in the mind of another (i.e. that he might 'get away with it').

Now, the human developmental literature suggests that children develop the ability to attempt deceit (though not necessarily with any accompanying success) at about 3–4 years of age (O'Connell, 1998). Moreover, this also coincides with their development of theory-of-mind abilities: hence, they come to understand that they can know something that their carer does not know; therefore, there is the possibility of managing information (*I didn't hit Mark, Mummy, Nicky did it!*).

Thus, when he engages in deceit, a deceiver seems to acknowledge (at least implicitly) that different agents can believe different things; he seems to understand (at some level) what philosophers call 'intentionality':

> *I know p.*
> *He does not know p.*
> *I know that he does not know p.*
> *Therefore, I may try to make him believe q.*

Clearly, there is the potential for some form of hierarchical regression here, receding 'into the distance' throughout individual minds or brains (with different levels of awareness and understanding) and also the mass of human communications, as we attribute different levels of intentionality to our own and others' mental states. Indeed, we may witness the distortion of such a process when a paranoid (in the 'psychotic' sense, deluded) patient attributes knowledge to individuals who do not possess it *(He knows what's going on)* or when conspiracy theorists tell us that the 'truth is out there' (*There are key players, the masons and templars, who know the truth, but they are misleading everyone else . . .*). There seems to be a notion that different, distant players in this game of deceit enjoy different levels of intentionality. (Indeed, this 'talent', for understanding and retaining multiple levels of intentionality, may be the stuff of which great writers are made [Dunbar, 2005].)

However, the crucial point, and one to which we shall return later, is that an episode of *attempted* deceit tells us something about the mental state of the deceiver; it denotes premeditation; it suggests 'intent'; hence, it informs our notions of their moral responsibility.

The evolution of deception

Although the use of camouflage and distraction has a very long evolutionary past, stretching back over millennia to incorporate relatively primitive organisms (Giannetti, 2000), some 'knowing' use of deception (apparently accompanied by a degree of insight into the deceived other's perspective) is a behaviour that appears to reach its apogee among primates. The work of Richard Byrne and his colleagues is particularly informative in this regard (e.g. Byrne, 2003). Hence, when human researchers observe non-human primate colonies, the subjects of such observation can sometimes be seen to engage in seemingly 'deliberate' deception of their conspecifics. The usual misdemeanours concern access to food and sex, and it seems as if some 'higher' primates can deploy normal elements of their behavioural repertoires in such a way as to mislead their opposition (to their own subsequent advantage). Such behaviour has been termed 'tactical deception' and, allowing for the frequency with which human researchers will have studied different primate species (and, hence, accrued positive observations), it seems that the frequency of such tactical deception increases in the evolutionarily more advanced primates (i.e. gorillas, bonobos, and chimpanzees, sharing a common ancestor approximately 12 million years ago; Fig. 89), and bears a statistical relationship to the volume of their neocortices (Fig. 90). Hence, Byrne (2003) writes:

'Simply knowing the ratio of the brain volume taken up by the neocortex, divided by the volume of the rest of the brain, enables us to predict 60% of the variance in the amount of deception that is observed in the species concerned.' (p. 51)

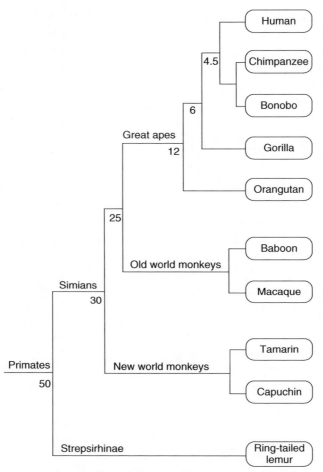

Fig. 89 A cladogram showing different primate species and the approximate times of their evolutionary divergence (in millions of years). Tactical deception is observed the most among those primates towards the top of the cladogram (specifically, gorillas, bonobos, and chimpanzees). The implication is that tactical deception will be even more prominent among humans! Reproduced from *The Social Brain–Evolution and Pathology*. Brune M, Ribbert H and Schiefenhovel W 2003. Copyright John Wiley & Sons Ltd. Reproduced with permission.

One implication is that 'higher' centres located within the primate brain facilitate this (relatively) recently elaborated behaviour: the 'knowing' use of deception (Byrne and Corp, 2004). Nevertheless, in the absence of direct access to other primates' mental states (i.e. their hypothesized consciousness), we cannot tell to what extent their actions are indeed 'conscious' or 'premeditated'. All we can say is that certain of their behaviours appear 'knowing' in their deployment.

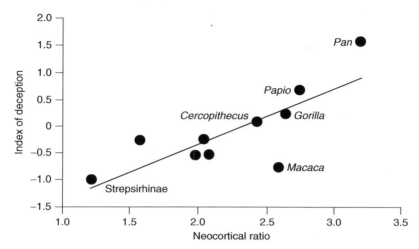

Fig. 90 Graph demonstrating a linear relationship between the frequency of observed tactical deception in different primate species and the neocortical ratio (an index of evolutionarily enhanced 'higher' centres in the primate brain). Deception becomes more common as the higher centres undergo relative expansion. (From Byrne 2003: 52). Reproduced from *The Social Brain–Evolution and Pathology*. Brune M, Ribbert H and Schiefenhovel W 2003. Copyright John Wiley & Sons Ltd. Reproduced with permission.

Another implication of such work is that it locates human behaviour at the end of an evolutionary trajectory; hence, human deception, in all its many guises, may be similarly supported by biological changes, and facilitated by adaptive changes in (relatively 'recent') cognitive neurobiological architectures. Moreover, if we hypothesize that this is the case, then we may extend our theory to suggest that 'higher' brain systems will also be engaged (and 'activated') when humans tell lies (Spence, 2004).

The psychiatry of deception

Now, from the first principles, it seems reasonable to posit that 'trust' and our human 'truth bias' will be most exposed (to error and/or exploitation) during those encounters in which the phenomena to be discussed by two or more interlocutors are inherently subjective, where only one party has direct access to the information concerned, such as when that material comprises the contents of their own (personal) states of consciousness. Hence, a discipline such as psychiatry, concerned as it is with abnormalities of phenomenology (the subjective mental state), must place especial emphasis upon enhancing the relationship between speakers (and their mutual veracity). Listening very closely to what others say is a central component of the medical process, but of course it can misfire. Differences in class, culture, education, and assumptions about life and the world may each lead to honest confusions—misunderstandings.

However, there will also be occasions when one or the other party sets out to deliberately mislead their interlocutor, or falls into such a procedure as a way of avoiding unpleasantness (an 'easier option'). Doctors have traditionally been accused of failing to disclose a patient's diagnosis, especially when its associated prognosis is poor; some have administered placebos, purportedly benignly but nevertheless paternalistically, in that they deliberately misled their patients (Sokol, 2006). Meanwhile, patients may conceal their non-adherence to treatments, their disagreement with the doctor, or their seeking of (simultaneous) opinions and treatments elsewhere, and sometimes, deception may be more integral to their state (Table 18, left column; see Hughes et al., 2005).

We may identify two categories of psychiatric syndrome that involve some element of deception:

1. Those where deception is *central* to the diagnosis itself (as in antisocial and psychopathic personalities, malingering, etc.), and

2. Those where deception arises as a *consequence* of something else, contingent upon another disturbance of functioning (e.g. as in the addictions or eating disorders, where patients may be embarrassed or ashamed of some of their thoughts and actions and therefore seek to conceal them).

Now, to acknowledge the possible occurrence of deception is not necessarily to make moral judgements regarding individual patients; rather, it is to acknowledge

Table 18 Psychiatric syndromes involving deception, directly or indirectly

Deception central to diagnosis	Deception a possible consequence
Conduct disorder	Eating disorders
Antisocial personality disorder	Alcohol addiction
Psychopathy	Substance misuse disorders
Munchausen's syndrome	Paraphilias
Munchausen's syndrome by proxy (factitious or induced illness [FII])	Obsessive-compulsive disorder
Malingering	
'Pathological lying'	
Instrumental psychosis	

There are other psychiatric concepts in which the question of deception is controversial, ambiguous, or the 'victim' is thought to be the subject herself: for example, in conversion and dissociation syndromes (hysteria), the 'Ganser' state, the psychodynamic 'defence' mechanisms, 'self-deception', and delusions.

that human communication may be complex and multilayered and that, although we do not wish to judge others, we may sometimes have to anticipate what they are thinking and doing. In some cases, the deception may harm the patient himself or herself (as when a suicidal intent is denied but then acted upon or a depressed patient collects potentially dangerous medicines from more than one treating physician, simultaneously, in circumstances where each is unaware of the others' existence, such as in 'private practice'). Sometimes, the harm is directed towards others (e.g. a sexual victim is being 'groomed' although intent is denied; a perceived persecutor is being stalked with a view to 'revenge'). There are many possible scenarios played out within the psychological and psychiatric treatment realms (Table 18).

Pathological lying

Now, if lying is a 'normal' aspect of human behaviour, can it ever be termed 'pathological'? Well, the literature seems to admit two broad possibilities:

1. Those cases where lying is repeatedly used to harm *others*, to con and to cheat them (e.g. Yang et al., 2005);

2. Those cases where 'stories' are told, which may be improbable or fantastic but which do not seem designed to gain any tangible reward. The tellers of such tales often seem to harm *themselves* by their habits; indeed, their motivations remain obscure (e.g. in Munchausen's syndrome, *pseudologia fantastica*; Bass, 2001).

There have been relatively few empirical studies of the biology of pathological lying, but one sequence of work has been especially informative. Adrian Raine's group have studied antisocial people living in the community in Los Angeles and have found that, compared with control groups, they exhibit reduced pre-frontal grey matter volume. However, among those antisocial people who also exhibit a pattern of repeated lying and cheating (e.g. in the context of fraud and malingering), they have found an excessive volume of prefrontal white matter (Yang et al., 2005), especially in orbitofrontal cortices (Yang et al., 2007), even when compared with other antisocials. Hence, given what we have alluded to with respect to primate evolution, and the sociological, game theory notion that psychopathy may represent a persistent, stable evolutionary strat-egy (if minimally represented in human societies [Mealey, 1995]), it becomes conceivable, as suggested by Raine's group, that antisocial pathological liars are somehow 'aided' in their deceit by a facility bestowed upon them by differ-ences in their prefrontal white matter structure. More white matter, more neural 'connections', might facilitate cognitive operations. Furthermore, this would be congruent with an older psychiatric literature suggesting that such liars exhibit enhanced verbal skills (Ford et al., 1988). This is a fascinating line of work and argument, with wide-ranging implications. However, we must acknowledge one possible caveat: at present, we cannot say definitively whether such prefrontal findings represent a 'cause' or an 'effect' (Spence, 2005). In other words, does (constitutional) brain structure predispose to lying or does repeated lying alter brain structure? At present, we cannot say, although Aristotle (1998) would seem to have favoured the latter scenario:

> '[M]en become builders by building, and lyre-players by playing the lyre; so too we become just by doing just acts, temperate by doing temperate acts, brave by doing brave acts.' (p. 29)

Pathological truthfulness

Whereas some psychiatric disorders are associated with a propensity towards deception, others may be associated with an apparent 'failure' to deceive. For instance, it has long been recognized that children with autism exhibit difficulties in deceiving others, which may be related to impairments in their abilities to 'mind read' or appreciate others' perspectives (deficits affecting their 'theory of mind'; e.g. Happe, 1994). Indeed, the existence of such a pathological scenario also serves to highlight the ambivalence manifest by human cultures with respect to lying (alluded to earlier): although deception is overtly discouraged and purportedly immoral, its relative absence may be indicative of psychopathology. Hence, intermittent dishonesty rather than consistent truthfulness is inherently acknowledged as constituting the statistical 'norm'. It is the person who is consistently truthful who comes to be labelled as 'abnormal'. Therefore, this is one case where morality and biology seem to be diametrically opposed (Spence, 2004).

However, although it is likely that the failure of cognitive processing revealed by pathological 'truthfulness', in the context of autism, implicates aberrant frontal lobe processes (e.g. Fletcher et al., 1995), autism is, of course, also associated with a great many other psychopathological disturbances and impairments of development (i.e. it is not solely comprised of 'pathological truthfulness'.) Hence, it would be potentially more informative to ask specifically whether pathological truthfulness can ever emerge *de novo* among adults who have previously evinced 'normal' development. There are two lines of enquiry that are informative here:

1. In some patients with orbitofrontal lesions, a behaviour termed 'pseudo-psychopathy' has been described, characterized by 'outspokenness', lack of 'tact and restraint', and being 'brash and disrespectful', 'open and frank' (Blumer and Benson, 1975).

2. There is also recent empirical evidence that such patients (with orbitofrontal lesions) are unnecessarily confiding, overly intimate in the details that they share with strangers (Beer et al., 2003).

Taken together, these strands of evidence (admittedly emerging from rather small literatures) point to a possible relationship between prefrontal (especially orbitofrontal) lobe function and a subject's veracity. Although those who lie to harm others may exhibit increased orbitofrontal cortex (OFC) white matter (Yang et al., 2007), those who experience lesions in similar regions (during adulthood) may be rendered 'tactless' and inappropriately truthful (Blumer and Benson, 1975). On the background of what we have learnt from non-human primate studies, it seems permissible to hypothesize that developments within orbitofrontal regions can be implicated in the emergence of the human capacity for bearing false witness.

Neuroimaging of deceit

To summarize, much of the evidence that we have considered thus far has relied upon 'natural experiments' for its acquisition: the observations of field researchers working among non-human primates, the consequences of brain damage to formerly 'normal' humans, or the unknown aetiology of those difficulties in communication encountered by people with autism. To rely on such sources of information in constructing a biological neuroscience of deception would condemn researchers to the protracted, opportunistic acquisition of 'special' cases; in other words, its advance would be largely stochastic. However, the recent advent, and widespread availability, of functional neuroimaging technology has afforded us the opportunity of studying deception in the healthy living brain in a planned, stepwise progression. Indeed, functional neuroimaging has allowed scientists to probe a vast array of cognitive processes and to rapidly gather information about candidate brain regions implicated in these and similar functions. There has been a radical expansion of the field of reasonable enquiry open to contemporary neuroscientists and the rate of data acquisition has been rapid. With modern brain imaging techniques, we really may begin to ask the question *which are the brain systems implicated in telling a lie?*

Therefore, in the following account, I am going to follow a line of research emerging from our own laboratory. Though I shall say very little about other neuroimaging groups' data, these have been the subjects of recent reviews and detailed accounts may be found in Spence et al. (2004) and Spence (2008).

Cognitive subtraction

To date, the methods of functional neuroimaging used in deception research have shared a common feature: they have all relied upon proxy markers of synaptic activity to infer changes in local neuronal function when subjects undertake different cognitive tasks, such as telling the truth and telling a lie. Local changes in synaptic activity are associated with changes in regional cerebral blood flow (rCBF) and also the oxygenation state of blood haemoglobin. Essentially, local changes in synaptic activity (resulting in increased local metabolism) precipitate an 'overcompensation' in the haemodynamic response, such that blood flow increases to the brain area concerned and the blood's haemoglobin goes from being relatively deficient in oxygen (deoxy-haemoglobin having increased, consequent upon the increased local synaptic activity) to accumulating a relative excess of oxygenated haemoglobin (oxy-haemoglobin). Such changes, accompanying local synaptic activity, are the parameters measured in positron-emission tomography (PET; where a 'radiotracer' such as Oxygen^{15} labelled water provides the signal through which changes in rCBF volume may be detected) and functional magnetic resonance imaging (fMRI; where the blood oxygen level-dependent [BOLD] response constitutes the proxy measure).

Hence, central to current studies has been the requirement that subjects are studied under more than one 'cognitive condition' (i.e. in more than one mental state), so that their proxy measures of synaptic activity may be contrasted in data analyses, through 'cognitive subtraction' (e.g. subtracting those brain images acquired when the subject was telling the truth from those acquired while he or she was lying), in order to reveal those brain regions exhibiting areas of increased neuronal response associated with the latter, lying, condition (relative to the truth condition):

[Lie scans] − [Truth scans] = Areas of activity associated with lying

Hence, this enterprise is targeted upon locating anatomical regions of physiological *difference* emerging between these cognitive states (i.e. in the preceding, the subtraction would *not* reveal those areas of brain activation *shared in common* by lying and telling the truth, though these might be elicited through other experimental designs).

Practical matters

It should be noted that the success of this enterprise depends upon many levels of information. These include the accuracy, sensitivity, and reliability of the brain scanners used; the validity of the experimental paradigm deployed (e.g. Is the subject *really* being called upon to 'deceive' anyone, and is deception the sole difference between the two, or more, cognitive conditions assayed?); the extent to which the subject performs the task accurately (and consistently); their compliance with other aspects of the procedure (e.g. not moving their head, as movement artefacts will degrade the image); the absence of other confounders (e.g. extensive dental work in the upper jaw of a subject undergoing fMRI); and the extent to which behaviour can be monitored and measured during the scan (e.g. Can response times [RTs] and accuracy be recorded?).

These steps are followed by a host of data-analytical steps (which may be broadly similar yet vary in their particulars between investigating laboratories): the options chosen as brain images are 'realigned' (so that they all are similarly orientated in space), 'normalized' (the warping of images, so that they all come to occupy an ideal, 'standardized', brain atlas space, at which point all images are rendered in the same dimensions—i.e. they are of the same 'size'), and 'smoothed' (essentially a way of improving images, minimizing any remaining variations between individual brain shapes and increasing the 'signal-to-noise' ratio). Hence, this science is inherently multidisciplinary: it requires collaboration between physicists, radiographers, and radiologists, physicians, psychologists, neuroscientists, mathematicians, and data analysts. The process may fail at many levels.

Human error

As an illustration, I offer one simple example. I do this not only so that the non-neuroimaging reader may gain some insight into the day-to-day travails of brain imaging but also so that they may understand how fragile this scientific endeavour can be, at times.

When we were carrying out a particular line of research, which involved MRI scanning in a radiology department on Tuesday mornings, we found that on some Tuesdays our data were very poor indeed: there was 'noise' scattered across the images and the data could not be analysed. Various possible sources of error were explored, local changes in electrical equipment investigated, neighbouring departments visited, and the scanner examined. In the end, we discovered that the ambient temperature of the scanning room was itself variable over time. We learned that on Monday afternoons there was a 'paediatric list' running in the scanner, during which children underwent anaesthesia so that they might be scanned without incurring movement artefacts. We then discovered that, for sound medical reasons, the anaesthetic team turned off the air conditioning in the scanner room while performing such procedures (in order to manage the children's circulation and body temperature more safely). However, they did not always remember to turn the air conditioning back on again when they had finished! Hence, the temperature in the scanning room could sometimes gradually rise over an ensuing Monday night, so that it was relatively high on the following (Tuesday) morning. Fortunately, our 'problem' went away when we enacted stricter temperature control procedures.

I offer this as one simple example of what can go wrong; the point is that this form of investigational technique (functional neuroimaging) must be conducted painstakingly, and sources of variation in data quality rigorously pursued and corrected.

Thus, the researcher wishing to elucidate neural evidence of 'truths' and 'lies', especially where that proposed investigation might impact a real-world problem and the fate of a living human subject, would be well advised towards caution. One feature of our own work has been the desire to replicate findings at each stage, to focus on the same brain regions again and again, and to see what will survive repeated scrutiny.

The Sheffield model

From the beginning of our work in this area (ca. 2000), we have followed a rather simple model, hypothesizing that deception is reliant upon the prefrontal cognitive executive for its execution. To be more specific, we have posited that key regions of the prefrontal cortex will be implicated in different aspects of the deceptive process:

1. We posited, on the basis of a wide range of basic neurological and func-tional neuroimaging data (demonstrating the contribution of the dorsola-teral prefrontal cortex [DLPFC] to the generation of novel responses or responses where the subject is granted latitude about what to choose; e.g. Spence et al., 2002; Chapter 2), that the DLPFC would be implicated when liars elaborate new lies, such as when they 'tell stories'.

2. However, we also posited that there was another process that was more basic to the execution of deception: an ability to withhold the truth. To consider this phenomenon, we posited that where a subject knows the answer to a question, that answer forms a relatively prepotent response to that question. So, in telling a lie, the liar must crucially withhold the prepo-tent response, the truth. Furthermore, we posited that such processes would be most exposed under those conditions where the liar is constrained to answering with either a 'yes' or a 'no' and where there is an emphasis on speed of response. Hence, we posited that inhibitory prefrontal regions should be implicated in this form of lying, and that the candidate region would be the OFC, most specifically the ventrolateral prefrontal cortex (VLPFC; an area known to be involved in response alternation and sup-pression; Butters et al., 1973; Iversen and Mishkin, 1970; Starkstein and

Robinson, 1997; Chapters 2 and 4). Indeed, as we have already noted, lesions of the OFC may render adults pathologically truthful.

3. Finally, we incorporated a finding that has long been recognized in the polygraph and social psychology literatures: lies often incur longer RTs than truths (Vrij, 2000). Indeed, perhaps the most compelling example of this finding was reported in a paper by Vrij and Mann (2001), in which the authors studied videotapes of an interrogation of a man accused of killing a child (in a country on the European mainland). This man eventually confessed and was convicted of the child's murder. However, when extracts of the interrogation tape were compared statistically, that is, the epochs during which the accused gave conflicting accounts of his whereabouts, actions, or clothing, it was found that during those epochs when he had lied he had exhibited fewer limb movements (the so-called 'motivational impairment effect'), longer RTs (i.e. longer delays in his speech), and more 'non-fluent' speech errors (i.e. more 'ums' and 'ahs'). Such findings are consistent with our model, in that we posit that 'higher' elements of the cognitive architecture are engaged during deception, their involvement incurring a *processing cost*, manifest as *increased RT*.

Placing all these elements in the model, we arrived at the framework shown in Fig. 91. In it, we move from developmental factors (on the left) to current neuroanatomy and physiology (middle), and on towards emergent behaviours (on the right). As in previous chapters in this book, we owe a debt of

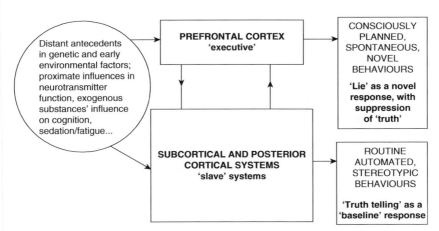

Fig. 91 Schematic showing the cognitive neurobiological basis of deceptive behaviour. Lies behave like executive-mediated responses in that they implicate higher brain systems and also involve longer response times. Truth telling appears to be the baseline function.

gratitude to Tim Shallice's (1988) concept of the supervisory attentional system (SAS; prefrontal executive and medial premotor regions modulating 'lower' motor centres, as compressed into the middle section of this framework; Chapters 4, 6, and 7), and we should also admit that the left-hand side of the model ('development') is theoretically underspecified, though we would foresee genetic and early environmental factors as contributing here. Indeed, it is between the 'development' and 'anatomy' columns that we should currently place the Raine group's work on pathological liars (who exhibit increased orbitofrontal white matter).

We should also make two further points:

a) The relationship between items in the middle and right-hand columns is merely functional and much simplified (e.g. the prefrontal cortex would not enact lies 'on its own': it must act 'via' other brain structures), and

b) The role of the executive (middle column, top) is both to facilitate certain behaviours and to inhibit others: it may bias the lower systems towards new, novel responses (via the DLPFC) or suppress their prepotent response tendencies (via the VLPFC).

Falsifying memories

The kernel of our approach has been to study subjects under conditions where their latitude for response is maximally constrained, to yes or no answers. Hence, we have chosen to focus very much on the information being probed at the expense of the interaction between subjects. This may be critiqued, as a potential weakness, but it is both expedient in the scanning environment, where interactions are mediated via a technological interface, and serves to emphasize the brain of the deceiver rather than that of their 'victim': that is, it focuses on information known and withheld, and thereby helps to establish a 'normal' database from which we might extend to more complex empirical designs in the future.

In our first experiment (Spence et al., 2001), we probed recent episodic memory. We asked subjects which of 36 very simple actions they had performed on the day that they were studied. Crucially, one of our team obtained these data *prior to* the neuroimaging phase of the study and retained a 'ground truth' template of those actions performed by each subject on that day (i.e. before the subjects learnt the relevance of these questions). Hence, we would be able to check the consistency of our subjects' responses throughout the ensuing scanning procedure. Each question was then asked repeatedly in the MR scanner, under a counterbalanced design, and subjects were instructed to give what they regarded as the truthful response in the presence of one cue and what they regarded as a lie in the presence of another (they pressed 'yes' or 'no' buttons on a keyboard). A 'stooge' in the observation room attempted to 'tell' which response sets were true and which were false. When we analysed our data, we found the following (Fig. 92):

1. RTs were significantly longer during lies than truths;

2. Prefrontal activity (especially in the VLPFC and anterior cingulate cortex [ACC]) was significantly greater during lies than truths; and

3. There were no brain regions where truths elicited greater brain activity than lies.

4. The results were replicated when the procedure was repeated (in the same subjects) using a slightly modified protocol (questions being presented aurally on this occasion, through earphones, rather than visually, on a screen; Experiment 2, Fig. 92).

These findings are consistent with our a priori hypotheses; they also support our basic theoretical premise: truthful responding comprises a relative baseline in human communication and deceit a superordinate function, requiring the intervention of cognitive 'executive' systems, thereby incurring a processing cost, manifest as longer RTs.

Can this method be applied to forensic questions?

In more recent experiments, we have had the opportunity of applying this simple methodology to address more serious questions—in people who assert that they have been the victims of 'miscarriages of justice'. Under such conditions,

Ex.1   Ex.2   Both experiments

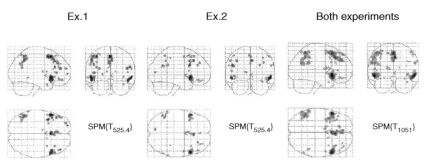

SPM{T$_{525.4}$}   SPM{T$_{525.4}$}   SPM{T$_{1051}$}

Fig. 92 Functional magnetic resonance imaging data taken from Spence et al., *Neuroreport* 2001; 12: 2849–2853. In experiments 1 and 2 (left and centre) normal males exhibit greater prefrontal activation while providing deceptive responses than with truthful responses. The areas of activity are greatest in the bilateral ventrolateral prefrontal regions, anterior cingulate cortex, and also the left parietal cortex. A combined analysis of both experiments (right) emphasizes the contribution of these specific areas. With permission from Wolters Kluwer Health.

if we are to apply our basic method, then each investigation becomes essentially a single-case study. This is because the prevailing 'ground truth' relates to a unique event: a crime, with its own particular circumstances and time lines. It follows that, apart from basic hypotheses regarding cognitive neurobiological architecture (e.g. the involvement of the VLPFC during lie responses), there can be no 'control' group or database for such a study (few others will have been implicated in precisely the same scenario as the subject whom we attempt to investigate). Here we are dealing with aspects of long-term episodic memory, but we can adapt our approach to ask questions regarding those specific points upon which there is disagreement (i.e. the conflicting views of the 'accused' and their 'accusers'). However, we are also dependent upon the impacts of several less predictable factors:

1. The availability of a clear central narrative of an event, which exists in two contested forms (avowed by the accused and their accusers);

2. Sufficient points of disagreement for us to be able to pose varied though related questions, in counterbalanced designs over the course of a brain imaging experiment (thereby reducing the potential for automation of the subject's responses, which might occur if only a single question was asked repeatedly);

3. A subject's account that is not weakened by what we might term 'narrative inhomogeneity'. If there are 12 key points to the narrative, the statistical power of our paradigm would be radically constrained if, for example, 3 points were actually falsifications; and

4. The events concerned should be describable in unambiguous terms (requiring the subject to recall a single, specific episode). Statements should be feasible in the scanner, of limited length but also highly content-specific.

In a recent study (Spence et al., 2008), we examined a woman who had been accused and convicted of harming a child in her care. We adapted our technique so that she might be scanned on four occasions, in a more sensitive MR scanner (at 3 Tesla), using a bank of 36 questions, administered in counterbalanced designs, while we recorded motor responses and timings. Details of the case were obtained on interview and through the use of trial-related transcripts. We invited the subject to respond to questions under two conditions:

1. Giving what she would regard as the 'truth'; and

2. Giving what she would regard as a 'lie' response (i.e. endorsing the view of her accusers).

We predicted that if the subject was essentially truthful, then there should be greater activation in the VLPFC and ACC, and longer RTs when she endorsed the views of her accusers (i.e. when she 'lied'). We posited that the opposite finding (i.e. greater VLPFC and ACC activation and longer RTs exhibited when she endorsed her *own* account) would be inconsistent with her claims of innocence.

Now, from a purely statistical perspective, the null hypothesis is highly likely to be borne out in such experiments: that is, there is a 95% probability that there will be no discernible difference between brain maps or RTs under each condition. Hence, such experiments may well 'fail'. Moreover, we have to state categorically that (at the moment) we cannot *prove* whether a subject is guilty or innocent. We are merely asking whether brain scans and RTs are 'consistent' or 'inconsistent' with that (index) subject's account of events.

Nevertheless, in this case, we were able to obtain clear-cut (statistically, highly significant) results, which suggest that our protocol has potential. When the subject endorsed the accusations against her (i.e. when she 'admitted guilt'), her prefrontal activity and RTs were significantly increased (Fig. 93). Hence, though we have not proven her innocence, we have demonstrated that her functional anatomical and behavioural parameters behave 'as if' she were wrongly convicted.

Accused's
Version

Accusers'
Version

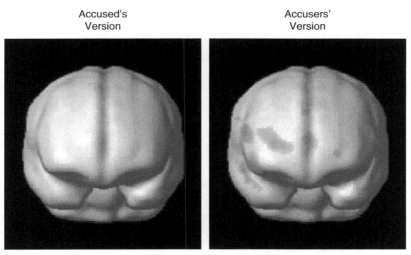

Fig. 93 Data derived from a single subject who was accused and convicted of harming a child. When the subject endorsed her accusers' versions of events (image on right), she exhibited increased activation of prefrontal regions relative to those scans in which she provided her own account of events. Although they do not prove that she is innocent, these data are consistent with her version of events. Reprinted from *European Psychiatry* 23. Munchausen syndrome by proxy or miscarriage of justice: an initial application of functional neuroimaging to the question of guilt versus innocense. Spence SA et al (2008) with permission from Elsevier Ltd. (See colour plate section).

In developing this line of work, we have generated future hypotheses on the basis of past experiments where we were able to determine which 'half' of the responses were *definitely* lies, either through the use of screening interviews prior to the procedure (as in Spence et al., 2001) or the retention of concealed testimonies (set aside during scanning and later decoded, post-scanning, as in Spence et al., 2004). Therefore, in research terms, as long as there is an adequate means of establishing 'ground truth', there is a way of discovering where the major changes in brain activity occur during lying. However, once we enter the forensic sphere, we are (almost by definition) unlikely to know the ground truth, so the logic of such experiments is radically reversed (and therefore much more difficult to execute):

> We go from asking what are the correlates of (known) lies to asking whether (predicted) neural patterns denote (unknown) lies.

Clearly, we are only at the very beginning of such a science.

Caveats and concerns: is there an ethical way forward?

Now, if we set aside our concerns regarding the validity and reliability of such techniques, and assume that empirical, technical issues may be 'ironed out' in the future, then there is still a further question that we must pose concerning the putative application of fMRI to lie detection. Because, if

> We *can* do it . . . ,

Then . . .

> *Should* we do it?

This is an inherently ethical question. Indeed, it is one for society at large to debate and decide about and it would be presumptuous to proffer conclusions here. However, we might say this: if one is really concerned with medical ethics and the proper treatment of human subjects, then one cannot foresee a situation in which it would ever be justifiable to scan people against their 'will'. It may be that the 'special case' of an alleged miscarriage of justice provides the appropriate medium for ongoing work, in the near-term future, though I must stress once again that subjects should be 'truly' free to volunteer to participate (and not exposed to subtle forms of coercion). We have to remain mindful that some of those affected by such 'miscarriages' (and imprisoned) may have enjoyed very limited prospects of case review; they may not have had a 'voice'; hence, they may be 'desperate' to clear their names (and thereby vulnerable to exploitation and manipulation). Nevertheless, the simple fact that we might even begin to ask such questions may offer hope to those who are genuinely afflicted.

> It's always as well to remember, when considering "miscarriages" of justice, as the authorities so neutrally and quaintly like to call them, that the framing of the innocent axiomatically involves the exculpation of the guilty. This is abortion, not miscarriage.
>
> (Hitchens, 2001, p. 8)

It is at least conceivable that we may wish to use fMRI lie detection as a means of reversing such calamities but so much depends upon our society's (i.e. our collective) 'will'.

A moral brain may behave immorally

The evidence that we have considered in this chapter, sourced from a variety of literatures, among them studies of non-human primate colonies, of human patients who have sustained prefrontal injuries, of others who have told 'pathological lies', and those, apparently healthy ('neurotypical'), people who have undergone recent functional neuroimaging experiments, all points to the centrality of prefrontal systems in the implementation of deceit. Humans and other 'higher' primates seem to possess the 'necessary' cognitive neurobiological apparatus that enables them to attempt the deception of their neighbours, their conspecifics. Furthermore, although human communities often profess moral values that abjure deception, closer scrutiny of their etiquette suggests that deception 'oils the wheels' of human discourse and interaction. Hence, deception provides an intriguing example of a situation in which professed morality and biological endowment seem to be at odds with each other. Indeed, were the 'norms' apparently professed on behalf of so many cultures and epochs actually to find themselves embodied within any real, living human agent, then it is quite conceivable that such a person would attract a pathological attribution, a 'diagnosis'. He might be called autistic. He might be called 'pseudopsychopathic'. By this I mean that the person who speaks the truth on all occasions, and without embellishment, is likely to run into difficulties (ironically, with his conspecifics, *the people he chooses not to deceive!*).

Furthermore, if we recall some of the issues that we rehearsed in Chapter 2 regarding the likely role of the OFC (and especially the VLPFC) in response reversal and suppression, on the basis of changing contingencies (i.e. response 'values'), then we may posit that the VLPFC becomes engaged during deception because the 'truth' must be suppressed and hence, concurrently, a 'value' readjustment must occur. It is as if the brain 'normally' accords truth the higher value, the 'baseline', default response (and one might posit sound evolutionary reasons for this, not least to do with accurate subjective appreciation of salient information), whereas under conditions of deceit it may adapt to 'value' falsehoods more 'highly'. Hence, deceit may become the more 'rewarding' response mode. Again (and as we hinted at in Chapter 2), ventral and medial brain systems seem to function 'as if' biology 'recognizes' valence, value, moral checks, and balances. It doesn't necessarily 'do the right thing', but it does seem to 'represent' what is right and what is wrong. It is the agent who 'chooses' what 'to do' next.

Chapter 9

Harming others

Squeeze a man hard and you'll always find something inhuman.[19]
  One can see the logic of dynamiting a [cell full] of suspects (women suspects: this happened in the Ukraine). But the more typical preference was to administer a slow death. There are many accounts of prison floors strewn with genitals, breasts, tongues, eyes and ears. *Arma virumque cano*, and [the culture of] Hitler-Stalin tells us this, among other things: given total power over another, the human being will find his thoughts turn to torture.[20]

Now that we have assayed the putative cognitive neurobiology of such behaviours as 'everyday' deceit and pathological lying, the time has come to extend our inquiries into the 'darker' side of human nature. Such a study is legitimate in the present context, for, if we wish to 'really' understand human beings and the extent to which they might enjoy volitional 'freedom', then our cherished notions and fragile hypotheses are likely to encounter their most stringent test here: when we look at the damage that adult human beings will (knowingly) inflict upon each other. Indeed, as we shall see, such a line of study reveals many of our assumptions and intellectual inconsistencies to be just what they are: useful 'rules of thumb' that may not survive closer critical scrutiny. In short, I shall argue that little is as clear-cut or as 'obvious' as it may at first seem. I shall also give some flavour of how difficult it would be to change the situation, as it applies, in 'everyday life'. In a nutshell, there is often too little evidence available for us to be able to 'think scientifically'.

---

[19] Antonin Artaud (cited in Hayman, 1996, p. 23). Hayman R. Antonin Artaud. In '*Antonin Artaud: Works on paper*', edited by M. Rowell. New York: Museum of Modern Art, 1996, 17-24.

[20] Martin Amis [*Koba the Dread: Laughter and the twenty million*. London: Jonathan Cape, 2002, 200-201.]

Three Questions

First of all, it is important to ask three questions, the answers to which are of central importance to our future progress. Though some of the terms that I shall borrow (from other literatures, below) may sound arcane, I hope that the reader may bear with me so that we might more effectively make a case for subtlety when (eventually) we come to consider the vexed issue of 'responsibility'.

What do we mean by 'moral evil' and 'natural evil'?

Well, first it may be helpful to clarify what we mean by the word 'evil'. The *Oxford English Dictionary* (OED) offers a variety of definitions, many of which might be applied to apparently 'purposeful' acts:

> Morally depraved, bad, wicked, vicious...
> Doing or tending to do harm; hurtful, mischievous, prejudicial...
> Depraved intention or purpose...desire for another's harm...
> What is morally evil; sin, wickedness.
> Anything that causes harm or mischief, physical or moral.

However, overall, the OED delineates two broad categories of 'evil':

1. Examples of the 'bad' in a 'positive' (one might say 'active') sense, as in morally depraved or wicked acts, doing or tending to do harm, having a malevolent intention, etc.; and

2. Examples of the 'bad' in a 'privative' sense (as the absence of the 'good'; essentially a 'negative' evaluation), as in a diseased organ, an unsound or corrupt form, something that is inferior in quality.

Notice, there is something quite different about these two applications of the word. For, as we have implied (above), the first sense can be applied to 'agents'; it describes the things that people may 'choose' to do, 'deliberately'. Indeed, if they choose to do these things, to perform these sorts of acts, then they seem to be 'opting' for evil. In contrast, the second sense of the word appears morally neutral, more a case of mishap, mistake, or happenchance. There is a disorder of 'formation', of the constitution of the object so described; somehow, things have 'gone wrong' in the natural world.

Such a distinction (between the positive and the privative) brings us very close to that which pertains between 'moral' and 'natural' evil, a theological dichotomy that has been reviewed recently by numerous authors, among them Peter Vardy (1992) and Susan Neiman (2002). So what do we mean by these alternative forms of evil?

'Moral evil' is essentially the evil that agents choose to do. It comprises the 'bad things' that people do when they know that they are 'doing wrong'. So, for instance, the torture alluded to in one of the quotations at the head of this chapter necessarily involves the knowing infliction of pain and suffering on another human being. Indeed, that sense of 'knowing' is most eloquently captured in the following passage from Antonio Tabucchi's *The missing head of Damasceno Monteiro*:

> ...I have a mania for remembering the names of torturers, for some reason remembering the names of torturers means something to me, and do you know why? [B]ecause torture is an individual responsibility, to say you're obeying orders from above is inexcusable, too many people have used that shabby excuse to shield themselves by legal quibbles, do you follow me?

(Antonio Tabucchi, Originally published in 1997)

(If you have detected any contemporary resonance in this quotation, at the time that you have come to read this passage (whenever that may be), then perhaps you have just encountered evidence of the 'stability', the essential repetitiveness, of human (im)moral conduct. Sadly, 'we' are forever harming each other).

Now, to the theological (or at least, 'believing' Christian) mind, the existence of moral evil is the price that we humans pay for our freedom of the 'Will' (our, as yet hypothesized, 'capacity for choice'; Chapter 2). For, in order to exercise choice, all options must be left open to us. Hence, on this view, God has permitted the existence of human, moral, evil because its selection (and subsequent execution) comprises one of the 'possible' outcomes inherent in our constitution as 'free agents'. Were we to be 'prevented' (in some divine, spiritual/neurological chimerical way) from performing evil acts, then we might 'appear good' to an external observer but this would constitute an illusion (i.e. a 'misinterpretation of a veridical stimulus'). For, without the 'possibility' of performing 'evil' there is no choice and if there is no choice then, no matter how 'good' we might appear to be, there is no morality. We become biological machines, 'obeying orders'. So, to an apologist for a deity, it is quite possible to 'defend God' (no blasphemy is intended), because God has given us freedom of choice, freedom to choose. Hence, all the moral evil at large in the world becomes the 'fault' of humanity itself. (Nevertheless, whether any amount of human freedom adequately compensates for the suffering of the innocent, even that of a single child, is a moot point, a raw nerve prodded again and again in Dostoyevsky's *The Brothers Karamazov*. It is also thoughtfully and seriously re-examined in Peter Vardy's (1992) text, where the author eventually concedes that Dostoyevsky's novel contains 'in my view, the most effective attack against God ever produced', p. 72).

'Natural evil', in contrast, describes the bad things that happen in the world that are not subject to human control or agency. Hence, Susan Neiman (2002) chooses as an example the 1755 Lisbon earthquake – a disaster that impacted the ways in which a number of contemporary intellectuals came to construe God.

For our purposes, we might propose that tsunamis, hurricanes, and earth-quakes all provide us with ample examples of 'natural evils', events which 'Nature' precipitates, and for which no human agent can be held 'responsible' (though at times, of course, one may consider whether human agents might have planned better for the future, e.g. in the adequate construction of other people's dwellings or the maintenance of river levees; nevertheless, one cannot accuse even the most incompetent official of having 'caused' a tsunami; though one suspects that some exponents of the 'Chaos theory' might think about it).

Now, as it happens, the perceived existence of natural evil presents even more of a problem for the apologist for a deity. For, while he/she might have defended moral evil on the grounds that it constitutes the 'price' that humans pay for freedom (above), there really does not seem to be a comparable justifi-cation for the natural phenomena that kill people and render survivors home-less. Vardy (1992) essentially admits that this is the case, and concludes (as have many others) that God is ultimately un-knowable. More vociferous responses accrue within Neiman's (2002) account:

> God is either willing to remove evil and cannot; or he can and is unwilling; or he is neither willing nor able to do so; or else he is both willing and able. If he is willing and not able, he must then be weak, which cannot be affirmed of God. If he is able and not willing, he must be envious, which is also contrary to the nature of God. If he is neither willing nor able, he must be both envious and weak, and consequently not be God. If he is both willing and able – the only possibility that agrees with the nature of God – then where does evil come from?

> (Pierre Bayle, cited in Neiman, 2002, p. 118)

As we have noted (in Chapter 8), the person who 'speaks his mind' may find that his popularity undergoes something of a depreciation. Pierre Bayle was a seventeenth-century Protestant who had to escape religious persecution in Catholic France: '[those] who tried to leave for more hospitable countries like Prussia or the Netherlands were sent to the galleys, if male, and to the prisons, if female, for the rest of their miserable lives' (Neiman, 2002, p. 117). Although Bayle managed to escape (to the Netherlands, where he published anony-mously), '[his] brother in France was arrested in his stead and presumably tor-tured to death in the prison where he perished five months later. Scholars hold this to be the signal event in Bayle's life, undermining any possible belief in a just God who rewards the righteous and punishes the vile' (Neiman, 2002, p. 117).

Natural evil poses something of a problem for a deity's apologists. Nevertheless, one straw that may be clutched at appears to be Immanuel Kant's conjecture that natural evil provides humans with even more opportunities to behave well (a proposition examined in Neiman, 2002). For, if the planet were to be without random calamity, if we always received our 'just dessert' in this life, then might we not come to behave 'morally' merely as a way of obtaining reward? We might behave well simply in the expectation that we should receive an existential 'pat on the back'. However, on a planet where there is no simple pattern of moral cause and effect, i.e. where 'bad things happen to good people', morality has to be practised for its own sake. One chooses the 'good' because one believes that it is the 'right' thing to do, not because one expects a reward that is really little more than a bribe. Indeed, upon reflection, does this not seem to mirror the plight of Job in the Jewish scriptures (the Christian *Old Testament*)? Time and again Job is made to suffer. Bad things happen to him, and around him in the world, yet he remains 'good'. His patience has been tried but he remains 'true'. This defence (of natural evil) has intellectual merits, but it does make one wonder about the proposed affect/morality of the originator of such suffering.

Now, why have I subjected the reader to this theological interlude? Have we wandered off track? I shall argue that we have not.

The relevance to our onward journey of the theological conceptions of moral and natural evil is that they force us to acknowledge our assumptions about the root causes of human behaviour. Indeed, the distinction seems almost too neat, too convenient: for, it lends us an 'easy' contrast between those 'bad' acts that are 'chosen' (by a 'free' agent) and those that happen by chance (mistakes, accidents, and oversights). So, on the face of it, we might even suspect that this moral distinction shores up a legal distinction that is routinely rehearsed in courtrooms: that between 'murder' and 'manslaughter'. For, in order for a verdict of murder to be returned, there must be evidence of '*actus rea*' (i.e. an agent performed an act; he unlawfully killed someone) and '*mens rea*' (i.e. the same agent intended to perform the act; he had 'malice aforethought'). This second condition is not satisfied in manslaughter, where the actor did not 'intend' to kill his victim. Hence, if taken at face value, we have a very simple dichotomy – one that may be explored and delineated within the courtroom, namely that differentiating intended, freely chosen, 'moral evil' (murder), from circumstantial mishap, manslaughter (e.g. the perpetrator states that he had not intended to kill his victim; yes, he had wanted to 'hit him' but an accident occurred: the victim fell and struck his head on the pavement; thus, moral evil was compounded by natural evil). Upon such a reading, manslaughter *always* incorporates an element of 'natural evil' (though the size of its relative contribution is likely to vary from case to case).

All this seems (conveniently) clear, albeit at a rather superficial level. However, there is a problem: the distinction does not always hold and it seems even less likely 'to hold' in the future, if it must withstand a rising tide of neurobiological 'advance'. What do I mean by this? Well, let me explain.

In order to defend a distinction between moral and natural evils, one has to believe that there is a clear line (or at least a convincing 'gradient') that divides the realm of human agency from the biological (and other forms) of determinism. In other words, you really have to accept some 'space' for 'Freedom of the Will' (without such freedom there would be no 'agency'). However, if you do not accept the concept of a 'Free Will', and you do not believe that humans make free choices, then you render moral evil (and, hence, moral accountability) incoherent. No organism can be held 'responsible' for a behaviour that has 'simply' been pre-programmed into it. To apportion blame under such circumstances would be rather like holding one's alarm clock 'personally responsible' for waking one up in the morning even though one had programmed it to do so! Therefore, if you are a hard-line determinist, whether in terms of biological, psychological, or social causation, you eject morality and responsibility from the human equation the moment you jettison 'freedom of choice'. *For if you contend that humans are not 'free' then you can hardly blame them for what they do.*

So, to be provocative, for the radical determinist (and indeed the rather unimaginative 'behaviourist') the distinction between murder and manslaughter is meaningless; all that matters is that a given organism killed another given organism; the mechanism by which that killing occurred is of little relevance, there was no 'intent' (it is an illusion), no 'choice' (it is an illusion); the salient 'diagnosis' is solely one of 'identity': which organism did it? What they were 'thinking of' at the time is of no consequence.

However, if you think that there is a problem with this approach, then you may wish to acknowledge some element of human 'control'; you may wish to apportion some degree of moral responsibility to human actors who engage in 'intentional' acts and, indeed (to the arch determinists out there), you may appear to be someone who is hankering after some sort of 'ghost in the machine' (see Chapter 4).

Now, is this not all rather unsatisfactory? We seem to have fallen into a situation where we have to choose between our 'selves' as constituting either automata or ghosts. The former have illusions, subjective mental states that seem real to them (and volitionally relevant), but which are purportedly *not* contributory to voluntary acts (after Libet); the latter enjoy a Cartesian existence, presumably 'acting upon' some kind of 'soft machine' through some form of 'thought control'. Is there a 'middle path' open to us? Might there be some form of compromise?

Well, one could argue for 'limited freedom'. Perhaps one could say that we all have a 'little elbow room' but that it is susceptible to constraint, by 'natural' processes. However, if you were to propose this line of argument, then one might anticipate another problem arising. For, if you were to allow 'extenuating' circumstances, 'mitigating factors', to be admitted as evidence, then something else would begin to happen.

As we offer such details as:

'The perpetrator was drunk at the time of the offence, he comes from a violent home, he was abused as a child, he has low levels of serotonin-metabolites in his cerebro-spinal fluid, he once suffered a penetrating head injury,'

What happens?

Well, what happens is that we diminish the domain of moral evil (i.e. we attempt to 'explain away' some of the perpetrator's 'intended' behaviours) and we 'replace it' with natural evil. In essence, we reverse the logic of Brutus' interlocutor in Shakespeare's *Julius Caesar*:

> The fault, dear Brutus, is not in our stars,
> But in ourselves, that we are underlings.

(This seems to me to constitute a refutation of 'natural evil', as applied to human ambition). However, nowadays the statement might become:

The fault, dear Brutus, is not in our 'selves',
But in our frontal lobes...our supervisory attentional systems...our serotonin metabolism...our upbringing...

Indeed, if we continue to add mitigating factors, if we add in purportedly defective genes, reported prenatal and perinatal events, then we might predict that in the future there may be absolutely 'no room left' for moral evil at all. All 'bad' behaviour would (eventually) comprise a concatenation of 'natural evils'. Indeed, there might never be the need to invoke the concept of a 'rational criminal', for reasoning itself would have been revealed to be the product of entirely specified antecedents. Hence, moral evil is (apparently) an ever-shrinking concept while natural evil is (apparently) an ever-expanding one. This appears to be the inevitable conclusion of a materialist volitional neuroscience.

Moreover, it is also worth noting that the prospects do not necessarily get any rosier for the 'offender' who is convicted and committed under such a system. After all, temporary incarceration as a form of punishment, rehabilitation, or as an 'example' to others only makes sense if based upon the assumption that people may change their behaviours. Its rationale (in these terms) is lost if the future is pre-determined and immutable. So, were one to become a radical determinist, then it might 'make sense' to 'simply lock people up and throw away the key' because they are 'faulty specimens' (not 'moral agents'). They are incapable of change, 'they have no choice'. If one really believes that antisocial humans are entirely determined, then the safest (and perhaps 'easiest') thing to do is to exclude them from society: a kind of quarantine for volitional 'failure':

> In the final state there can be no more 'human beings' in our sense of an historical human being. The 'healthy' automata are 'satisfied' (sports, art, eroticism, etc), and the 'sick' ones get locked up... The tyrant becomes an administrator, a cog in the 'machine' fashioned by automata for automata.
>
> (Alexandre Kojeve, writing in 1950, cited by Mark Lilla, 2001, p. 135)

The impact of such a radical version of determinism is actually rather similar to the situation that one might anticipate emerging consequent upon an uncritical incorporation of Benjamin Libet's findings into the praxis of 'Law and Order'. If you really believe that no action is 'freely chosen', then murder and manslaughter become indistinguishable; perceived 'intent' does not matter anymore.

What do we mean by 'instrumental' and 'reactive' forms of violence?

Now, if we move from an attempted ethical account of humanity's 'bad behaviour', towards a more phenomenological account of one of its exemplars – namely violence, then we encounter a rather similar dichotomy, one that bears a structural resemblance to those pertaining between moral/natural evil and murder/manslaughter. For, within the forensic psychological and psychiatric literatures there is often a distinction drawn between 'instrumental' violence and violence which is 'reactive' or 'impulsive'. What is 'violence' and how do these terms differ? Well, the World Health Organization (WHO, 1996) defines violence in the following way:

> The *intentional* use of physical force or power, threatened or actual, against oneself, another person, or against a group or community, that either results in or has a high likelihood of resulting in injury, death, psychological harm, maldevelopment or deprivation (italics added).

Note: the behaviour is intended; it is a voluntary behaviour on the part of the perpetrator (the WHO, at least, seems to apportion 'Free Will' to human actors). However, we may further define what the perpetrator is actually doing (below).

'Instrumental violence' has a specific 'end in sight'; it is, by definition, 'premeditated'. Hence, there may be a very many exemplars of such violence, e.g. that occurring during bank robberies, boxing matches, sadistic killings, militarily aggressive procedures (e.g. pre-emptive 'air-strikes'), and following the knowing pursuit of 'victims' (e.g. those identified on the basis of some 'external' characteristic such as gender, ethnicity, dialect, or accent; i.e. those carrying 'marks' of difference that are sought out by aggressors; Komar, 2008).

Instrumental violence is 'knowingly' applied. The agent cannot reasonably claim to have been unaware of what he was doing throughout the course of what may have been a very long sequence of (consciously mediated) purposeful acts; a trajectory the outcome of which was apparent from the start. A pilot took off, knowing that he was carrying bombs. A sadist locked his hostage in the basement, knowing that he would later return to torture her.

Nevertheless, we should acknowledge that 'instrumental violence' does not 'simply', 'always', or even 'necessarily' equate to 'moral evil', for, depending upon one's ethical standpoint, not all instrumental violence may be 'wrong'. The pilot defending his country may be said to be performing a moral 'good', a boxer may be engaged in 'sport'. Those senior German military officers who attempted to assassinate Hitler might ultimately have been construed as having behaved heroically, saving many other citizens from suffering and death (had they succeeded). Indeed, some politicians in our own time have even attempted to exonerate those who torture for them because they assert that these agents, soldiers, and 'private contractors' are fighting a 'war on terror'. So, although one may hold quite contrasting views concerning the morality of such exploits, the point is that a simple 'collapsing' of conceptual boundaries (between 'moral evil' and 'instrumental violence') would probably be inaccurate.

In clinical forensic practice, instrumental violence is often the mark of the personality-disordered individual, especially the antisocial person (exemplified in their most extreme form by the psychopath): someone who is unencumbered by concern for 'others' (Tables 19–21). Such people are hypothesized to lack 'empathy' – that immediate visceral awareness that one may experience of another's pain and suffering. Indeed, perversely, such suffering is often what the psychopath seems to be seeking (we shall say more about personality disorders in due course).

'Reactive/impulsive violence' is, by its very nature, contingent. It is precipitated rather than planned, retaliatory (on some occasions) rather than motivated *a priori*, and its relation to morality may be even more ambiguous (than that of instrumental violence; above). We see reactive violence in a host of 'normal' and 'abnormal' situations, often where an urge towards destruction (of the self, others, or inanimate objects) is prominent: In English city centres on Saturday nights, when the inebriated perceive themselves to have been slighted, when those whom they hit respond with retaliation, when the intoxicated and addicted lose 'control of themselves', when an abused woman finally 'breaks' and stabs her abusive partner, when a romantic partner finds that they have been cuckolded ('something snapped'), when those with organic brain states lose their inhibitions (e.g. consequent upon frontal lobe lesions and

Table 19 Medical conditions that may present with 'violence'

Category	Exemplars
Organic mental states	Structural deficits (e.g. frontal lobe lesions, frontal lobe dementias, Huntington's disease)
	Seizure-related activity (e.g. frontal and temporal lobe foci)
	Episodic dyscontrol (aetiology and status uncertain)
	Alcohol and substance-related disorders (e.g. intoxication with alcohol and withdrawal [delirium tremens]; in response to alcoholic hallucinosis)
	Suspicion and 'paranoia'; psychosis secondary to amphetamines, cocaine
Functional psychiatric disorders	Schizophrenia
	Bipolar affective disorder, especially in the manic or hypomanic phases
	Delusional disorders, especially 'pathological jealousy' (Othello's syndrome) and erotomania (de Clerambault's syndrome)
Personality disorders	'Cluster B', especially antisocial, borderline, and narcissistic personalities
	'Cluster A', especially paranoid personalities
	Psychopathy, best understood as a subgroup, a severe manifestation, of antisocial personality disorder

dementias, and late in the course of Huntington's disease), and in those who are experiencing radically disordered perceptual states (e.g. in the context of alcohol withdrawal/delirium tremens, acute psychosis, complex-partial seizures (also known as temporal lobe epilepsy) and, sometimes, the acute sequelae of head injuries).

The point is that each of these episodes may be regarded as less the consequence of the deliberations of a perpetrator's (hypothesized) 'Will', and more a case of their having 'lost control'. Though the situations vary markedly, and not all of them are as 'innocent' or as 'mis-adventurous' as each other, in each case there is an element of the misunderstood, the unforeseen, and unintended (hence, the contrast with the premeditation inherent in instrumental violence, above). Nevertheless, not all exponents of reactive violence deserve the medical equivalent of a Monopoly game's 'Get out of jail free' card: we bear some responsibility for the situations into which we launch ourselves, so, while the person with Huntington's disease or a frontal lobe dementia is hardly responsible for their plight, the drunken reveller and the disinhibited aggressor, 'high' on crack cocaine, *have* contributed to their own present mental state. Hence, in the terms of E.W. Mitchell (1999), they are 'meta-responsible' for their ensuing predicaments. Note again, however, how this last statement also

Table 20 The personality disorders as classified according to the *Diagnostic and Statistical Manual*, 4th edition (DSM IV)

Category	Personality disorder (DSM IV category number)
Cluster A	Paranoid (301.0)
	Schizoid (301.20)
	Schizotypal (301.22)
Cluster B	Antisocial (301.7)
	Borderline (301.83)
	Histrionic (301.50)
	Narcissistic (301.81)
Cluster C	Avoidant (301.82)
	Dependent (301.6)
	Obsessive-compulsive (301.4)

Source: From the American Psychiatric Association (1994).

Table 21 Characteristics of an antisocial personality (DSM 301.7), according to the *Diagnostic and Statistical Manual*, 4th edition (DSM IV)

Criteria

A: *There is a pattern of disregard for and violation of the rights of others occurring since age 15 years, as indicated by three (or more) of these features:*

> Failure to conform to social norms with respect to lawful behaviours as indicated by repeatedly performing acts that are grounds for arrest;

> Deceitfulness, as indicated by repeated lying, use of aliases, or conning others for personal profit or pleasure;

> Impulsivity or failure to plan ahead;

> Irritability and aggressiveness, as indicated by repeated physical fights or assaults;

> Reckless disregard for the safety of self or others;

> Consistent irresponsibility, as indicated by repeated failure to sustain consistent work behaviour or honour financial obligations;

> Lack of remorse, as indicated by being indifferent to or rationalizing having hurt, mistreated, or stolen from another.

B: *The individual is at least 18 years of age.*

C: *There is evidence of Conduct Disorder with onset before 15 years of age.* *

D: *The occurrence of antisocial behaviour is not exclusively during the course of Schizophrenia or a Manic Episode.*

Conduct Disorder (312.8), although a diagnosis of children, is very similar in its criteria to antisocial personality disorder in adults. It is characterized by a 'repetitive and persistent pattern of behaviour in which the basic rights of others or major age-appropriate societal norms or rules are violated ...'

Source: From the American Psychiatric Association (1994).

becomes incoherent if one posits that there is no such thing as 'Free Will' and that perceived intentions are irrelevant (above). According to such reasoning, the plight of the person with Huntington's disease becomes somehow 'equivalent' to that of the Saturday night reveller. Is this 'just'? (I suspect that even the most radical determinist may have difficulty defending such a breach of 'common sense').

Nevertheless, the perpetrator of such (reactive/impulsive) violence is generally held to be *less* responsible for their behaviour (than the instrumental aggressor), either because overwhelming environmental factors had supervened (e.g. they were attacked) or else because their 'inner balance' had been perturbed by organic factors (e.g. the effects of a frontal lobe tumour).

Hence, one might posit the following:

a) That if the really 'big problem' facing humanity is that of 'moral evil' – those acts that we 'choose' to do even though we 'know' that they are wrong – then the focus of our attention may, at least initially, be most profitably directed towards 'instrumental' antisocial conduct.

b) When we come to consider 'reactive/impulsive violence' we are more likely to be dealing with a 'full' or 'partial' variant of 'natural evil' (i.e. behaviour that is, to some extent, beyond an individual agent's current volitional control).

c) While humanity itself may by characterized, though not 'diminished', by the sorts of changes of behaviour that accompany a defined organic pathology, a 'natural evil' (e.g. such as when a frontal lobe tumour precipitates disinhibition, aggression, and insensitivity towards others; humans are, after all, prey to many such pathologies), it (humanity) *does* often seem 'diminished' by the occurrence of moral evil (e.g. when a ruling elite attempts to exterminate a group it designates as 'other'; when a man holds his daughter hostage in a basement for decades, repeatedly raping her; when 'sex tourists' from wealthy countries 'holiday' in poor countries in order to gain access to vulnerable children). Such behaviours say a lot about 'humanity' and where its moral 'baseline' may be located (below).

d) Hence, in very simple terms, natural evils inform us as to how an individual human actor may 'breakdown' under certain pathological conditions, while moral evils tell us something more about the limits of 'normal human action'; they tell us what 'we' are capable of, 'as a species'.

e) Therefore, to reiterate, our bigger problem as a species is 'moral evil'. One might even speculate that this is what will ultimately 'limit' our survival, our 'future'.

f) However, and seemingly paradoxically, 'moral evil' is a category that is apparently contracting all the time: it may become increasingly subsumed within 'natural evil', as more and more 'explanations' are found for instrumental (premeditated) violence.

g) So, if 'moral evil' were ever to collapse entirely into 'natural evil' (i.e. if the two categories were to be subsumed into one 'natural' category), then we would gain not only an accurate (deterministic) understanding of 'bad' behaviour but also a full understanding of 'human nature'; and if that was the case then we might be forced to conclude that humans do not 'choose' to perform bad actions in any meaningful sense (i.e. 'intentions do not matter'); we are, instead, 'inherently flawed' (in the sense of a 'natural evil'; according to the OED, the embodiment of a 'privation' of the 'good'). If this is true then we, as a species, constitute 'an unsound or a corrupt form' (Question 1; above).

Where is humanity's moral 'baseline'?

Notwithstanding all of the above, if we take the view that there is 'something wrong' going on when human beings torture, rape, maim, and murder each other, then we are necessarily endorsing an evaluative statement; we are making a judgement about the events that we have observed. These (let us call them) 'extremely antisocial' behaviours clearly deviate from what we would regard as 'normality'. However, a question arises as to whether our judgement of 'normality' is primarily 'moral' in its orientation, evincing a concern with what human beings 'should do', what it is that constitutes 'correct' human conduct (in terms of values such as 'good' and 'evil', 'right' and 'wrong'), or whether it is essentially 'statistical' in orientation, evincing a concern with events that are relatively uncommon ('un-usual' in terms of their frequency, etc.); events that are remarkable solely because of their rarity, their apparent deviation from statistical 'norms' of human conduct. (Actually, we may experience an intuition that *both* modes of judgement are alive and well within us, but let us try to hold on to this distinction for the time being, in order to consider the following line of argument).

If my judgement of such matters is primarily 'moral', evincing a concern with how humans 'should' behave, then it is likely to invoke some form of moral standard and the judgements that I make may well incorporate notions of 'moral evil' (i.e. if I believe that human beings may behave 'morally', then it is likely that also I believe that they may behave 'immorally'). I may hold that individuals are responsible (answerable) for their actions because their 'bad' actions emanate from the choices that they have made (and, hence, at a specific moment 'preferred'). I accord these subjects the status of 'moral agents'.

However, if my judgement is more 'statistical' in its intuition, if I am responding to whether or not an event is infrequent, then I may be more inclined to view those deeds recounted (above) as statistical aberrations, 'outliers', and hence, indicative of some kind of 'disturbance' of function. In other words, I may be more likely to invoke some form of 'natural evil' (i.e. something has gone 'wrong' within the agent or in their external environment). Moreover, I am likely to accord such a subject a reduced capacity for moral agency (i.e. a 'diminished responsibility'). This line of argument may sound strange, but it often forms the core of a 'psychiatric defence' when an offender with a personality disorder does something so 'bad' that the press and the public wish them to be severely punished for it, while psychiatric opinion favours their incarceration in a 'special hospital' (arguing for a 'medical' disposal). A sceptic might posit that the 'diagnosis' here comprises solely a description of some very bad behaviour: the antisocial person performs antisocial acts 'because' he has an antisocial personality; the grounds upon which his antisocial personality is diagnosed comprise a history of antisocial acts; this is a tautology (and see Pincus, 2001, p. 78).

What I believe about the nature of the act performed (the alleged 'offence') is very likely to be influenced by the interaction of such ethical and statistical factors (Figure 94). What do I mean by this? Well, consider the following examples:

1. Take a hypothetical environment in which rape is a rare occurrence (so: a 'bad' act is also a 'rare' act). When it does occur we may be more likely to

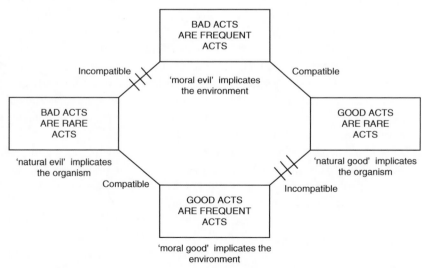

Fig. 94 Cartoon illustrating the understanding of good and bad acts in the context of specific environments where such acts are frequent or rare. When such acts are rare they tend to be interpreted as 'natural' phenomena; when they are frequent they tend to be interpreted in 'moral' terms. See text for details.

countenance 'abnormality' on the part of the perpetrator, e.g. we might ask 'what is *wrong* with him?' 'Has he got some form of personality disorder?' Further, if we identify such a 'cause' then we are effectively substituting 'natural evil' for 'moral evil'. In other words, we make the 'moral' 'natural'. At a very simplistic level, we might deduce that 'he did a bad thing because he has a bad (i.e. an unsound or corrupt form of) mind/brain'.

2. Now consider another environment in which rape is a frequent occurrence (hence, a 'bad' act is also a 'frequent' act). When an army rapes a civilian population, do we look for an individual perpetrator's abnormality? Do we look for personality disorder? No, we probably accord the environment some role in these events (given overwhelming numbers and overwhelming arms, its effect is one of 'facilitating' 'what can be gotten away with'; or else, we might say that it was, to some extent, 'understandable' that an individual soldier 'followed the crowd'). However, afterwards, we are likely to make moral claims upon such perpetrators (or at least to attempt to do so). We may hope to 'bring them to book'. As a human community we will probably see this form of behaviour as an instance of 'moral evil'. (If you doubt this, then ask yourself this question: Would you seriously offer justifications for, or accept 'excuses' from, those who commit such mass rapes?)

3. Conversely, consider an environment in which altruism is a common occurrence (i.e. where a 'good' act is also a 'frequent' act). Do we invoke 'abnormality'? No, why should we? In this case, the index behaviour is morally desirable and statistically 'normal'. So, we may feel that there is no need to look for explanations since we are not often called upon to 'explain away' what is 'good'. We may be completely uninterested in attempting to posit a distinction between a 'moral good' (what the subject chooses to do, knowing it is good) and a 'natural good' (what is determined by non-agentic factors). However, I suspect that while we would recognize an individual subject as behaving well (performing 'moral good'), we would probably also apportion some of the credit for his 'goodness' to his environment or society at large (though this involves assumptions that we shall explore further, below). We might feel that his environment facilitates his 'goodness'. Indeed, we might even posit that this is precisely why some people will to choose to live in a specific milieu (e.g. a convent, monastery, retreat, or commune) so that their environment may assist them in leading moral lives (though we should not overlook the human tensions that exist within such communities). Consider then, another issue that arises: For if 'everyone is good' in such a situation, the presence of natural goodness (i.e. a 'good society') may actually diminish the role of 'moral goodness' in our index individual; it may be 'easier to be nice if others are nice'; also, the

social influence is there to urge conformity. Such a critique is not without precedent: 'If you love those who love you, what credit is that to you? For even sinners love those who love them. And if you do good to those who do good to you, what credit is that to you? For even sinners do the same. And if you lend to those from whom you hope to receive, what credit is that to you? Even sinners lend to sinners, to receive as much again' (Luke 6: 32–34). One way of parsing such a critique is to suggest that altruism is 'easier' if and when others are altruistic. One behaves morally. However, the severest test awaits those residing in the fourth category (below).

4. What is happening in an environment in which altruism is rare (hence, 'good acts' are 'rare acts')? How should we regard an exponent of kindness in such a place? In a brutal prison or concentration camp how might we evaluate the person who 'retains' her 'humanity'? Do we have any interest in invoking the dichotomy conjectured between 'moral good' and 'natural good'? Well, clearly, such a special person constitutes both a 'good agent' and a statistical outlier (i.e. she is statistically highly 'abnormal'). Indeed, had she (our altruistic, good agent) instead constituted an extremely anti-social agent in an altruistic environment (category 1, above) then we should probably have searched for evidence of 'natural evil' (i.e. pathology). Hence, in the current case ('goodness in a bad place'), should we not be searching for evidence of 'natural goodness'? What is it that makes our agent so good in such a bad place? However, maybe we also experience an intuition that such a search for 'natural' explanations would detract from our agent's 'goodness'. If she had 'good genes' and a 'good frontal lobe', would her goodness be less moral and more natural? Would it matter? Well, if all that we have said so far about 'evil' is reasonable (above) then we may simply have to face the fact that 'goodness' is another area where moral agency may gradually succumb to natural explanation. Indeed, if we are pessimists, we may believe that we have just thrown the baby out with the bathwater (i.e. in seeking to explain away 'evil' we have just jettisoned the 'good'). However, if we are optimists then we may believe that should we ever be fortunate enough to find a cause of 'natural goodness' then at least it might allow us to engineer a better future for all humans. Maybe we could 'make' everyone 'good'. Now, if your intuition is that you do not accept this argument (that there might be such a thing as 'natural goodness', which is capable of incre- mentally displacing 'moral goodness'), then (once more) you are opting for leaving open a space for moral action, moral agency. Hence, you are opting to preserve a space for human freedom.

Now, to continue: What I believe about an action, its 'valence' in both ethical ('good/bad') and statistical ('rare/frequent') terms, is likely to be heavily influenced, indeed to be underpinned, by my assumptions about the moral 'baseline' evinced by humanity, in general:

a) Should I believe that human beings are potentially 'perfectible', that in their 'natural state' they would behave well, that they might even be 'restored' to 'grace' (potentially), then I am more likely to see the antisocial (in all of its many forms) as a manifestation of some sort of perturbation (or lack) within the offender: in other words, I am more likely to believe that he could and would have behaved differently (i.e. better) had he not suffered a 'fall', whether in terms of his moral or material (physical, psychological, or social) well-being. If his bad actions are really quite extreme, then I may feel that they are both morally and materially/statistically aberrant. Nevertheless, crucially, because I believe that humans may be 'perfected', I may come to think of the perpetrator as abnormal, a 'victim' to some extent; he has deviated from the optimal path of human development. (However, notice also, that on this reading of the human condition, *everyone* becomes a potential victim, because all of us are demonstrably imperfect, so no one has achieved the (hypothesized) optimal state of humanity and hence: all of us only ever hold (at best) partial or, indeed, (at worst) no responsibility for our plight; i.e. in a 'better world' we would all have been 'better persons', better agents.) The inspiring aspect of this thought is its corollary: *all are flawed, therefore, all might be improved.*

b) However, what would happen if I were to adopt a different baseline assumption? Imagine that I accept that humans are 'merely' another product of evolutionary processes, natural selection, constituting essentially 'just' another higher ape. Hence, because we are animals who have had to survive in very many hostile environments, I come to believe that our nature is, by definition, a predetermined 'mixed blessing': we are not 'perfectible' because we do not have 'perfection' within us (there is no perfect moral 'place' from which to 'fall'): we are animals who can and will behave 'well' and 'badly', according to our needs and desires; according to our circumstances. So, if I believe this to be the case I may be much less inclined to invoke moral evil; I may accept that human behaviour incorporates a large amount of natural evil; and I may conceptualize the 'normal' moral parameters of 'normal humanity' as admitting a great many 'bad' acts ('because people will vary in their 'morality', just as they vary in their height, hair colour, and blood pressure'). A really deviant act would then constitute an extreme example of some very abnormal (i.e. statistically aberrant) phenomenology, something whose 'particular badness' comprises its sheer rarity or bizarreness of execution. However, I might still believe that most antisocial conduct is in fact 'normal', for a portion of the population (just as playing the guitar or liking poetry is 'normal' for some of the population), a product of natural variation; I might only look for indications of especial pathology in the most 'statistically abnormal' acts. Indeed, were I to do so, I would probably be 'looking for' specimens of natural evil, causes of a 'broken agent'.

So, it appears that an enormous amount depends upon my assumptions about where the optimal human moral 'baseline' lies. If humans are animals exhibiting a distribution of 'good' and 'bad', similar to that of any other physiological property then I should expect bad acts to be committed, I should not naturally assume that they represent the outcome of moral evil, rather I should regard them as instances of natural evils constitutive of the species. When I see a particularly bad act, I may entertain the notion that this represents a particularly large statistical variant upon the background of normal variation, among human agents, and I might search for the (natural) cause of such an apparently 'broken agent'.

Moreover, under this assumption (of natural moral variation) it follows that if I hope to 'improve' human conduct, while assuming it to be 'normally' distributed, then I should not imagine that I am 'restoring' humanity to its 'rightful place' (because there is not one; its 'natural place' is where it is already). Instead, I am engaging in some form of 'engineering'. I am hoping to 'push' the distribution of human evil in the same way that I might hope to 'raise levels of literacy', 'increase rates of immunization against measles', or 'improve dentition'. Please note, I am not criticizing the desire to 'improve humanity', I am merely giving it its correct title: the quest is one of human 'improvement' via bio-psycho-social engineering; it is not about 'restoring' humans to their 'natural state'.

However, remember that there is also another way of thinking about humanity. According to this contrasting construction, one might suggest that we are indeed 'perfectible' agents, that in our 'normal' state we would all be ethical agents, the producers of exclusively 'good acts'. Hence, all of us 'should' (ultimately) occupy the same ethical space. On this argument, everyone is (at least potentially) perfectible, hence, there must be 'reasons' for their moral failures and these comprise two (by now, familiar) possibilities:

a) There is a natural evil, that impacts upon our 'perfectible' neurobiology;

b) We have 'Free Will' and we have chosen ('moral') evil on occasion, even in the presence of 'perfect' neurobiology.

Does any of this matter? Well, it matters a great deal when we come to think about what we may realistically achieve with respect to human nature. Furthermore, it underpins our use of terminology (are we engaged in 'restoration' or in 'engineering'?). It asks us to question how honest we are being when we use words to describe our endeavours.

Furthermore, as I have implied repeatedly, whether we think humanity is not operating at optimal morality or is operating at its best 'possible' level (because it is naturally, inherently flawed), where we locate its 'usual level of functioning' depends a great deal upon what we think 'normal' people are doing. How 'bad' can people be while still constituting part of a 'normal' sample?

So, how 'bad' is still 'normal'?

On a weekend in 2003, I conducted a highly artificial (and equally anecdotal) experiment (one which the reader might very easily attempt to replicate tomorrow): I made a note of all the stories contained within a British Sunday newspaper (a 'quality broadsheet'). Here is a selection of what I found:

1. Two sons of a Middle East dictator were described at length; their reported conduct included the routine torture and rape of their subordinates and the beating to death of transgressors in front of multiple witnesses (who did nothing to stop them);

2. Another story concerned the exhibition of this pair's corpses to the media; they had been killed by military forces;

3. A different story concerned the conduct of groups of healthy, affluent young men (aged 20–30 years), in a Far Eastern country, who routinely enjoyed the gang rape of prostitutes; they experienced this sort of behaviour as a form of 'bonding';

4. There was an account of the indiscriminate bombing of families, including the elderly, women, and children, who were sheltering in a church in a disintegrating state in West Africa;

5. There was a debate concerning whether a 'double agent', acting on behalf of domestic security services, was allowed to kill with impunity while operating 'under cover';

6. A man was described who had spent periods of time in a mental hospital before becoming a recluse, repeatedly brandishing firearms, and finally shooting a teenage burglar in the back; he had found him (the 'victim') in his (the gunman's) house late at night;

7. There were descriptions of killings connected to a 'human-trafficking' operation; this involved young girls who believed that they were entering the United Kingdom in order to make 'Bollywood' films but who, in reality, were coming to be sold into prostitution;

8. An account of a European terrorist group that had lately taken to using children to plant their bombs in tourist destinations;

9. There were the protracted, tawdry recriminations that followed the flood of alleged lies and counter-lies that led up to a country being taken to war (by a government, making its case, on the basis of a 'dodgy dossier').

All of this is happening in the world at large. All of it is happening 'now'. Where does the limit to 'normal' human morality lie? How 'bad' must bad behaviour be before it becomes 'abnormal'? What does not seem to be in doubt is that humans may do a great many terrible things without there being any evidence of 'disease', of mental illness, of natural evil... . In many such cases, the only 'natural evil' present seems to be humanity itself.

Biological accounts of 'abnormal' violence

Notwithstanding our concerns regarding the extent of 'normal' human 'evil' (whether it is 'moral' or 'natural' in aetiology), let us start to construct an account of purportedly 'abnormal' events; an account that is primarily based upon hypothesized biological determinants. In the following sections, I shall examine some of the notable papers that have emerged within this field, papers that are often cited when authors provide mechanistic accounts of human violence. For the most part, the violence described here falls within the category of 'reactive/ impulsive' (above) though as we approach the end of this section we shall encounter further cases that might, at least potentially, inform our knowledge of 'instrumental' violence. Throughout this section the pertinent question is:

To what extent do the 'special' data reported 'explain' the behaviour described and to what extent was the perpetrator of a deed 'responsible for their actions'?

A strange case, associated with abnormal brain structure

A paper by Relkin and colleagues (dating from 1996) is often cited in this context. It concerns the case of a 65-year-old man (the improbably named 'Spyder Cystkopf'), who, in the context of a domestic argument, killed his (second) wife of 10 years. Although the couple were reported to have enjoyed a good relationship, there arose an altercation during which Cystkopf's wife did something that she had never done before: she scratched his face (while simultaneously shouting at him and criticizing him for his 'lack of emotionality'; Relkin et al. 1996, p. 173). Cystkopf denied that this assault elicited any emotion within him, but he likened his subsequent actions to 'pulling my hand from a hot frying pan' (p. 173). 'I found myself hitting her again and again with my right hand' (p. 173). His wife fell over and Cystkopf then put his right hand over her neck, leaning down on her with his full weight 'until her body became lifeless'.

Afterwards, he attempted to remove any evidence of the struggle then he threw his wife's body out of a window (they lived in an apartment block in Manhattan), trying to make it seem like suicide, before collecting his briefcase, and beginning his journey to work. He was apprehended.

What do we make of such a case, such a bizarre series of events?

Well, when the suspect was later evaluated he was found to be an intelligent man who had no history of violence or addiction. There were no prior forensic activities. He had enjoyed a stable family life: his first marriage had lasted 25 years, yielding two children, and only ended when his first wife had died of natural causes; his second marriage commenced a year later. He had also achieved a notably successful career as an advertising executive. Cystkopf was, for the most part, cognitively intact; however, he exhibited a restricted and, at times, inappropriate affect (he did not exhibit remorse for his wife's killing, he talked about it in a 'matter of fact' way) and he also exhibited subtle impairments in his right-hand function (he was dextral, but his execution of fine motor performances was slightly slower with the right hand than with the left). Furthermore, he exhibited some very interesting findings on brain imaging (see Figures 95 and 96).

His brain scans revealed that Spyder Cystkopf had a large arachnoid cyst lying between his left frontal and left temporal lobes, so that the former was displaced upwards while the latter was displaced downwards. Furthermore, the state of his skull and records of a cerebral angiogram, performed some years earlier, suggested that although this man had been born with his cyst it had probably only increased in size over his later adult years. Indeed, the reason that he had undergone the earlier angiogram was because of the occurrence of transient neurological symptoms in the past (and the cyst had not been discovered then).

Hence, Cystkopf exhibited a demonstrably abnormal brain 'structure' (Figure 95) and he could also be shown to have abnormal brain 'function': Figure 96 shows a positron emission tomography (PET) scan demonstrating clear evidence of reduced metabolism in his left frontal and left temporal lobe regions. Moreover, the patient evinced abnormal autonomic (sweat) responses to emotionally laden visual stimuli, findings that are consistent with those seen in patients with bilateral orbitofrontal cortical lesions (Relkin et al. 1996).

Now, if we recall some of the properties of the orbitofrontal cortex (OFC) that were touched upon in previous chapters of this book (especially Chapters 2, 4, and 8), then we might expect that an orbitofrontal impairment, secondary to a locally expanding lesion (in this case a cyst), might well impact upon an agent's ability to control his actions. In other words, it is conceivable that Cystkopf killed his wife as a consequence of his inability to control his reactive response to her assault. Is this feasible? Furthermore, if it is, is he guilty of murder or manslaughter, 'not guilty by reason of insanity', or simply 'not guilty'? Does he bear *any* responsibility for his actions?

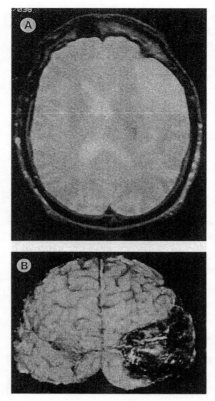

Fig. 95 Magnetic resonance image scan relating to the patient Spyder Cystkopf. This patient exhibits a large lesion in the region of the left frontotemporal lobes. From Relkin N, Plum F, Mattis S, Eidelberg D, and Tranel D. Impulsive Homicide Associated with an Arachnoid Cyst and Unilateral Frontotemporal Cerebral Dysfynction. In *Seminars in Clinical Neuropsychiatry*, 1996. Courtesy of Damasion H, University of Southern California.

Actually, there is little 'closure' to be offered in this index case, for, not only did Cystkopf apparently accept a 'plea bargain', thereby accepting a conviction for manslaughter (the consequences of which he seems not to have fully understood; remarking that he planned to 'return to work' after a long period of incarceration, commencing after the age of 65 years), but he also declined a surgical excision of his lesion. So, not only was his 'responsibility' never tested in court but also we shall never know whether he might have 'improved' (or been 'restored to normal') following surgery.

Nevertheless, what do we make of this case? The published account is couched very much in terms of a clinical lesson, a didactic exemplar: that alleged offenders, who exhibit psychiatric or neurological abnormalities,

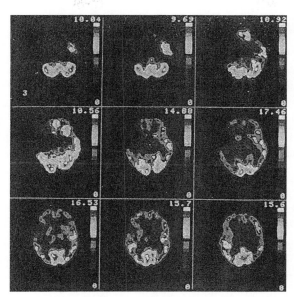

Fig. 96 Positron emission tomography scan relating to Spyder Cystkopf. These data show reduced activity in the region of the left frontotemporal lobes. (Left is; left in these images). From Relkin N, Plum F, Mattis S, Eidelberg D, and Tranel D. Impulsive Homicide Associated with an Arachnoid Cyst and Unilateral Frontotemporal Cerebral Dysfynction. In *Seminars in Clinical Neuropsychiatry*, 1996. Courtesy of Damasion H, University of Southern California.

should be fully investigated prior to trial (and, hence, disposal). However, I think its potential lessons are of even wider significance: for, this case demonstrates that the existence of organic evidence actually makes judicial decision-making far more complex than it might otherwise have been (assuming such findings are taken seriously). Consider the following:

1. On the face of things, at the time of his arrest, Cystkopf appeared to be a callous offender: he evinced little or no remorse for his actions, he was unresponsive to emotional stimuli (indeed this was the accusation that his wife had fatefully levelled against him), his behaviour following the killing evinced an attempt at deceit (cleaning up the apartment and continuing with his preparations for work), and the way that he treated his wife's body was shocking (throwing her out of the window);

2. Nevertheless, the very abnormality of such conduct, arising as it did in the late adult life of a previously 'normal' individual, points to something having 'gone wrong';

3. Furthermore, there was evidence of neurological dysfunction and gross organic disturbance.

4. So, the question is whether Cystkopf's behaviour and his pathology were meaningfully related. Was it all a bizarre coincidence or did his arachnoid cyst influence this man's behaviour on the day that he killed his wife? Can we ever know for certain? Well, we can never 'prove' a 'null hypothesis', so, by definition, we cannot prove that the behaviours and the lesion are totally coincidental, unrelated. Conversely, even though we have a plausible sequence of events, we cannot 'prove' that the lesion caused the event to happen (i.e. we cannot state unequivocally that the lesion 'did it'). Eventually, we are likely to decide on the basis of probabilities (less graciously construed as a jury's intuition). What would a jury of 'reasonable people' decide in such a case?

5. Furthermore, even if the jury were to decide, 'yes, his lesion had something to do with his behaviour', what should its verdict be? 'Murder' seems an unwarranted conclusion: Cystkopf (apparently) lacked premeditation. Yet, how do we choose between 'manslaughter' (technically possible), which can, again, seem overly harsh (if he 'lost control' because of a lesion he did not choose to have residing within his brain), and 'not guilty by reason of insanity' (again, a technical possibility)? Indeed, even Cystkopf's reported behaviour after the killing does not help us here, for while his apparently callous disposal of his wife's body might demonstrate to an unsympathetic jury that his was a calculated intent to deceive (a 'conclusion' especially likely if the accused had never undergone a brain scan), to a more sympathetic jury might it not provide 'merely' another instance of his impaired emotionality? His emotions seem to have been grossly disturbed although 'cognitively' he was clearly 'aware' of what he had done.

6. What does one 'do' with the subject when he is convicted? Does the existence of his lesion mean that he is a 'risk to the public' or might we posit that with his particular 'risk history' it is very unlikely that that specific risk situation might ever arise again (perhaps Cystkopf would have to endure attempted assault before any new threat would arise, within him)? Should he get a long sentence, a short sentence, a suspended sentence ('the loss of his wife is punishment enough') or should he reside in a psychiatric hospital for the rest of his life (because he may never be of 'low-risk' to society)?

The real lesson from this case is that even when there is a gross disturbance of brain structure and function, ample evidence of 'natural evil' (according to the OED), the 'correct' course of action, the 'correct' judgement remains difficult to discern unequivocally. Indeed, even knowing all that we think we know we still cannot prove ('scientifically', rather than legally) that at the time of his actions Spyder Cystkopf was subject to *any* influence from his lesion. We may 'believe' that he was, but how can we 'prove' it?

> In the final analysis no human action is ever fully explicated (to the level of certainty): our provisional understanding is always contingent upon what the subject actually 'says' (even if we do not believe them).

> (Spence, Chapter 8)

An unusual genetic endowment

Another source of biological data is provided by a subject's genetic endowment, their 'genotype'. On the face of it, this provides a biological substrate that may be even more pervasive in its influence (and, indeed, 'earlier' determined) than that arising from a discrete brain tumour (above). A key paper in the history of genetic accounts of violence is that of Brunner and colleagues (1993) who described a very rare genetic abnormality affecting a large Dutch family. The genetic abnormality comprised a point mutation on the gene that codes for the structure of the enzyme monoamine oxidase A (MAOA), an enzyme that we have encountered previously (in Chapter 4): it is implicated in the catabolism (i.e. the breakdown) of the neurotransmitters dopamine, noradrenaline (norepinephrine), and serotonin. The effect of the point mutation is to precipitate a 'complete and selective' deficiency of MAOA (Brunner et al. 1993), so that none of these neurotransmitters is metabolized (hence, at a simplistic level, they might each be expected to reach 'higher than normal' levels in the brains of those affected). Furthermore, such a sequence of events would be predicted to result in lower levels of 5-HIAA (a metabolite of serotonin) in the affected subjects' cerebrospinal fluid (a finding that is itself associated with reactive/impulsive violence; see Chapter 4).

Now, another feature of this mutation is that the affected MAOA gene 'resides' on the X chromosome of the human genome. Therefore, while a male (XY) individual who receives this gene from his mother suffers the consequences of this unopposed abnormal gene (because he has only the one X chromosome, and it is carrying the mutant form), women (XX) who receive the gene are (at least, in this family) heterozygotes, i.e. all women have two X chromosomes so those affected by this mutation have one affected X chromosome (carrying the mutation) and also one normal (i.e. unaffected) X chromosome. Hence, while women may carry the abnormal gene, they seem not to express it (i.e. they are probably 'saved' by their 'normal' copy of the MAOA gene, residing on their 'other' X chromosome). Men, however, with only the abnormal X chromosome, exhibit signs of a 'phenotype' related to their mutant MAOA gene.

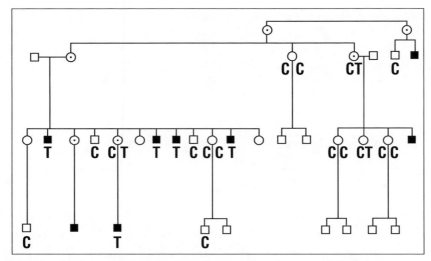

Fig. 97 A family genogram taken from the paper by Brunner et al. (1993). Those males carrying the normal 'C' allele did not exhibit abnormal violence. Violence was exhibited by those carrying the 'T' mutation.

In this Dutch family, males who carried the abnormal gene exhibited a syndrome characterized by borderline 'mental retardation' (now termed 'learning disability') and behavioural abnormalities, the latter comprising 'impulsive aggression, arson, attempted rape, and exhibitionism [i.e., exposing themselves]' (Brunner et al. 1993, p. 578).

The family tree is shown in Figure 97. Because the family, the 'kindred', is relatively large there are sufficient relatives for the investigators to have been able to demonstrate a clear association between the abnormal behavioural syndrome (above) and the gene's mutant form: there were five affected males, all of whom carried the mutation and all of whom exhibited the syndrome, and 12 unaffected males, none of whom carried the gene or manifested the syndrome. Moreover, in those who underwent further investigations, there was evidence of a disturbance in their enzyme activity (as hypothesized, above).

So, if taken at face value, we seem to have a very clear indication that an abnormal gene, a mutant form of the gene coding for the structure of MAOA, impacts human development so that not only is an affected male rendered 'learning disabled' but also impulsively aggressive. A number of comments might be made:

1. The association between the abnormal gene and the abnormal behaviour is plausible since we 'already' know that the neurotransmitters likely to be impacted by such a mutation are themselves likely to impact voluntary behaviour and especially impulsivity (a case could be made for 'high levels'

of dopamine and noradrenaline and 'low' levels of serotonin being involved in impulsivity).

2. Clearly the gene and the behaviour 'coincide', they co-occur within this kindred, and there appear to be no exceptions to this 'rule'.

3. There is little information given regarding the behaviours involved, other than their (generally) impulsive nature (for instance, we do not know to what extent the incident(s) of attempted rape or exhibitionism were planned or 'reactive'). However, the authors themselves noted that 'it should be stressed that the aggressive behaviour varied markedly in severity and over time, even within this single pedigree'. This suggests that a static genetic lesion (a point mutation) was of varying impact upon behaviour, or subject to varied salient environmental interactions over time.

4. Finally, it is conceivable that the association with 'violence' *per se* is a red herring. For, as the authors noted, all the affected males had learning disabilities and much of their disturbance arose in the context of 'a tendency toward aggressive outbursts, often in response to anger, fear, or frustration' (Brunner et al. 1993). Hence, a counter-argument here would be that their problem is mainly one of learning disability, associated with poor coping skills, and that the impulsive violence reported is actually a consequence of such a failure to cope. In other words, the association 'holds up' not because it is primarily to do with violence but because the abnormal gene co-segregates with learning disability, within this particular kindred.

So, once more, we have what could be seen as a compelling association between a biological factor (a 'natural evil') and a form of violence (apparently impulsive in its character), though we can see that there are caveats. Nevertheless, the paper remains informative because it prompts us to consider what we 'should' do with such information.

Supposing, for the sake of argument, that the genetic mutation in this family is the root 'cause' of the male violence reported. What is our response? Are these men 'free'? Are they 'responsible' for what they do? This is a moot point in a sample of people residing on the borderline of learning disability since, even in the absence of violence or further abnormal features, we would probably hold that they are likely to experience reduced capacity in certain areas of life, in certain situations, *a priori*. However, we lack the information to take this line of inquiry any further here.

Nevertheless, assuming that violence is associated with an abnormality of the MAOA gene, we might posit that:

1. Subjects may be less able to control their behaviour for 'organic' reasons (a 'natural evil');

2. Therefore, they might be held 'less responsible' for their antisocial acts;

3. However, the very fact that such acts are intermittent suggests that there are periods during which (and environments within which) affected individuals may exert 'sufficient' control over themselves.

4. So, what should society 'do' with such people? If they offend should they be given more lenient sentences (in the legal system) or potentially longer terms (in hospital settings)? If they have not offended, but carry the gene, should they be 'watched closely', 'tagged' (as suggested by one recent reviewer; Moosajee, 2003), or detained indefinitely (clearly a breach of their civil liberties)?

5. An enlightened, though perhaps rather paternalistic, response might be to 'manage' the environment (so-called 'nidotherapy'). If an individual of limited capacity only becomes violent under very specific circumstances, following very specific 'provocations', then perhaps their environment can be adjusted to help them (and us) remain at peace: there are ways of circumventing some disabilities, which may be relatively straightforward to arrange, e.g. supported accommodation, direct debit payment of bills, provision of meals, and protected social activities. Naturally, this will depend upon the extent (and funding!) of the services available.

I do not pretend to know the answers to these questions, concerning Brunner's patients; I do not know the people concerned. Yet, I rather suppose that even if I did know them I should still find it hard to decide. Ultimately, it is for societies to make choices using (or perhaps ignoring) biological data, but the point that we return to once again is this: biological information does not necessarily, or entirely, explain 'what has happened', nor does it assist that much in specifying 'what should happen, next'.

A bad early life and the variation within a gene

What one may assert with greater confidence is that recent advances in experimental design and data analytical techniques have facilitated the performance of evermore ambitious and sophisticated studies concerning the emergence of complex human behavioural traits under a variety of potential, partial, competing influences. Our next example is a particularly sophisticated study that benefits from the availability of immense resources and a very long period of 'follow-up' (the duration over which human subjects were observed and intermittently assessed). This study is by Caspi and colleagues (2002) and it derives from the highly productive Dunedin Multidisciplinary Health and Development study, conducted over recent decades in New Zealand. The basic design of the study involves a cohort of 1037 children 'enrolled' at birth (of whom 52% were male) and followed-up at ages 3, 5, 7, 9, 11, 13, 15, 18, 21, and 26 years (by which time the cohort was still 96% intact; Caspi et al. 2002). Various forms of data have been collected and multiple investigations performed on this sample, and it has yielded much that is of interest to psychiatrists. However, in the present context, we are interested in an observed association between measures of a particular genetic variant (a 'functional polymorphism' that is distributed across the 'normal' population), accounts of childhood maltreatment, and assessments of antisocial conduct among the cohort's males as they entered adulthood (specifically, those males having four Caucasian grandparents, thereby reducing the sample's genetic heterogeneity).

Once more, the gene involved is the one encoding for the MAOA enzyme (located on the X chromosome at Xp11.23–11.4). However, in contrast to the Brunner study (above), in the present case we are dealing with the effects of 'more or less' of the enzyme being expressed (synthesized), rather than its complete absence (as was the case following the point mutation described above). Hence, all males were tested for their genotype (their version of this single gene on their sole X chromosome) coding for higher or lower levels of MAOA expression, and this value was computed with their childhood experience ('absent', 'probable', or 'severe' maltreatment) and their subsequent patterns of antisocial conduct during adolescence and early adult life.

Fortunately, the records accrued in the course of this study were sufficiently detailed for investigators to be able to derive four measures of antisocial conduct among these males:

1. Diagnoses of adolescent 'conduct disorder' (essentially the childhood antecedent of adult antisocial personality disorder (ASPD)), defined according to *Diagnostic and Statistical Manual of Mental Disorders (DSM IV)*;

2. Convictions for violent crimes (identified via the Australian and New Zealand police database);

3. A predisposition towards violence as assessed at interview when they were aged 26 years; and

4. Symptoms of ASPD as obtained from third-party informants (again, when the subjects were aged 26 years).

The study's central finding was a fascinating one. Increasing levels of childhood maltreatment correlated with increasing levels of later antisocial conduct (on all four measures, as would have been predicted *a priori*) among those with 'lower' levels of MAOA expression; however, this effect was apparently suppressed among those with higher levels of MAOA expression. Hence, there was evidence of a gene–environment interaction. Whereas, childhood maltreatment increased the likelihood of an antisocial adulthood among those with one form of the functional polymorphism, it did not produce such an outcome among those with the other form.

These findings are particularly striking when one examines the impact of the (maximally) affected group in terms of their 'volume' of antisocial activity: this 12% of the male birth cohort accounted for 44% of the cohort's violent convictions; furthermore, among those with the low-activity MAOA genotype who were severely abused in childhood, 85% would go on to perform some form of antisocial behaviour.

This is a remarkable finding and it suggests that for a small (absolute) number of people relatively few predictive factors may be informative of their future life trajectory. The sample number in each of the pivotal analyses in this paper was well over 400, though the 'core' group of offenders (in the analyses displayed) was often 12 or 13 men. This is perhaps the best example of a study defining a ('determined') risk of violence.

However, there is also another way of construing the data. For, enzyme expression in itself (i.e. on its own) did not determine who would go on to offend: 'the main effect of MAOA activity on the composite index of antisocial behaviour was not significant' (Caspi et al. 2002). So, had this been a study of purely genetic risk, it might have produced a negative finding (cf. Brunner et al. 1993). Conversely, it was early life experience that was the major cause of later antisocial conduct: 'the main effect of maltreatment [alone] was significant'. Hence, although one's attention may be drawn to those males who would end up offending in adulthood, the remarkable group are actually those males who were severely abused in childhood, but did not go on to offend (they number 18–20 in many of the analyses presented). High MAOA expression appears to have ameliorated the effect of severe maltreatment in childhood (and this may relate to the role of neurotransmitters in modulating stress responses; Caspi et al. 2002).

So, if one is faced with a population of children, one might search for genes to establish who might be at risk of later offending. One might look for genes that protect some of them from the effects of abuse. Alternatively, one might create a society in which children were not abused in the first place. As this study demonstrates, a lack of abuse would impact adult rates of antisocial conduct.

Again, as in the earlier study of group data, it is difficult to express an opinion as to whether individual subjects are 'free' or 'responsible' (we do not know the specific details of the offences recorded). For the arch determinist, their conduct would seem to be specified by antecedent factors and events (genes and abuse) – powerful forms of 'natural evil'. However, even here we are confronted with the impact of human agency. For, after all, who was it that performed such abuse?

Furthermore, this study links us to a theme that runs throughout several studies of young adults who are 'living' on death row in North American prisons (see Pincus, 2001, for a review). Such offenders, who have committed violent crimes, have often been subjected to severe abuse themselves in childhood, and subsequently have accrued a variety of neuropsychiatric and neuropsychological impairments. One study by Lewis and colleagues (1988), of 14 juveniles held in four states in the United States of America (40% of those juveniles in jails across the country who were awaiting execution at that time) revealed that nine had major neurological disorders, seven were psychotic, seven had organic impairments, only two had IQs greater than 90 points, and 12 had been subject to brutal abuse (five had been sodomized by members of their own families). Now, one might argue that all of this represents a concatenation of 'natural evils', impacting human cerebral control systems, yet one might also pose the question:

What is the 'rational' response of a developing agent towards a society of other agents that has allowed it (the developing agent) to undergo protracted abuse and suffering, without protection? How does even a 'normal' agent respond to such circumstances?

One possible disadvantage of our current, albeit understandable, enthusiasm for mechanistic accounts of the brain and psychological function is that it may obscure the necessity for less technical and more 'humane' modes of intervention. It may also allow society at large to sidestep a rather inconvenient question: when one lives in a civil society, what is the nature of one's obligation(s) to one's neighbour? Or, to invoke an older literature: 'Am I my brother's keeper?'

Behaving badly, in the community

As I have already mentioned, on several occasions, it is widely recognized that there is an association between frontal lobe impairment and overt violence. In people who have undergone frontal injuries in childhood or adulthood, violent conduct is more common (Anderson et al. 1999; Grafman et al. 1996) and, conversely, among offenders who have committed violent crimes 'frontal' impairments are more often elicited on neuropsychological testing (see Brower & Price, 2001; Blair, 2003; Pincus, 2001; Raine, 1993). There have been several studies of incarcerated antisocial people examining the structure and function of their brains (e.g. Raine et al. 1997b). However, whenever we encounter a 'life-long' condition, as opposed to the consequence of a defined, specific lesion, arising at a defined moment in an individual's life, there is often a question concerning the contribution of possible confounding variables: antisocial people have often sustained head injuries along the way, abused illicit substances and alcohol, and they may have experienced co-morbid psychiatric and neurological disorders, so it can be difficult to obtain unequivocal findings (i.e. findings which relate solely to their 'personality disorder').

However, a landmark study in this area is that of Adrian Raine's group examining antisocial people living in the community in Los Angeles (Raine et al. 2000). Raine posited that such community-based individuals would provide a more valid representation of antisocial people in general, in contrast to those who have been studied while incarcerated. He also studied several control groups, i.e. not just 'healthy' people (who might, of course, be expected to differ from 'antisocials' in multiple ways), but also people who exhibited substance misuse disorders and others who carried psychiatric diagnoses. Hence, in this study there were three 'control' groups.

Raine and colleagues recruited participants from employment agencies located in Los Angeles and assessed them on a great many measures. Pivotal to this process was the elicitation of 'honest' accounts of past misdemeanours – something of a delicate topic if a potential subject had yet to be apprehended for an 'offence'. So, the investigators took steps to guarantee that any details that might be divulged to them would remain confidential, without incurring the prospect of prosecution:

> To help minimize false negatives (denial of violence by truly violent offenders), a certificate of confidentiality was obtained from the Secretary of Health, Education and Welfare, Washington, DC, that protected the research investigators under section 303(a) of Public Health Act 42 from being subpoenaed by any federal, state, or local court in the United States to release the self-reported crime data. Consequently, subjects were protected from the possible legal action that could be taken against them for crimes they [had] committed and admitted in the interview, but which were not detected and punished by the criminal justice system.

> (Raine et al. 2000, pp. 120–121)

All the participants underwent structural MRI brain scans and also underwent a skin conductance experiment, one that probed their autonomic (sweat) response when they had to read aloud a 2-minute long, self-composed statement about their personal faults. The groups studied comprised 21 people with ASPD, 34 healthy subjects, 26 subjects with substance misuse disorders, and 21 'psychiatric controls'. All the subjects were male.

What were the behaviours that the ASPD group admitted to? Well, there were some very serious offences (and, hence, offenders) among them:

- 52.4% reported having attacked a stranger and having caused bruises or bleeding
- 42.9% reported having committed rape

- 38.1% reported firing a gun at someone

- 28.6% had attempted or completed homicide.

Such a list makes for stark reading, though it is worth recalling that the total ASPD group size is 21, so that this is still quite a small group of offenders (in terms of absolute numbers).

What were the findings? Well, Raine and his colleagues found that ASPD subjects exhibited a specific reduction in the volume of the grey matter within their prefrontal cortices (as a whole, they did not compartmentalize the cortex into specific regions), and this reduction was significant in comparison with each of the control groups studied. Furthermore, ASPD subjects exhibited a significantly reduced skin conductance response when reading out their faults, i.e. they exhibited less autonomic responsiveness (this is in keeping with previous studies). Indeed, the magnitude of their reduced responsiveness correlated with the reduction of their prefrontal grey matter volume (suggesting, once again as hypothesized, that the prefrontal cortex plays a role in modulating stress response).

Hence, Raine and colleagues obtained evidence for a prefrontal lobe deficit being linked to the performance of violent antisocial acts, and they managed to control for many of the confounding variables that usually undermine such studies. Therefore, the implication is that those with ASPD may have been hampered in their ability to modulate their behaviour, particularly their ability to suppress inappropriate responses, and that this impairment is linked to reduced prefrontal cortical grey matter volume.

Such a study provides another example of a scientifically meticulous design, and a method, an approach, that managed to access a marginalized group of people (antisocial subjects, living in the community). So it may seem mean-spirited to mention one caveat. However, this is just to clarify what must be acknowledged: that the study is cross sectional, it examines subjects at one point in time. Therefore, on its own, it cannot tell us whether the effects seen constitute 'cause or effect'. Do people with ASPD exhibit behaviour that is caused by their brain findings or are their brain findings the consequence of their lifestyles? We cannot say, but we should acknowledge that Raine et al.'s findings are consistent with what should have been expected on the basis of childhood development studies: his Los Angeles sample tended to be taller than their controls and they exhibited lower resting-state heart rates (these are findings that have also been reported in children who later go on to become antisocial; see Raine, 1993). Hence, it seems as if people 'destined' to develop ASPD deviate from 'normal' rather early in their lives (though this in itself does not tell us whether that deviation is genetic, environmental, or social in origin, or indeed a combination of all three).

Constructing an antisocial brain

By now, it will have become apparent that there are some very accomplished studies in this field, performed by investigators attempting to elucidate why it is that some human beings grow up to become 'antisocial', to be the 'kinds of people' who will repeatedly harm others. The four papers that we have just examined in some detail represent only a selection of 'highlights' drawn from across this field, though their findings are indicative of an emerging consensus: that antisocial people exhibit biological differences relative to the 'normal' population, that such differences may arise very early in life (our exception, above, was the case of Spyder Cystkopf, an example of what might be called 'acquired sociopathy'; Blair, 2004), and that (in general) an account may be offered of such differences implicating brain systems that are concerned with impulse control and response regulation, especially under conditions of stress. When authors specify a relevant prefrontal region it tends to be the OFC (below) and when they examine neurotransmitter systems these tend to be the major systems that we have reviewed in Chapter 4: the serotonergic, dopaminergic, and noradrenergic systems (and see Nelson & Trainor, 2007).

Hence, by way of summarizing what is a very large field, I ask the following question:

If one were to be perverse enough to actually want to 'create' an antisocial individual then how might one set about doing such a thing?

Well, sadly, there are a number of 'positive' leads to go on. Table 22 presents what we might glean from the work of major researchers in this field, not least the groups of Adrian Raine, Avshalom Caspi and Terri Moffitt, Jonathan Pincus, James Blair and others, together with data arising from such diverse projects as the UK Government Home Office's 2003 Crime and Justice Survey, and the Project on Human Development in Chicago Neighbourhoods. If one considers the list of possible antecedents to an antisocial adult life, then one thing seems very clear (to me): that there are very few items over which the young, developing agent has any direct control. Where he is born and to whom he is born are predetermined (relative to his life). His genetic endowment, by definition, precedes 'him'. The conduct of his ancestors, his parents, his neighbours, even the youths in his neighbourhood is largely beyond his control. When one looks at the combination of biological, psychological, and social endowments that 'predict' the emergence of an antisocial man, a second point also becomes obvious: if he has any freedom at all then it arises within very narrow constraints. I do not claim that he is not free. I merely speculate that his 'freedom', if it exists, is likely to be very limited.

Table 22 How to make an antisocial person

Empirically based suggestions
Take a male child.
Have him born unwanted, possibly following a failed termination of pregnancy, separate him from his mother in the first year of life.
Give him antisocial parents and/or a family history of criminal activity.
Raise him in close proximity to an antisocial father.
Raise him in a poor household, in a disruptive neighbourhood; make sure it is a neighbourhood with low levels of 'informal social control' and diminished 'collective efficacy'; make him a victim of crime.
Give him delinquent peers.
Make him tall for his age at 3 years (and also malnourished).
Give him a low resting heart rate and reduced autonomic responsiveness to alerting stimuli or threats at 15 years.
Give him a personality with 'callous traits'.
Expose him early in life to drugs and alcohol (do the same to his friends).
Bestow upon him a low IQ, attention deficits; later on, add a severe mental illness and multiple head injuries.
Abuse him from an early age.

Sources: Blake et al. (1995), Brennan et al. (1997), Eisenberg (2005), Farrington (1995), Ishikawa et al. (2001), Jaffee et al. (2003, 2004), Lewis et al. (1988), Liu et al. (2004), Luntz and Widom (1994), Lyons et al. (1995), Mullen (1992), Pincus (2001), Raine (1987, 1993), Raine and Venables (1984), Raine et al. (1990, 1994, 1995, 1996, 1997a), Struber et al. (2008), Viding et al. (2005), UK Home Office (2003) and Chicago Neighbourhoods Project. (See Sampson, 1997 and Sampson et al., 1997).

Furthermore, one might well predict that someone emerging with a 'full house' of such factors (as shown in Table 22) would exhibit very little empathy towards others. If empathy has to be learned from socialization (as posited by James Blair, 2004, and Paul Mullen, 1992), then where do the opportunities for such learning arise within such a pathological matrix?

Putting emotion and action together

Despite the many social and psychological adversities that are likely to have impacted the developing antisocial brain, there is a case that can be made for postulating a relevant biological substrate, a system, via which abnormal aggression may manifest itself, later, during adult life. In this account I shall draw very much upon the work of James Blair, a British psychologist now working at the National Institute of Mental Health, Bethesda, United States of America.

Blair (2004) utilizes the distinction (that we have already outlined) between reactive/impulsive violence and violence that is 'instrumental' or premeditated.

While antisocial people and those with other 'Cluster B' personality disorders (such as 'borderline' personality disorder) exhibit increased rates of reactive/impulsive violence, psychopaths are generally distinguished by exhibiting *both* reactive and instrumental forms of violence (especially the latter (Table 23)). Indeed, their crimes are classically 'cold-blooded' (Woodworth & Porter, 2002). So, what is it that might be capable of linking, while also potentially differentiating, the neurological bases of such different modes of violence? Blair posits the contribution of the 'reactive aggression system', a system with a long evolutionary past, discernible within many animal species and also, crucially, 'present' within humans (Figure 98). This system comprises key subcortical elements, including:

1. The medial nucleus of the amygdala (located within the temporal lobe),

2. The medial hypothalamus (pivotal to the autonomic system), and

3. The dorsal periaqueductal grey (PAG).

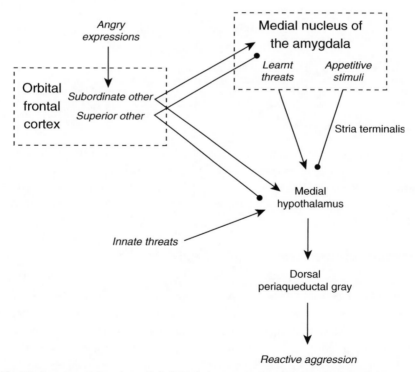

Fig. 98 A cartoon taken from Blair (2004) demonstrating the organization of those brain regions involved in aggression in the mammalian brain. See text for details. Reprinted from *Brain and Cognition* 55/1. The roles of orbital frontal cortex in the modulation of antisocial behaviour. Blair RJR (2004) with permission from Elsevier Ltd.

Stimulation of such areas in animals can precipitate aggression (Treiman, 1991) and it is thought that they constitute a neurological hierarchy, i.e. whereas the emergence of aggression originating within the amygdala 'relies' for its expression upon the lower structures being intact, they (e.g. the PAG) may generate aggression without necessarily involving the amygdala. However, both the OFC and the amygdala may exert influences over the lower centres (though their influences are of different types, see below).

The 'amygdala' plays a crucial role in the organism's relationship to aversive or threatening stimuli within its external environment. Hence, there are many brain-imaging studies demonstrating that human subjects 'activate' their amygdalae when they are exposed to angry faces (whether or not they are consciously attending to those faces). The implication is that the amygdala provides a 'fast', subcortical, implicit means of recognizing threats in the environment, as a consequence of which the organism may be better prepared to respond appropriately. In animal models, a low level of stimulation (e.g. consistent with a distant threat) will cause the organism to freeze. As the threat approaches, or stimulation increases, the organism will attempt to escape its environment. When the threat is very close and escape becomes impracticable, the organism will respond with reactive aggression (see Blair, 2004, for a review of the relevant animal literature).

However, the amygdala is also implicated in 'learning' about threats and learning the appropriate response to dangerous situations. Hence, in 'aversive' conditioning an organism learns that a particular behaviour will elicit painful consequences (i.e. it will be 'punished'). Hence, the organism learns not to perform that behaviour! In passive avoidance learning, the organism learns not to respond at all to certain stimuli (because such, evoked, responses would also incur punishment). Blair posits that in the human condition we expose ourselves to aversive conditioning when we hurt others. So, if a young child is in the playground and he hits another child, let us call him 'Johnny', then it is likely that Johnny may respond by crying (this constitutes the 'unconditioned' stimulus). The perpetrator, if 'normal', perceives such a response as aversive, unpleasant; if he is capable of empathy then he might experience an element of distress himself. Under normal conditions, such a course of events may form part of his 'moral socialization':

> Moral socialization is the term given to the process by which [caregivers], and others, reinforce behaviours that they wish to encourage and punish behaviours that they wish to discourage. Importantly, the unconditioned stimulus (US; the punisher) that best achieves moral socialization as regards instrumental antisocial behaviour is the victim of the transgression's pain and distress; empathy induction, focusing the transgressor's attention on the victim, particularly fosters moral socialization.
>
> (Blair, 2004, p. 202)

Table 23 Key features of a psychopath

Social deviance items ('factor 2')	Emotional/Interpersonal items ('factor 1')
Impulsive	Glib and superficial
Poor behavioural controls	Egocentric and grandiose
Need for excitement	Lack of remorse or guilt
Lack of responsibility	Lack of empathy
Early behavioural problems	Deceitful and manipulative
Adult antisocial behaviour	Shallow emotions

Source: Adapted from Hare (1993, p. 34).

Now, Blair posits that psychopathy, especially the application of instrumental violence, is an outcome of failed moral socialization (Mullen, 1992, similarly posits a failure of 'moral development'). What is central is the notion that the amygdala is abnormal in developing psychopaths. Hence, they will not learn from aversive conditioning (i.e. punishment does not 'work'). Nor do they develop empathy for their victims (because empathy is also reliant upon amygdala function). Indeed, some of the observational data that have been alluded to in the work of Adrian Raine (above; another British psychologist working in the United States of America), and deployed in Table 22, are consistent with this position: notice how often future offenders (even in childhood) are found to have low heart rates and to be less autonomically responsive to emotional or distressing stimuli. Indeed, such a lack of responsiveness was also detected in Spyder Cystkopf (a case of 'acquired sociopathy'; above).

Furthermore, there are emerging brain-imaging studies of adult psychopaths that show structural and functional abnormalities of their amygdalae (see Kiehl et al. 2001; Tiihonen et al. 2000). So, if the amygdala is dysfunctional in psychopaths, then this may help to 'explain' why they are capable of instrumental violence: they do not 'feel others' pain', they do not learn from punishment, and they may not recognize fear or distress in their victims (they themselves exhibit deficits in facial affect recognition). In essence, violence proceeds (and may be premeditated over variable periods) because there are no 'brakes' upon its execution.

In contrast, the forensic relevance of the OFC is specifically connected to its role in modulating 'reactive' aggression. Blair stresses that this need not be solely inhibitory in nature, for there are times when aggression or violence is contextually appropriate. What is important is establishing such 'appropriateness'. He posits two modes of operation at the level of OFC that are likely to impact reactive/impulsive violence:

1. We know from a large literature (parts of which we 'sampled' in Chapters 2, 4, and 8) that the OFC is implicated in changing, reversing, or withholding

responses to the environment, especially when response contingencies have changed, i.e. when the 'reward value' of specific behaviours has altered. Hence, the OFC forms a crucial link between action and expectation. Moreover, if the OFC is involved in monitoring reward values and reward expectations, then it may experience a 'mismatch' when a formerly rewarded behaviour is no longer reinforced (by receipt of a rewarding stimulus). Blair (2004) posits that such a mismatch may form the neurobiological/computational equivalent of our phenomenological experience of 'frustration'. Hence, an organism that has behaved in certain ways in the expectation of a reward may become frustrated, and react aggressively, when such a reward is not forthcoming. We might think of a great many situations, especially those connected with hedonic experiences, where such 'disappointments' may precipitate violence (think of the man who rapes a woman with whom he had expected to have consensual sexual intercourse but who, in the course of a 'date', received an explicit warning that she would *not* be consenting after all). Hence, the OFC may be implicated when organisms respond aggressively to 'not getting their own way'. Notice also, how this takes us back to a distinction that we rehearsed in Chapter 2: that between the motor performance of an act (i.e. its mode and accuracy of 'execution') and the meaning or 'moral value' of that act. While acts that are abnormal in their execution often implicate the dorsal brain systems (e.g. the abnormalities of parietal and premotor cortices associated with the dyspraxias), actions which are aberrant in their 'values', i.e. immoral acts, often seem to implicate medial and ventral brain systems. This is something also intimated by Blair (2004): "'It is unlikely that elevated levels of instrumental [aggressive] behaviour in specific individuals are due to abnormalities in any of the systems for motor behaviour; individuals presenting with heightened levels of instrumental aggression do not show general motor impairment. Instead, it is likely that such individuals show elevated levels of instrumental behaviour because they have been reinforced, and not punished, for committing such behaviour in the past' (pp. 201–202). Nevertheless, we should not suggest that the aggression that follows such 'violations of expectations' is always pathological in nature; there may be situations where this sort of response is 'necessary' for ensuring 'fair play'. When organisms live within communities, when they are situated within reciprocal relationships, there may well be a need to monitor social interactions, social exchange (something that became obvious in Chapter 8, when we examined the human behaviours of deception, 'free-loading' and cheating).

2. A further nuance to the OFC's contribution to the regulation of violence, especially in the reactive context, is its relevance to social hierarchical arrangements within primate colonies (something that we also touched

upon with respect to OFC and serotonergic systems in Chapter 4). Blair posits that the OFC is involved in a process of 'social response reversal' (SRR), essentially a means by which an organism may execute actions that are hierarchically appropriate. Hence, if one is situated low down the social order and one receives a threatening glare from one of one's superiors, then it may be advisable to cease performance of whichever action it was that provoked their censure, i.e. it is time to change one's own behaviour, while also suppressing any signs of reactive aggression. Responding aggressively to a superior primate is likely to elicit further punishment. However, if one is relatively high up within the hierarchy and one receives a glare from a subordinate, then it might be entirely appropriate to emit some form of reactive aggression oneself, in order to 'keep them in their place'. Such behaviours may be studied and elicited in non-humans primates and there seem to be grounds for believing that something rather similar might apply among humans (indeed, this proposition may have immediate resonance with a number of readers who are working within hierarchical organizations). Intriguingly, alcohol and benzodiazepines (drugs such as diazepam) may specifically impact SRR behaviours while serotonergic drugs may impact behavioural change in response to changing reward contingencies (i.e. 1, above), again specifically, suggesting that different neurotransmitter systems may be implicated in modulating different aspects of reactive violence (Blair, 2004).

So, are we any the wiser now? Well, we have just delineated a brain system that is pivotally involved in the execution of violence and which may be modulated by relatively 'higher' centres with different behavioural 'remits'. Indeed, we can see that there may be a host of situations in which different forms of aggression or violence may be 'required' or 'appropriate' within an adult primate's life, and where 'abnormal' neural substrates may have disrupted what it is that 'should have happened next'. Lesions of the amygdala may render humans hypo-aggressive, so that they fail to respond to threat when they might be expected to do so (appropriately), or hyper-aggressive, so that they respond to a threat that is mis-perceived. Lesions of the OFC may render an agent unable to control the 'appropriateness' of their aggression, reacting 'badly' to frustration, making the 'wrong' response within a hierarchical system.

Indeed, all of this coincides rather well with recent insights into the 'human condition' that have arisen from neuroimaging studies exploring the relationship between gender and violence (reviewed by Struber and colleagues, 2008). It transpires that there is a higher ratio of OFC grey matter to amygdala volume among women compared with men; indeed, both sexes have the same size amygdala but the OFC is larger among women (Gur et al. 2002). Furthermore, other authors have found that there is lower 'functional connectivity' (i.e. less temporal correlation across distant neural activities) between the OFC and amygdala in men than in women (during a face-matching task), suggesting that OFC regulation of the amygdala may be weaker among males (Meyer-Lindberg et al. 2006). Hence, it may be the case that there are organic, biological reasons why men are more often aggressive and violent than women. There may be biological 'reasons' for their lesser ability to 'control' their reactive/impulsive aggression.

Pathological states

So, to conclude, Blair's (2004) model suggests that reactive violence is primarily a consequence of the OFC's inability to modulate aggressive responding under emotionally charged conditions, while the instrumental violence typical of 'developmental psychopathy' is more a consequence of problems connected which the amygdala (which may be demonstrated to be small or hypo-functional among selected groups of psychopathic offenders). Blair suggests that while the reactively violent fail to 'control themselves', the instrumentally violent have undergone inadequate 'moral socialization'. How did the latter situation come about? In theory, it came about because an abnormal amygdala rendered the developing psychopath incapable of appreciating the aversive consequences of their antisocial acts (during their development). They were unable to appreciate (or recognize) the distress of others; hence, they did not learn to moderate their conduct towards them. Indeed, they could not learn from punishment (because they did not respond to aversive stimuli; a position congruent with the lower heart rates and impairments of skin conductance response to stress, observed among the antisocials in Raine et al.'s, 2000, paper). Furthermore, as life proceeds, such children ('destined' to become psychopathic) accrue the positive reinforcements associated with rule-breaking behaviour. So, while they cannot be 'punished' they, nevertheless, receive the 'benefits' that may accrue from 'breaking the rules'.

This is a compelling model and it serves to explain in neurological terms how interactions between humans may be modulated or not according to the state of very specific brain regions and circuits. It offers up the possibility of further empirical studies (to confirm or disconfirm the central 'links' in this causal chain) and it also provides a rationale for discarding punishment as a mode of influencing children carrying such 'callous' traits. Nevertheless, a problem remains: what can be done to ameliorate their social, emotional, and moral limitations?

Returning to 'normal'

Before we end this chapter it seems appropriate to retrace our steps, to consider what it is that we have found.

We stated at the outset that there were certain important questions that we needed to answer because our answers would serve to highlight the assumptions that we habitually 'permit' ourselves to make with regards to the 'nature' of human behaviour. Is it chosen or is it caused? Is there a difference between murder and manslaughter? Will moral evil eventually be replaced by natural evil when we have 'explained away' all of human misconduct? I think it would be fair to say that these questions remain open, although we have perhaps 'pushed' our reader well along the road to 'determinism':

1. We may simply accept that all human behaviour is 'determined' and hence, conclude that harmful behaviour directed at others is ultimately entirely the product of 'natural evil(s)'. Furthermore, such natural evil may incorporate variations within genes concerned with neurotransmitter metabolism, aspects of prefrontal cortical or amygdala development, the impact of lesions in the brain, or else aberrant influences located within the experiential and social spheres: being abused, unwanted, exposed to antisocial behavioural patterns exhibited by others, or the 'natural evils' constituting alcohol or drugs (see Table 22).

2. Within the context of a natural species, itself the outcome of evolutionary processes, it is only to be expected that different organisms, different subjects, will receive different genetic endowments, and though this may reflect a 'natural evil' (in theological terms) it may also simply reflect 'normal' (biological/behavioural) variation across the species.

3. Under optimal conditions some human beings may appear to lead what appear to be moral lives, which only become morally aberrant when pathologies supervene (e.g. the brain tumour exhibited by Spyder Cystkopf, or the personality deterioration that may result as a consequence of a frontal lobe dementia or Huntington's disease).

4. However, the characterization of 'normal' still depends upon our assumptions about what it is that 'most people' do, and what they may be expected to do under certain, specified circumstances.

5. So, might we learn more about human nature's 'moral baseline' when the 'normal' environment shifts, drastically? Well, we might.

Exposing the normal

There are many examples that might have been chosen to demonstrate how fragile the 'normal' state of human morality is. For, while our bio-scientific research paradigm is largely focussed upon those who have become 'offenders' within stable, civil societies (Figure 94), there is a whole other area of endeavour occurring within social psychological fields of inquiry and those concerned with recent history that broadens the scope for characterizing 'normality'. What these lines of inquiry have in common is that they expose the more unpleasant aspects of 'normal' people. Here I shall close on only two such examples:

1. What people do when they have 'permission' to punish another human being, a stranger, unknown to them;

2. What normal people do when their society descends into barbarism.

The Milgram experiments

The reader of this text may already know of the seminal experiments conducted by the late Stanley Milgram and his colleagues at Yale University during 1961–62, and first published in 1963, concerning the 'obedience' of apparently normal people to perceived 'authority'. These experiments cast a rather dim light upon human conduct, what we can expect to happen when we are 'on our own' in the presence of authority; when we think that we may punish an unknown stranger, without fear of reprisal. Furthermore, this is a body of work that has been replicated by other investigators on many occasions (inside and outside the United States of America; see Blass, 2004).

The central conceit behind Milgram's study was that a sample of 'normal', healthy adults, was recruited from the local community via a press advertisement, inviting them to take part in an experiment concerning memory. People would be paid a reasonable sum of money 'up front' for their participation (plus travel expenses) and they would receive their payment irrespective of what transpired during the course of the study.

Each volunteer was studied over an hour, on their own. However, they were deliberately given the impression that they were one of two volunteers meeting with an experimenter for the first time. In fact, both the 'experimenter' and the 'other volunteer' were members of the study team (i.e. they were Milgram's confederates).

The experimenter was dressed in a grey lab coat. This was the result of a specific decision: Milgram had not wanted to use a white coat as this might have conveyed the air of a medical experiment. The experimenter read from a precise script and, although the 'real' volunteer did not know it, the events that were about to unfold had already been rehearsed, scripted, and certain vocal responses taped (below).

Early in the process, the two 'volunteers' were given envelopes indicating which of them would play the part of a 'teacher' and which the part of a 'learner'.

In fact, the selection was predetermined and the experimenter's confederate always played the part of the learner. Hence, the 'real' volunteer thought that they had been selected to play the 'teacher' purely by chance.

What transpired then was that the learner went into another room, from which he was able to converse, via a microphone, with the experimenter and the teacher (i.e. the 'real' subject of the experiment). The learner would subsequently have to learn (apparently) new material (word lists), and provide correct answers when asked to recall items. If his answers were incorrect then he was to receive an electric shock, apparently dispensed via an apparatus that was in the same room as the experimenter and the teacher. It was the 'teacher', i.e. the 'real' volunteer, who was called upon to administer such 'shocks' (in fact, no shocks were dispensed though the teacher did not know this).

The apparatus that Milgram had had constructed for the experiment appeared to be a convincing metal box with switches, dials, and flashing lights. It allowed the (apparent) administration of ascending doses of electricity, and carried the following gradations:

'SLIGHT SHOCK

MODERATE SHOCK

STRONG SHOCK

VERY STRONG SHOCK

INTENSE SHOCK

EXTREME INTENSITY SHOCK

DANGER: SEVERE SHOCK' (Blass, 2004, p. 79).

Two final switches were simply labelled 'XXX'.

As the reader has probably anticipated by now, the real purpose of the experiment was to see how far the 'real subject', i.e. the 'teacher', would allow the experiment to proceed before they ceased to participate, before they terminated their compliance. For, as the 'learner' (apparently) made more and more errors, it was they (the 'teacher') who were called upon to administer the electricity, in response to instructions from the 'experimenter'. This remained their apparent remit even after the learner had begun to express his (apparent) distress, becoming increasingly vocal, progressing onwards through shouts and screams, until an ominous silence ensued.

So, when would a 'normal' person stop electrocuting a stranger, someone taking part in a behavioural experiment, someone who could quite easily have 'been them' (apparently), on the basis of a chance dealing of envelopes at the very beginning of an experiment?

Well, 65% of people taking part in the experiment (the initial sample comprised 40 people) would have continued electrocuting the subject until he apparently collapsed or died. Indeed, even among those who finally objected, none had done so before they reached the level of 'INTENSE SHOCK' dispensation (Milgram, 1963).

In subsequent experiments, conducted inside and outside of the United States of America (by 19 groups of investigators between 1967 and 1985) the average percentages of subjects who would have gone on electrocuting their 'learners' 'until the end' have been 60.94% (among USA samples) and 65.94% (among other samples including those from Italy, South Africa, Germany, Jordan, and Austria; see Blass, 2004), respectively.

What does this tell us about 'normal' human behaviour? Well, it provides us with empirical evidence that under the 'right' (i.e. wrong) conditions approximately two-thirds of 'normal' humans would severely damage a total stranger, in apparent obedience to 'authority'. When they are granted permission to punish, most subjects keep going. Any moral superiority that one might feel with regards to the 'abnormal' antisocials we have described (above) would, therefore, appear rather premature. Much depends upon context, 'situation' (at least according to Milgram).

Ordinary people

Hence, it may come as little surprise that we should turn our attention to non-experimental settings wherein 'normal' people have done terrible things to their neighbours, when the situation has allowed them to do so. I shall not labour the point at length but I shall draw on a recent, key text by James Waller (2002).

Waller is a social psychologist who has examined the gross destruction of human life occurring in the context of genocide, mass killing, and 'ethnic cleansing' (Waller, 2002). He provides examples from many theatres of cruelty: the concentration camp at Mauthausen, the massacre at Sand Creek in 1864, the Armenian genocide, the massacre at Babi Yar, the invasion of Dili (East Timor), the Tonle Sap massacre (in Cambodia), the 'death of a Guatemalan village', the church of Ntamara (in Rwanda), and the killings in the 'safe area' of Srebrenica (in former Yugoslavia). Waller is explicit in his conclusion that there is very little that is abnormal about those who commit such atrocities; indeed, when psychologists and psychiatrists have examined certain high-profile offenders (such as the Nazi defendants at Nuremberg) they have found little to comment upon (as we might have anticipated: see Figure 94). Waller's conclusion is that the propensity for extreme cruelty is a common human attribute, one that is found in all settings and is revealed by the dissolution of normal societal constraints.

> I believe that there are acts so vile that our task is to reject and prevent them, not to try to understand them empathetically.

> (Waller, 2002, p. 15)

In such situations, personal ambition, prejudice, and complicity, 'rational self-interest', allow 'ordinary people' to 'turn a blind eye' or else to join in:

'First the girl had to dig out a hole in the field, while her mother, who was 7 months pregnant, had to watch while chained to a tree. They slit open the stomach of the pregnant woman, ripped out the unborn child and threw it into the hole in the ground. Then they threw the woman in as well and the small girl too, after they had raped her first. She was still living when they covered the hole.' This is an eyewitness account by one Angela Hudurovic, recounting how the Ustashi militia (a Croatian nationalist group) tortured her sister and mother to death during the Second World War (see Rose, 1995, 'text 52', p.119).

Perhaps all that one can conclude from such material is that there is such a thing as 'latent morality': we simply do not know what 'normal' humans are capable of while we encounter them within relatively safe, predictable, stable cultural milieu. The base state of human morality is not necessarily apparent under stable conditions, in universities and labs. Terrible as it may seem, the true 'baseline' in human moral conduct is most likely revealed when humans enjoy power over others, when they outnumber their victims, when they may literally 'get away with murder'.

Furthermore, if we take the work of Milgram and others to be accurate (and valid), then we must conclude that when we look into our mirror we encounter the face of someone who is at some considerable risk of 'latent immorality'. For, on strictly statistical grounds, each of us carries within us a greater than 50% probability that we would actually torture someone else, were a permissive situation to arise; were an 'authority' figure to grant us 'permission' to do so. Fortunately, civil societies usually spare us this realization. Perhaps they 'protect' us from ourselves.

Chapter 10

Human response space

> If the paths I had followed had been inked in, it would have seemed as though a man had kept trying out new tracks and connections over and over, only to be thwarted each time by the limitations of his reason, imagination or will-power, and obliged to turn back again.[21]
> > It ain't why, why, why,
> > It ain't why, why, why,
> > It ain't why, why, why,
> > It just is . . . [22]

A recurring theme, running throughout the course of this book, has been the constraints that delimit human behaviour. In each chapter, there has been an anatomical, physiological, psychological, or social boundary to the trajectory of unimpeded human 'action', volition. This is unsurprising: we are material beings living among a community of other material beings, all of us inhabiting a material world. Nevertheless, it may be helpful to rehearse the variety and extent of these constraints before going on to consider how we might lessen their purchase upon us (assuming that we should 'wish' to do so). Indeed, if we understand these constraints well enough, then we might ask whether or not we really retain any volitional 'room for manoeuvre' at all?

The ties that bind

In the Prologue, we began by confronting one of the biggest limitations impacting our perceived 'freedom of the will', namely our limited awareness of our own immediate (very-short-term) intentions to act. In Benjamin Libet's classic

---

[21] W.G. Sebald. *Vertigo* (translated from the German by M. Hulse). London: Harvill Press, 1999 (first published in German 1990), 34.

[22] Lines from Van Morrison's song '*Summertime in England*', on the album '*Common One*'.

experiments, the central finding was that human actors only became aware of their intentions to perform a voluntary act 'freely, spontaneously', after an identified physiological process had already commenced, a process that was detectable by experimenters using electroencephalography (EEG) to measure electrical activity emerging over the subject's scalp. The subject was aware of 'intending to act' but only *after* the neural train of activity (leading to that act) had begun. In other words, the train had already left the station!

Furthermore, we saw that in the context of other experiments that Libet and his colleagues had performed (with congruent findings), a picture emerged of the human conscious mind 'requiring' a finite period of neuronal processing in order for it to become subjectively aware of its own volitions or sensory experiences. The figure arrived at by Libet was in the region of 500 ms. However, from our perspective, the absolute value of this period of 'neuronal adequacy', subjective 'delay', is not crucial; what matters is that there is a finite delay between neural events happening in the brain and their subjective correlates impacting consciousness (in the form of what philosophers might call 'qualia'). So, once again, we have a finding that is consistent with our view of ourselves as material beings, composed of physical processes: the emergence of conscious qualia from the biological substrate of our brains takes a finite time, something on the order of some hundreds of milliseconds. Hence, we are always experiencing 'the past'.

In Chapter 1, we considered the basic anatomy and physiology that allowed a human agent (your author) to move his right index finger. Much of this 'wiring' is so well understood that it constitutes canonical knowledge; it is the bedrock upon which much of clinical medicine is practiced, yet it also serves to show us how intricate, and fragile, is the instantiation of human 'action'. There are many links in a 'causal' chain that are invoked by my seemingly 'simple' decision to move my finger, 'whenever I wish'. These links must be (proximately) *causal* for, if there is a neurological mishap at any step along the way (within the brain, the spinal cord, or 'out' at the periphery), the movement does not emerge: I am paralyzed. I may still 'wish' to move but my actions are impeded.

We saw also that the state of my anatomy sets the limits within which my body, my organism, may 'wish' to move. I happen to be capable of making a discrete index finger movement, but this is not a very common undertaking across the breadth of the animal kingdom; it owes much to the particular arrangement of my corticospinal neurons, and the richness of their connections with alpha motor neurons located in the ventral horns of my spinal cord; it also relies upon a relatively discrete muscular distribution to the joints of that same finger. I may only become aware of my motor limitations when something goes wrong, when an injury or lesion further restricts the motor options open to me, but the fact is that my options are always to some extent 'set' by the 'design features' of the human organism. Indeed, such features include a host of reflex procedures, to which I do not even have to attend; these processes protect and assist me, throughout my 'ambulatory life'.

In Chapter 2, we 'stepped forward' within the frontal lobes in an attempt to establish how it is that the behaviours that I may execute (utilizing the mechanical components of my body) might be elaborated in such a way as to appear 'volitional' or 'willed'. Even if we are radical determinists and we believe that there is no such thing as 'free will', we must accept that very often humans give us the impression that they are 'free': taking decisions, making plans, or doing things that have not been 'scripted' before, in the world (e.g. having conversations, or finding solutions to new problems).

As we moved forward through the frontal lobes, we noted two 'regularities'. First, there is often the emergence of what appears to be a hierarchy in neurological terms (the motor cortex is subject to the premotor cortex, the premotor cortex is 'downstream' of the prefrontal cortex, Broca's area is 'downstream' of the dorsolateral prefrontal cortex [DLPFC], the motor centres of the [dextral] right hemisphere are subordinate to those of the left, and even supplementary motor area (SMA)-proper is 'downstream' of the 'pre-SMA'), a hierarchy which may be exposed and revealed when 'things go wrong'. Second, there is a detectable 'gradient' arching over the cortical mantle, from the lateral systems implicated when an action is 'mechanically wrong' (e.g. in the dyspraxias) to the medial or ventral systems implicated when an action is 'morally wrong' (out of keeping with the agent's previous action choices or society's assessment of what is 'right'). The constraint we faced in Chapter 2 was that of knowing that some of our most cherished skills and judgements, our 'drive' and our 'intentions' (our 'memories of the future'), are crucially dependent upon the adequate functioning of such 'higher' frontal systems. The man sustaining a lesion in his frontal poles (Brodmann area [BA] 10), even if he appears intellectually intact, may suffer a drastic disorganization of his ability to construct and order his own future. He may not even be able to sequence a simple shopping trip or follow a simple recipe.

Furthermore, we saw that in certain frontal regions the processes underpinning consciousness were of limited capacity. The most obvious example was that of 'working memory', our ability to retain items of data within our conscious awareness, so that we might then manipulate them in order to generate new sequences of data, that is, 'novelty'. In the experiments of Marjan Jahanshahi and others, we saw that the DLPFC seemed to be pivotal to this process, and that interfering with its function could render the emerging behavioural sequence stereotypic. This is a subject that we shall return to: the tension that exists between our ability to 'automate' (i.e. to condense behaviours into stereotypic 'routines', manageable quanta of data that may be 'run', as programmes) and our desire at times to generate what is different, complex, or difficult.

In Chapter 3, we returned to some of the issues raised by Benjamin Libet and found them to have been further explored by Patrick Haggard and others. With respect to 'constraints', the issue that emerged here was the complex arrangement of the neurophysiological architecture that seems to underpin our (very-short-term) awareness of our intentions and 'willed' movements. We found that intentions were, in some sense, 'tagged' to processes occurring later in the chain of volition than was our 'awareness of movement'. Whereas our awareness of our intentions seemed to implicate the activation of the lateral premotor and primary motor cortices (as reflected in the 'lateralized readiness potential'), awareness of action seemed to implicate the SMA. Hence, the earlier subjective experience is 'tagged' to the later neurological event and vice versa.

Although we may now say a great deal about the structures and the processes that underpin the emergence of voluntary action, it seems that the emergence of our 'awareness' of agency (in the very-short-term) is still rather obscure. Certainly, it implicates medial premotor systems: if the SMA is stimulated, then the subject feels an 'urge' to move. If the SMA and/or the anterior cingulate cortex (ACC) are destroyed, then the subject may experience no 'will' at all; they may have literally 'nothing to say'. Medial premotor and prefrontal systems seem pivotal to what we might conceive of as 'the will', if by this we mean some intrinsic 'drive' to engage in new thoughts, or new behaviours. A patient who is akinetic and mute certainly appears to be deprived of their 'will': this would appear to be the ultimate constraint upon volition (short of actual death).

In Chapter 4, we attempted to refrain from thinking of human brains as collections of focal functions and instead invoked wide-ranging 'systems', on the basis of basal ganglia–thalamocortical loops, key neurotransmitter systems, the psychological understanding of defined ('controlled' and 'automated') processes, attributable to Tim Shallice, and the distributed systems that paralyze us in our sleep, specifically when we 'dream'. That chapter assayed a very rich and complex literature, from across several diverse fields. What features did we encounter? Well, we saw that the 'logic' that seems to underpin the loop systems is elegant in its precision and apparent order. Again and again we encountered loops that seemed defined by domains of function (motor, executive, emotional or limbic, response reversal or withholding, and eye movement control), and that diaschesis was a logical consequence of this arrangement (i.e. if a loop functions together, in unison, then any 'break in the chain' may precipitate a similar impairment; something we shall return to later).

We saw also that cortical function might be modulated 'up or down' by neurochemical events within the loop and that such modulation was subject to medical manipulation, specifically in the cases of Parkinson's disease (where the desire has been to enhance thalamocortical projections to the SMA, via exogenous dopaminergic manipulation) and psychosis (where the desire has been to reduce thalamic outflow to the cortex, through the use of antipsychotic medications). We saw that neurotransmitters radically impact what might be called the 'space' of human action: dopamine enhances action when present in optimal concentrations. When depleted (as in Parkinson's disease), deficiency of dopamine is associated with deficiency (a lack) of action, a radical constraint upon volition. The response 'space' is shut down. Conversely, we saw that serotonin seems to constrain response space. It facilitates control on the part of the organism. Deficiencies in serotonergic tone are associated with impulsivity, an inappropriate widening of the response repertoire, a tendency that may be associated with harm arising to the 'self' and others. Furthermore, we saw that a range of neurotransmitters (and the drugs that impact their systems) could shift the human agent towards action or inaction (as when we assayed some of the interventions deployed for catatonia and hysteria).

Again, with the Shallice model, the question was, 'How might any organism escape the constraints of a habitual response repertoire located within a familiar environment?' We saw that the environment could 'trigger' motor responses from us and that although these might be quite useful at times (i.e. when we are running on 'automatic pilot'), there would be occasions where a 'captured schema' constitutes an error. Remember Shallice finding himself in a familiar room, reaching for a light string that was not there. The tension returns: it is efficient to be able to 'run' automated routines (source schemata, containing component schemata) in a familiar, predictable environment, but the problem for human agents is that the environment is often unpredictable; we are often called upon to do 'new things', to 'break our habits'. At times, we need to exert control and this seems to implicate the 'supervisory attentional system' (SAS; though, as we have seen, very many authors have invoked similar control processes, under many different names). When we are fatigued, distracted, or attempting to do 'two things at once', we are more likely to lapse, to allow 'rogue schemata' to escape our control. We have a limited capacity for cognitive control. If this is 'freedom', then it is finite, and fragile.

Finally, in Chapter 4, we examined what it is that is happening to the body while we sleep. We found that we are (unknowingly) constrained via our reticulospinal pathways while we dream: we are paralyzed. Such paralysis prevents us from 'acting' out our dreams. It protects us (and those with whom we sleep!). We mentioned that this cast a rather oblique light on the question of consciousness and freedom. It suggests that although we may have doubts concerning the impact of our waking consciousness upon our 'volitions', our 'freedom' (i.e. post-Libet, we may believe that consciousness is 'not the initiator of our acts'), our bodies do not seem to share our uncertainties! They paralyze us in order to prevent our dream-consciousness from converting virtual actions, 'as if' movements, into the real thing. This is especially fortunate given that we may not 'wish' to do the things that we see ourselves doing in dreams. Indeed, the consequences for humans of a breakdown in such nocturnal (neurological) synchronization are dramatically apparent in those who experience rapid eye movement (REM) sleep behavioural disorder. Men strike their partners and hurt themselves while engaged in strange nocturnal narratives.

In Chapter 5, we began a rather more protracted assay of the things that may 'go wrong' within the cerebral motor systems. We found that 'parts' of the agent (hands, arms, and legs) may 'do only what they wish to do'. We borrowed the fictional character of Dr. Strangelove and found that his right hand's motor 'routines' were involuntary while they seemed to reflect his former life's voluntary behaviours. The problem for people exhibiting anarchic and alien limbs is that their own agency has undergone massive constriction; it no longer extends to the margins of their own physical bodies. Some element of their motor machine, their neurological hierarchy, has become 'independent' (of them, the subject or agent). However, the anarchic limb is not 'truly' independent, for, as we saw demonstrated by several investigators, what drives the limb is not an 'inner' drive but the stimuli offered by the external environment. It is the proximity of distracting objects and the waning of executive control, during the performance of other complex procedures, that 'releases' the limb. Again, the external environment 'captures' movements from the limb, movements that the 'true agent' can only control by subterfuge (e.g. tying the limb to her body, sitting on it, putting its hand in a glove, etc.) Hence, the lesson of the anarchic limb is that (at some level) we are living in equilibrium with our physical environment all the time; there are potential 'movements' within us that are not 'actions', we have not chosen them, yet they may be evoked by the environment if we fail to concentrate, if we sustain neurological lesions (especially within our medial premotor systems), or if we fail to 'control ourselves'.

Furthermore, our sense of agency is itself susceptible to even more radical intrusions, as when the somatoparaphrenic patient thinks that a limb of hers belongs to her mother or when people with schizophrenia experience their thoughts and actions as being externally controlled. We saw that in several contexts it is the parietal cortex (especially on the right) that is implicated when 'subjective control' is 'lost'. In some ways, this seems an 'unnecessary' psychopathology. Why do we not 'just' experience a 'loss of control', an 'absence of agency', without the intrusion of what is clearly a very powerful (pathological) experience of 'someone else' being involved. Even if we manifest a failure of 'forward modelling', why does the experience 'feel' as if there is someone else implicated? Remember, it is not 'just' that the patient reports a loss of control; it is not 'just' that the environment is tripping them up, or that accidents are occurring in their motoric control; it is that a force, a being, a 'cosmic string', or the 'thoughts of Eamonn Andrews' are entering their minds. I have no answer to this question but one might conjecture, albeit rather tentatively, that these symptoms seem to acknowledge (admittedly in a highly disordered way) our essential relatedness to each other. They almost seem to posit that 'if I am not moving this limb, then someone else (another agent) must be moving it'.

In Chapter 6, we assayed the correlates of avolition and apathy, verifiable 'absences' of action. We recounted the case of the young man who had lived on the streets, who spoke very little, did rather little, rocked on his chair, and sought out a video of 'Saturday Night Fever'. His behavioural repertoire was, objectively, very narrow. Indeed, although we treated some of his psychotic symptoms (the voices that commented upon his actions), we were largely unsuccessful in ameliorating his essential 'lack' of action. Nowadays, post-rehabilitation, he is a little better. He speaks more (but not a great deal; his sentences are still very short), and honours his sessions in a patients' shop. I see him walking. He is better kempt. Has this man regained his 'freedom'? Well, he is living in the 'community' now. He is out of hospital. He does the things that he wants to do; there is no coercion applied. He has also returned to a 'community' in another sense: he has lived in the one place for some years, he is no longer wandering the streets, moving from town to town, and he recognizes people, remembers them. He is among 'others'.

The avolitional syndrome renders people very limited in their responsiveness to their environment. One gets the impression, although it is difficult to know for certain, that thoughts are reduced, plans diminished. We saw that frontal systems are repeatedly implicated (both functionally and structurally) and we saw that the anterior cingulate loop was especially pertinent to the neurology of apathy, when formerly 'volitional' subjects were rendered avolitional by a lesion. Again, diaschesis was demonstrable: lesions might affect any part of that loop and still cause essentially the same picture, a radical lack of 'will'. Hence, again, the avolitional or apathetic syndrome is one of the most severe constraints that may impact a human agent. It demonstrates, once again, the materiality of human volition. A 'simple' discrete lesion, of the ACC, or caudate or thalamic nucleus, may turn us from an agent into a silent presence. If we wish to defend 'freedom', then we probably have to accept that whatever freedom we have is crucially dependent upon such pivotal brain systems.

In Chapters 7 and 8, we gradually invoked the role of yet another constraint upon human freedom. This was social rather than physical: the presence of other people. How do we negotiate a world full of other actors, other agents? How do we ensure that we get to do what we 'want' to do? Is there a social space for freedom? Well, much of the answer to that question depends upon where (and when) one lives. Casting an amateur historian's eye backwards, over what is known of the human past, it might not be unfair to posit that for the majority of human beings life has involved much regulation by others, control by their human 'conspecifics'? Maybe things were different when our distant ancestors lived among small packs, eking out a hunter-gatherer existence. However, if one considers the impact of 'civilization', of large numbers of people living 'cheek-by-jowl' in urban conurbations, staking out their claims to land, living within tribes, kingdoms, and empires, and surviving as slaves, surfs, and peasants, then it seems reasonable to posit that for many of our ancestors there might often have been a requirement to 'do as you are told to do'. Indeed, Adenzato and Ardito (1999) argue that having to exist within such systems is what fosters the necessity for deception: without the ability to withhold one's thoughts, to conceal one's activities, one might never have the opportunity of even brief episodes of 'freedom'. Indeed, if one jumps forward in time to more recent (and modern) totalitarian states, then one might well understand how an ability to withdraw from 'honest' communication renders survival possible.

When we dealt with hysteria or conversion disorder, we saw that this remains an intriguing concept, requiring seemingly clairvoyant powers on the part of the doctor (who must be able to 'tell what her patient is thinking')! Doctors are asked to decide whether a failure to move is biological, intentional, or 'unconsciously mediated'. Most intriguing of all is the finding that the maintenance of hysterical symptoms seems to involve the contribution of the cognitive executive. The patient must attend to her paralysis in order for it to persist. So, the constraint to which she is subject is the converse of that which impacts the patient experiencing an organic syndrome for, whereas the latter must try to keep 'attending' in order to ameliorate his impairment (i.e. if he 'concentrates', he can make his movements better, though not necessarily 'normal'), the hysteria patient must attend to maintaining her symptom (i.e. failing to attend leads to the re-emergence of 'normal' function, what Lacan and Zizek might have called the Real).

However, there is another constraint that stalks the patient exhibiting signs of hysteria or conversion disorder: the presence of other agents. For, it seems to matter whether other people are present, and it seems to matter what the physician 'does'. Furthermore, such interpersonal influences seem to have reached their apogee in the conduct of Jean-Martin Charcot and the culture of the Salpêtrière Hospital in Paris towards the end of the nineteenth century. We saw how Charcot's impact on people (and their motor systems) appeared almost miraculous at times (remember the coachman blessing himself when the 'paralyzed' girl began to walk). Hence, once again, the presence of the environment, in this case the interpersonal environment, impacts upon the actions of human agents: it seems to constrain their possibilities. However, the ways in which such 'impact' is conveyed through us (through our sensory systems) is currently obscure.

In the case of frank deception (Chapter 8), we see that the salient constraint is at first internal: that is, it is very much subsumed within the ability of the agent to withhold information. The more difficult the deception, the more the agent seems to inhibit motoric activities: movements are reduced (the motivational impairment effect), speech becomes slower, and there are more nonfluent interruptions ('ums . . . ahhs . . .' etc.; Vrij and Mann, 2001). Indeed, does the existence of deception not provide us with an opportunity to enquire the following of the radical determinist?

> Is deception not one of the most compelling arguments for human freedom? After all, it necessarily involves the 'knowing' manipulation of information towards an intended end. The agent does it deliberately (by definition). They are deliberately withholding or suppressing the 'determined', the specified, the prepotent response, that is, the 'truth'. What more could one ask for as a defence, a proof, of 'freedom'?

Again, the practice of deception provides us with evidence of a cognitive processing system that is of limited capacity. Withholding the truth often takes more time than telling it; the response time during lying is often prolonged. There are likely to be constraints upon an individual's ability to 'keep the deception going'. Hence, some commentators have suggested further increasing the cognitive load placed on prospective liars: questioning for longer periods, requiring greater and greater detail about 'factual occurrences', and asking the witness to go through the entire narrative in *reverse order*! All these procedures may make it more difficult to withhold the truth (a recent review is provided by Aldert Vrij [2008]). Furthermore, during attempted deceit, especially under 'high-stake' conditions, we see the capacity for human cognitive control pitched against the ingenuity of other humans, embroiled in counterargument and interrogation, another example of environmental constraints impacting human action (Vrij and Mann, 2001).

In Chapter 9, a chapter that necessarily assayed a wide range of literatures, we 'pushed' the notion of constraint about as far as it might go, for we were dealing with the most profound constraint of all: whether human agents are ever 'free', whether the bad things that they do to others are 'chosen' or 'determined', and whether they constitute instances of 'moral' or 'natural evil'. We argued that if one is a materialist then, ultimately, all evil collapses into the 'natural evil' category. If one rejects freedom, then all the bad things that happen in the world, whether or not they are proximately related to 'agents' or 'objects', are ultimately merely natural 'events'; they are not 'actions'. Hence, murder collapses into manslaughter, and the violence of the man suffering the terrible predations of Huntington's disease is no more 'natural' (i.e. no less 'voluntary') than the drunken violence executed on a Saturday night. All is 'natural'; no one is 'responsible'.

Furthermore, as we accrue more and more biological data that seem to suggest that people who harm others are themselves 'deviant', in a biological sense, maybe in terms of their prefrontal grey matter, maybe in terms of their neurotransmitter metabolism, or maybe in terms of their genetics, we expand the perceived (objectively defensible) contribution of 'natural evil' to forensic behaviours; we remove 'blame', and we exonerate 'wickedness'. Nevertheless, we also argued that the presence of an aliquot of 'natural evil' does not tell us the *full extent* of its contribution to human behaviour or at least not with any degree of precision. As we saw in the case of Spyder Cystkopf, it is very hard to know what significance to apportion a given biological abnormality. To what extent can one 'prove' that a given parameter, a specific lesion, somehow 'caused' a human behaviour? One cannot simply 'run the experiment again'. Obviously, the 'proof' required by a court of law is of a different quality to that required by science and, in many ways, this is reasonable, for the law must make far more practical decisions: 'What does one do now? How should the accused be treated?' Biological reductionism seems only to help us if we wish to think about these cases simplistically; however, as soon as we start to question the evidence, to probe alternative possibilities, life becomes far more complicated (again!).

So, when we approach the harm that human beings will do to others, we confront multiple constraints (impacting our hypothetical investigators):

1. Trying to decide upon the 'nature' of human nature (is it inherently 'flawed' or potentially 'perfectible'?);

2. Trying to decide upon the extent of the suspect's volitional control (admittedly only relevant if you are prepared to 'allow' a degree of 'freedom');

3. Trying to decide the extent of his conscious awareness (a subject's knowledge of their own causation);

4. Trying to discern the extent to which the perpetrator's consciousness admits 'feelings' (i.e. does a deficient amygdala 'really' constrain emotional experience, affective recognition?);

5. The extent to which one human can 'read' another ('we' cannot 'tell' what someone else is thinking; 'we' are poor at detecting deception);

6. The extent to which we can conceive of understanding other people's lives (how do a judge and jury 'judge' or 'understand' the agent who has emerged from the life trajectory that we sketched out in Table 22?);

7. The extent to which we acknowledge and might even 'measure' the 'control' that a 'normal' society exerts upon a 'normal' individual or that is 'removed' from an actor living in an abnormal culture (e.g. in the context of genocide); and

8. What do we estimate to be the limit of 'normal badness' within 'normal people' (if we take seriously the empirical evidence provided by Milgram and others and the 'real-life' evidence of countless atrocities, reviewed by Waller)?

The human capacity for volition, for voluntary control, or the apparent expression of 'willed' actions is subject to multiple constraints, summarized in Table 24. These constraints are anatomical, physiological, neurochemical, psychological (especially in terms of cognitive, computational processing resources), emotional (in terms of our ability to 'feel'), interpersonal, and social (our conspecifics and our hierarchies hold us in check, unless we reside at 'the very top' or 'the very bottom').

Expanding the response space

So, if one accepts that we may conceive of such a concept as 'human response space', a 'space for freedom', albeit one that is bounded by multiple physical, psychological, and social constraints (Table 24), then the question arises as to whether such a space might be 'expanded'. Can we increase the space of freedom, if only for a little while? What follows is not a systematic survey of any given field but instead a selection of some of those instances in which human beings (your author included) have tried to bring about such an 'expansion'. They range from the strictly medical, to the 'everyday' attempts of healthy human agents to 'change their habits', to the activities engaged in by some creative artists in order to attempt to prevent themselves from 'repeating themselves'.

Table 24 The limits of freedom (factors which determine the boundaries of the human response space)

Limit	Exemplars
Social ('agentic') environment	Facilitation of good or bad conduct by the company we keep; the state of 'society'. The worst aspects of our characters (our 'latent morality') may be held in check by societal constraints (Chapter 9).
	'Others' may also impact the expression of 'unconscious' symptoms and signs in hysteria (Chapter 7).
Physical environment	Sensory features of the external environment may 'capture' motor routines if the agent is distracted or impacted by medial premotor cortical lesions (see Chapters 4 and 5).
Body anatomy	This constrains the range of movements that may be undertaken by the agent (e.g. the limits of joint rotation, limb extension) and also the dexterity that may be exhibited (e.g. as a consequence of the ratios between corticospinal upper motor neuron axons and alpha lower motor neurons, located in ventral horn of spinal cord; see Chapter 1).
Brain anatomy	Specific, gross pathologies may impact critical brain regions, thereby impacting such features of volition as drive, motivation, and the 'will', especially following medial premotor and prefrontal cortical lesions. 'Strokes' or other lesions of the internal capsule will paralyze the contralateral side of the body. Left-sided frontal lesions will variously affect language (Chapter 2).
	Similarly, the basal ganglia–thalamocortical loops involving the anterior cingulate cortex and supplementary motor areas (SMAs) may reduce responsiveness. Lesions of the orbitofrontal cortex may 'release' inappropriate behaviours (see Chapters 2, 4, 6, and 9).
	Lesions of the medial premotor cortex and corpus callosum may render an agent susceptible to 'capture errors' (exhibited by an anarchic limb; Chapter 5).
Neurochemistry	A number of neurotransmitters impact the expanse of the human response space: optimal levels of dopamine facilitate the emergence of voluntary actions, whereas serotonin is implicated in constraining the emergence of impulsive, harmful behaviours (Chapter 4).
	Thus, the impacts of dopaminergic and serotonergic deficiencies are to impede and 'release' voluntary behaviours, respectively.
	It follows that neurotransmitter modulation through drug therapies may potentially restore the response space (see Chapter 10).
Physiology	Humans undergo paralysis of their 'voluntary' musculature at night during rapid eye movement (REM) sleep, when they dream. This involuntary constraint prevents harm emerging if/when humans 'act out' their dreams (occurring in REM sleep behavioural disorder; see Chapter 4).

Table 24 (continued) The limits of freedom (factors which determine the boundaries of the human response space)

Limit	Exemplars
Psychology (cognitive executive function)	Our capacity for information generation is limited, as is our capacity for retaining material in consciousness (in 'working memory'; Chapter 2).
	Our limited cognitive capacities are exposed in creative situations (through repetition and the emergence of artistic 'style', really a form of stereotypy) and during deception (when the liar evinces longer response times and greater activation of 'higher' brain centres during attempted deceit; Chapter 8).
	Distraction, sedation, and having to 'dual task' all impact the ability of the agent to generate novel information, deceive, or maintain hysterical phenomena (Chapter 7).
Phenomenology	The temporal delay inherent in 'neuronal adequacy' means that we are always experiencing 'the past' (see Prologue). Our sensation and intentions are perceived 'late'.
	Attention (concentration) may enhance motor performance in the context of organic pathology but is likely to worsen performance in cases of hysteria (Chapter 7).
	There may be 'limits' on the ability of certain agents to 'feel' emotions, to experience empathy for their victims, if their amygdalae are abnormal (e.g. in developmental psychopathy; Chapter 9).
Genetics	This is the ultimate constraint, setting the 'outer' limits of our anatomical/physiological structures and neurochemical parameters (e.g. the impact of the COMT genotype on perseverative errors [Chapter 2], the impact of the MAOA genotype on the exhibition of violence and antisocial conduct [Chapter 9]).

The human response space is likely to be inherently multidimensional because of both the multiplicity of potential influences on the limits of human volition/action and the multiple parameters susceptible to such influences (e.g. speed, angle, force, identity of motor response).

A cure for apathy

I begin with what is my favourite example of this endeavour. It is my favourite because I think it amply sums up what a 'perfect' medical intervention might look like (or at least begin to look like). For, if we allow ourselves to believe that the medical process is about restoring agency to another human being (restoring their 'independence'), so that they might overcome adversity and continue on 'their way' towards the completion of whatever life project it is that is 'theirs' to complete (over the course of a finite human existence), then what should we want from medicine? Should we not seek the restoration of 'freedom', the restoration of 'internally initiated' human acts?

In a paper published in 1991, Ken Barrett described four cases of 'abulia' (apathy) caused by different neurological diseases, each of which had rendered one his four patients incapable of voluntary action. Typically, they were rendered apathetic, sitting 'doing nothing' all day. They were very similar to some of those cases that we have reviewed in Chapter 6.

Barrett's first case ('case 1') was that of a young man suffering from Wilson's disease, a progressive disorder impacting the basal ganglia. Initially, he had presented with a depressive illness, but subsequently he descended into an apathetic state with marked neurological impairment; he exhibited 'severe hypertonia of the upper limbs and face, severe dysarthria, and became increasingly blunted emotionally and volitionally' (Barrett, 1991, p. 719). The patient lived with his parents, needed to be prompted to attend to basic hygiene and self-care, and spent much of the day watching TV, though he had little concern over what he saw.

Barrett gave this man a trial of a dopamine agonist (bromocriptine). The rationale was one that we have rehearsed in Chapter 4, namely that increasing dopaminergic tone would facilitate transmission within the 'direct' pathway of the basal ganglia–thalamocortical loop systems and hence increase excitatory neurotransmission between the thalamus and such output centres as the SMA and ACC. Such a sequence of events 'should' increase 'action'. What actually happened?

> 'An increase in his initiative began at 7.5 mg [of bromocriptine per day] and increased as the dose was increased. He read the newspapers for the first time in several years and became more discriminating over the TV programmes he watched; [he] selected his own videotapes. He started to go for walks and visited the local pub where he played games.' This improvement persisted.

Barrett's 'case 3' was an older man, a former miner who, in the past, had suffered from both a psychosis and repeated strokes. At the time of presentation, he was 57 years old, doubly incontinent, and answering only 'yes' or 'no' to questions. He would 'sit or stand unmoving if not prompted. He only ate with prompting, and would sometimes continue putting spoon to mouth, sometimes for as long as two minutes after his plate was empty.' A computed tomography (CT) scan of his brain revealed multiple vascular lesions throughout both internal capsules and the right caudate nucleus. Again, Barrett treated this man with bromocriptine:

> 'His first spontaneous activity, dressing without prompting, occurred at 20 mg. At 30 mg he started to initiate conversations with other residents, but there was considerable day-to-day variation. As the dose increased, he washed, dressed and ate his meals without prompting and was not perseverative.'

What do we make of these cases? They seem to provide instances of men who had been rendered unresponsive to their environments (apathetic, abulic, or avolitional, according to one's terminology) as a consequence of verifiable organic brain lesions being returned to some state of volition, to being able to make choices for themselves again. They 'returned' in some sense through the use of a medication, in this case a dopamine agonist, mimicking the effects of cerebral dopamine. These responses are impressive. They suggest that even an apathetic patient may 'come back'; furthermore, they seem to imply some kind of 'resumption' of activity. We do not know if the young man (case 1) made similar choices to those that he had made prior to his illness, but it is intriguing to think of an elevation of dopaminergic function impacting his ability to have preferences for one TV programme over another. In case 3, the improvement is even more surprising, given the very severe disability of the gentleman described. Is it fair to say that Barrett has increased the 'response space' open to his patients? My impression is that he has.

I would suggest that this is the sort of change that we should like to be able to bring about in a great many cerebral pathologies, that is, a meaningful return of voluntary behaviour, a capacity for volition. It is reminiscent of the achievements reported in Oliver Sacks' (1982) famous book, *Awakenings*, recording the therapeutic responses of his patients who had been left akinetic in the wake of the Spanish 'Flu' epidemic that swept the world in the early twentieth century. Sacks' patients, who suffered from a post-encephalitic form of Parkinsonism, were 'restored' in some sense following the administration of L-DOPA, a precursor of dopamine. Hence, in keeping with all that we have rehearsed (earlier in chapter 4) regarding Parkinson's disease and the restoration of 'internally initiated' actions with dopaminergic therapies (and their impact upon the medial premotor system), it is clear that modulation of the dopamine system may enhance volition. It expands the (potential) response space, the space for responses. Whether or not this constitutes 'freedom of choice' in the libertarian sense, and whether or not we are 'determinists' (i.e. reductionists), it would be fair to say that those patients who have had their 'volition' restored (even if only temporarily so) by dopaminergic interventions appear to be a lot less 'determined' (in the reductionist sense) than they had been while they were apathetic, or avolitional. A response space appears to have been 'opened'.

Restoring space to avolition

A problem for those of us wishing to restore 'response space' to people manifesting the avolitional state in schizophrenia is that the use of dopaminergic agents may well aggravate the schizophrenic illness itself: precipitating psychotic relapse, and the re-emergence of so-called 'positive' symptoms (delusions and hallucinations). So, investigators continue to look for alternative compounds that might restore function while not worsening such symptomatology.

One option, which presented itself to our group in the early 2000s, was to investigate the possibility of using modafinil to enhance cognitive control in people with chronic but stable schizophrenia. Modafinil is a drug that has been licenced in the United States and the United Kingdom as a treatment of narcolepsy (a condition characterized by excessive daytime somnolence, sleepiness). The drug provides an alternative to other treatments of narcolepsy, including the amphetamines, which are themselves activating but have the drawback that they may precipitate psychosis (and may of course become addictive). Modafinil is a novel 'wake-promoting' agent: it helps keep people awake. However, the problem with this drug is that it is active across so many neurotransmitter systems that one cannot say for certain which system is responsible for its beneficial effects—increased alertness without addiction. The drug has also been shown to enhance some aspects of executive function in healthy controls (and people with schizophrenia), so there have been hopes that it might evince 'restorative' properties if administered to people with severe neuropsychiatric disorders (see Turner and Sahakian [2006] for a recent review).

We performed a randomized double-blind placebo-controlled crossover trial to examine the acute effects of a single, small dose (100 mg) of modafinil in a group of people with chronic schizophrenia, studied on two occasions, one week apart. On each occasion, the drug (or an identically prepared placebo) was administered at 8 a.m. and the patient was scanned while performing a battery of cognitive tasks for less than an hour between 10 a.m. and noon (coinciding with the peak plasma levels of the drug). Then, they were observed on a research ward until 8 a.m. the following morning. While they were with us, all patients wore an Actiwatch, a wrist-worn device that provides an objective measure of how much they had moved around over the course of that day.

Hence, patients were essentially compared with themselves, on two occasions, once on modafinil and once on placebo (the order of administration being counterbalanced across subjects). What did we find? We found that

1. Patients 'moved around more' on the days when they had received modafinil. Hence, the drug did appear to have an activating effect, which could be seen to accrue over the day (see Fig. 99; Farrow et al., 2006);

2. During the performance of a motor task, which required patients to exert deliberate control over the timing of their own movements (executed with their right index fingers), there was a change in activity in dorsolateral

prefrontal regions (the bilateral DLPFCs), the magnitude of which corre-lated with the success of their performance. Those who exhibited greater increases in the modulation of their own movements (in response to modafinil) also evinced the greater increase in response in the left DLPFC in particular. These were also the patients who had exhibited worse verbal fluency performance at baseline (a proxy measure of left prefrontal cortex cognitive performance; see Chapter 2). Hence, modafinil seemed to enhance executive control among those patients who were initially most impaired: its effects on cognition might therefore be characterized as potentially 'restorative' rather than 'enhancing' among this particular group of patients (see Fig. 100; Hunter et al., 2006).

Thus, we have some preliminary evidence that modafinil might be able to impact the response space of those who are most severely incapacitated by schizophrenia. They may move more; they may evince more 'control' over their movements. Such are the prerequisites for an intervention that might allow subjects to 'sculpt' their own response space. However, much more work is needed in this area.

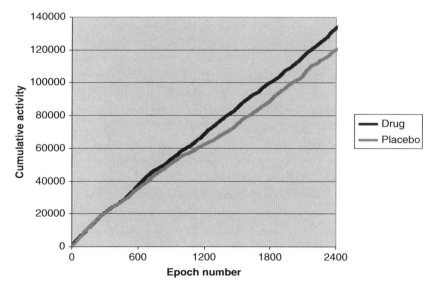

Fig. 99 Graph demonstrating daytime activity in a group of people with chronic schizophrenia. In the course of a randomized double-blind placebo-controlled trial, patients exhibited greater activity on the day that they received the drug modafanil than on the day that they received the placebo. Reprinted from the *British Journal of Psychiatry*; 189: 461–462. Farrow TFD et al, 2006, with permission from The Royal College of Psychiatrists. (See colour plate section).

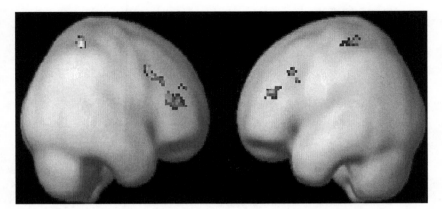

Fig. 100 Functional magnetic resonance images obtained from patients using modafinil showing increased prefrontal activation during the course of a motor task that required patients to control their own behaviours in time. Those exhibiting increased activation while on modafinil also exhibited better behavioural performance. (From Hunter et al., *American Journal of Psychiatry* 2006; 163: 2184–2186).

Is 'self-control' a muscle?

A completely different literature, but one which is also highly informative in the current context, is that found within the field of social psychology. Authors such as Roy Baumeister and his colleagues have entertained the notion that self-control, our ability to alter our habits, to change our behaviours, and to resist temptation, is analogous to a muscle. In other words, it is of limited 'strength'; it will become fatigued if exercised without rest; it may recover after a period of relaxation and, in the long-term, may even grow stronger with repeated application (exertion, exercise). Is this feasible?

Well, the literature derives largely from studies of cohorts of healthy people who are attempting to change something about themselves: keeping to a diet, giving up smoking, ceasing their use of alcohol, or trying to control their emotions. A recurring theme is that periods of time spent in environments that demand much of the subject are more likely to precipitate a relapse (in the undesirable behaviour) *later on*. Hence, if they spend periods in noisy rooms, if they are subject to random interruptions or disturbances, over which they have no control, or if they must tolerate discomfort, unpleasant smells, or overcrowding, then they are less likely to persist in their subsequent attempts to perform difficult cognitive tests administered immediately following the stressful situation. And, if they have been refraining from some undesirable behaviour prior to that point, they are then more likely to relapse: having a cigarette, taking a drink, 'giving in to temptation' (think of coming home, 'after a long day'). The point is that the 'control' processes hypothesized to reside within human agents constitute a finite resource (another one of our recurring themes); subjects can only 'put up a fight' for so long. Hence, those who are giving up smoking and who may be succeeding consistently in this quest may be relapsing in terms of their chocolate use. They seem unable to repress all their habits at once or at least for long (see Muraven and Baumeister [2000] for a highly accessible review).

> 'Consistent with the main prediction of the strength model [of self-control], we found that after an act of self-control, subsequent unrelated self-control operations suffer. After coping with stressors that may require self-control, people's subsequent self-control performance suffers. Coping with stress is also likely to lead to diet breaking and smoking relapses. Similarly, when coping with negative affect and (presumably) trying to make themselves feel better, people are poorer at delaying gratification and other self-control tasks. After resisting temptations, people perform more poorly on tests of vigilance and are less able to resist subsequent temptations (e.g. dieters who quit smoking eat more).'

> (Muraven and Baumeister, 2000, p. 254)

However, there is the tantalizing possibility that those who practice self-control may get better at it, over the longer term. So, although their 'control' may undergo fatigue in the short term, there is the prospect that perseverance helps. Muraven and Baumeister (2000) present evidence from other experiments demonstrating that students who have followed various self-control procedures over successive weeks exhibit greater effort on physical tasks when tested later compared with students who had not been required to practice 'self-control'.

This is an intriguing literature; maybe it constitutes an empirical base upon which to ground an intuition that we might have garnered anyway, from everyday life: 'changing ourselves' is difficult and demanding, and it may be a source of much struggle, but we can get 'better' at it, if we 'try'. However, if this is true, then what does it tell us about our putative 'response space'? It suggests to me that there are times when (if we try very hard indeed) we may sculpt that space, to suit our longer-term purposes (our 'goals'; Spence, 2008b). We might even alter the things that we do 'automatically' (e.g. 'stop reaching for a cigarette in times of stress and go for a walk instead').

The notion that one might manage one's future, as one might manage a budget or a bank account, is one that is also discernible in other psychological and psychiatric literatures. Thus, some authors talk of 'implementation intentions': the pacts we make with ourselves that will keep us on the right track in future situations. Such intentions follow an 'if-then' format. So, for instance, if I am attempting to give up my use of alcohol, then I may be most successful if

I anticipate what I shall need to do in 'tempting' environments should some-one offer me a drink:

> 'If I am offered a drink, then I shall ask for an orange juice.'
> 'If Joe suggests going for a drink, then I shall say I need to get home on time for dinner.'
> 'If Sue asks me to the party, then I shall say that I am working late.'

The point of these scenarios is that I might be more likely to succeed in my abstemiousness if I can say something 'automatically' that extricates me from a potentially risky situation. (In a sense, in each of these scenarios, I am taking advantage of what it is that BA 10 lends me: the attribute of a 'prospective mem-ory', a 'memory of the future'; for, it is only possible to plan ahead if I can con-ceive of such an 'ahead' in time; see Chapter 2 and the work of Paul Burgess).

A similar management style is espoused by George Ainslie (2001), another leading author in the field of 'self-control'. He has proposed a model to explain how and why we 'let ourselves down' when we opt for a short-term temptation in preference to a long-term goal (e.g. taking the drink that is offered rather than remaining abstinent). However, his important insight regarding our short-term temptations is that we are better off if our decisions can be constructed as dichotomous variables, that is, if we can put a 'clear white line' between what we 'should do' and what we do not wish to happen. Hence, for Ainslie, it is easier and more reliable to opt for abstinence over 'controlled' drinking because there is a clear distinction between having no alcohol at all and having a drink. Conversely, 'controlled' drinking exposes us to the dilemma of where to draw the line? If we allow ourselves 'one or two' drinks, then we are already on our way to taking a third. It may be more difficult to abstain then because we have already begun the suboptimal behaviour concerned and (as the chemical effects of alcohol accrue within us) our resistance may wane. Hence, 'grey' boundaries are more difficult to police than clear white lines (Ainslie, 2001).

Each of these approaches relies upon a belief that we may influence our future conduct, that we may prepare our future decisions, *before* life delivers us to the middle of our next predicament. In each of these cases, the actor is attempting to specify the limits of their response space ahead of time, prospec-tively (this would appear to be 'responsible'; Spence, 2008b).

Giving creativity a 'helping hand'

So much of this text has, necessarily, been concerned with what can 'go wrong' within our brains (i.e. with the volitional impairments with which human agents must sometimes have to cope) that it makes something of a pleasant excursion to consider what might be 'going on' when human agents are engaged in activities that express the very height of our species' volitional capabilities.

Many examples might have been chosen, but here I shall focus on only one: the lengths to which improvising musicians may go to try to provoke themselves into 'creativity'. Such a topic is large and might have been prefaced with many detailed modes of introduction. However, I shall offer just a very simple perspective, one that follows on from the issues that we have been discussing in this text, one that places its emphasis on the proposed generation of novelty:

1. An improviser undertakes to create a new sequence of behaviours in a context that may be more or less 'structured'.

2. That structure may comprise the themes derived from a predetermined piece of music, within which he or she is improvising, and/or the presence of other musicians who are also acting or sharing in the same virtual (i.e. musical) 'space'.

3. Such structures may impose a limit upon the improviser: for example, only certain notes and certain rhythms may 'fit in' with the predetermined theme; there may be 'turns' to be taken when other musicians are present.

4. An improviser might be especially 'free' when he is playing entirely on his own.

5. However, he might also choose to deliberately constrain himself, deciding to use only a part of an instrument, certain notes, and so on.

6. If one reads the comments of improvising musicians, there is often a reported emphasis on avoiding 'routines', avoiding what is 'predictable'; one gets the impression that when they play in ensembles, they are 'watching out' for indications of repetition or preparation among their peers, activities that are often frowned upon!

Consider the following extracts, drawn from the improvising literature. The first is taken from the late Derek Bailey's (1993) seminal account, *Improvisation: Its Nature and Practice in Music*:

> 'In 1968 I ran into Steve Lacy [the late soprano saxophone virtuoso] on the street in Rome. I took out my pocket tape recorder and asked him to describe in fifteen seconds the difference between composition and improvisation. He answered: "In fifteen seconds the difference between composition and improvisation is that in composition you have all the time you want to decide what to say in fifteen seconds, while in improvisation you have fifteen seconds."

> (Bailey, 1993, p. 141)

The rejection of repetition emerges in another exchange with Lacy:

> 'Jazz got so that it wasn't improvised any more. A lot of the music that was going on was really not improvised. It got so that everybody knew what was going to happen

and, sure enough, that's what happened. Maybe the order of the phrases and tunes would be a little different every night, but for me that wasn't enough.'

(Quoted in Bailey, 1993, p. 55)

Next, the pianist Paul Bley describes his approach to improvisation, in the light of his hearing the great alto saxophonist Charlie Parker ('Bird'):

'In hearing Bird's ability to anticipate what was coming and always thinking ahead, I've tried to extend that idea to listening for three things before I start playing a phrase:

One: What was the last phrase that was played, and what was the last note of the last phrase that was played, and what should follow that?

Two: What music has been played throughout the history of jazz that has to be avoided, leaving me only what's left as material for the next phrase?

Three: Where would I like to get to by the time my playing is finished?

All that in a split second during a pause in my phrasing.'

(From Bley and Lee, 1999, p. 35)

Next, consider the drummer Gunther Muller, attempting to limit his alternatives when he assembles his drum kit:

'At the moment I often play with just a snare on my left, a floor tom on my right, and a cymbal between them. I change the acoustic elements regularly so that I'm forced to learn new ways to play, and this gives me new ideas. It enables me to avoid automatic movements. Playing drums is a wonderful thing, but if you get used to fast sequences of automatic movements it becomes hard to really make music, rather than winding off your licks [routines] all the time.'

(Gunther Muller, quoted in *The Wire*, April 2000, p. 17)

He also takes a dim view of predictability:

'In the end, when a musician knows that an audience comes to his concert expecting to see special tricks, the concert becomes a kind of cabaret and has only little to do with music.' (p. 17)

Finally, here is another saxophonist, Lol Coxhill, talking about improvisation; notice how the same themes surface again:

'I can get more involved in it [free improvisation] as a listener than most other music. The very fact that it's open and you don't know what's coming next, you can't decide beforehand what's coming. Well, unfortunately, very often you can, but not when it's the real thing. There are a lot of people around who you know are going to play specific things as opposed to really try and get on with it and cliff-hang. You can't avoid having phrases. You don't look for them, but recognizable things emerge—nobody would know who they're listening to otherwise.'

(Lol Coxhill, quoted in *The Wire*, November 2001, p. 22)

On trying to be 'unrecognizable' himself, he says: 'It's the way you avoid playing the same things all the time! I know I can be listening back to something I've done and I think it's all right, [but] then I hear a phrase that I know I must have played a thousand times before and it really pisses me off [laughs]. I sometimes use phrases to get to somewhere else, not preconceived, but at a moment something briefly happens that is going to take it somewhere else. You get in and out of it. I loved Charlie Parker when I heard him at the age of 11, but so many recordings are available it becomes the opposite of what free improvisers try for.'

Hence, according to these 'witnesses', the practice of improvisation places very great emphasis on novelty generation, thinking in the instant of creation itself, and importantly, editing or suppressing that which is 'routine' or has been previously rehearsed (or played).

When I first became interested in the phenomenology of this type of music, what struck me was the very great resemblance to a particular cognitive procedure, one that formed the basis of a classic paper by Alan Baddeley in 1966. Baddeley reported a series of experiments in which healthy subjects had been asked to generate 'random' responses. In other words, they had to generate novel information, under changing conditions, each of them imposing different levels of constraint. Hence, if subjects were called upon to generate random sequences of letters or numbers, the following patterns emerged:

1. The faster they had to go, the more stereotypic their sequences became. The subjects generated less variety in their response sequences and hence, in the language of information theory, they exhibited greater 'redundancy' (i.e. less information).

2. If subjects were called upon to perform another executive task at the same time as generating information (randomness), then, as the former task become more taxing, randomness performance declined; in other words, their redundancy increased.

3. Finally, as the set size of response exemplars increased, that is, as the pool of alternatives from which a response might be chosen grew larger, the rate at which randomness could be generated increased at first but then underwent a levelling off until it reached a 'plateau'. There came a point at which the subjects could not generate information any faster.

Taken together, the conclusion drawn from Baddeley's (1966) experiments was that the human capacity for information generation behaved like a process of limited capacity: if you made it go 'faster', its performance declined; if you made it 'dual-task' (i.e. made it 'share' its resources with another executive task), its performance declined; and even when it was 'running' optimally (i.e. as the process became 'easier' with larger sets of exemplars to choose from), it eventually reached a level of maximal performance, beyond which it could not progress. In other words, the human capacity for generating novelty was finite, and its parameters tangible.

So, might we not expect rather similar constraints to apply to the creative brain, to the mind of a musician trying to be 'original', composing in 'real time', but afforded just a 'space' of 15 s to create (as was Lacy)? It seems to me that these improvising musicians are attempting to define a response space under the most trying of circumstances. Note that they also privilege 'control' above 'routines'; in the language of Tim Shallice's 1988 model (see Chapter 4), they appear to be using their SAS constantly; the last thing they want to hear from themselves is the emergence of recognizable 'schemata', phrases that they have played before. And yet, their project is surely doomed to failure, for ultimately they must impact the limits of their own processing capacity, mustn't they?

Well, both Bley and Coxhill made reference to the playing of the progenitor of bebop, Charlie Parker (1920–1955), a man who is widely recognized as having been a genius in his field, a player of immense speed, dexterity, and harmonic invention (Fig. 101). However, even here, there is something that

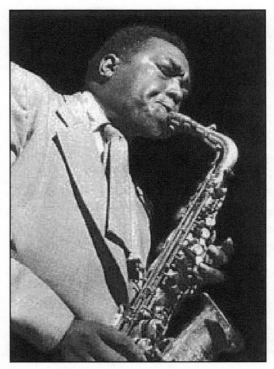

Fig. 101 The bebop pioneer Charlie Parker.

can be said regarding the limitations of human information generation. In the following, I am most indebted to a book by a Professor of Music, Thomas Owens, *Bebop* (1995).

Because Charlie Parker was so prolific and because there are so many extant recordings of his performances, it is possible for modern music academics to analyse his playing style (at least among those physical traces that remain). Having done so, it becomes apparent that even the great Charlie Parker's style is subject to dissection and critique. Analysts may not only spot the phrases that he borrowed from foregoing pioneers in the field of jazz (e.g. Lester Young) but also characterize how he used such materials, especially when playing at speed (recall: we should expect repetition, redundancy, to intrude upon the saxophone solo the faster it is played, for it becomes more difficult for the agent, the musician, to suppress the emergence of stereotypies; see Fig. 102).

> 'Because Parker's recorded legacy is extensive it is possible not only to compile a list of Parker's favourite figures [improvised phrases] but [also] to see how he used these figures in different contexts. A study of his hundreds of choruses of the blues in B♭, F, and C and dozens of choruses of *I Got Rhythm, What Is This Thing Called Love?, How High The Moon*, and others shows that his improvising was largely formulaic. The specifics of the theme were rarely significant in shaping his solo; instead, he favoured a certain repertory of formulas for the blues in B♭, a slightly different repertory for the blues in F, a much different one for *A Night in Tunisia* in D minor, and so on. Some phrases in his vocabulary came from swing, either unchanged or modified; others he created. But whether using borrowed or original melodic formulas, his way of combining and organizing them was his own.'
>
> (Owens, 1995, p. 30)

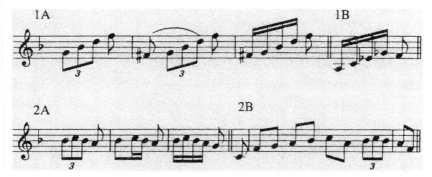

Fig. 102 Musical notation taken from the book Bebop: *The Music and its Players*. These patterns were particularly prevalent among Charlie Parker's improvised solos. (From Owens T. (1995), with permission from Oxford University Press).

Trying to 'act'

Much of this book has been concerned with the physical, psychological, and (to a lesser extent) social elements that must be in place in order for an 'agent' to 'act'. We have seen that such processes may be described but also that they seem to comprise a finite resource. If the human agent possesses any 'freedom' at all, then it is a freedom that is expressed under certain 'optimal' conditions, be they structural, neurochemical, interpersonal, or situational (Table 24). Phenomenologically, we certainly give the impression of being free, some of the time, but there are a great many circumstances that may serve to deprive us of such freedom.

In this chapter, we have sketched just a few of the ways in which human agents have tried to expand the space 'allowed' them for responses. This project manifests itself in its starkest form when we attempt to ameliorate the effects of neuropsychiatric disease (e.g. as when Ken Barrett utilized dopaminergic agents to help abulic patients). However, as we have just seen, much of what gives a creative life its edge, its 'purpose', is the desire to push one's 'self' further, to try to do what has never been done before. Any human being might only ever succeed in such an undertaking on very rare occasions. Nevertheless, it seems to be one of the things that keep us going.

Epilogue: Raising a fist

Certeau examined commonplace activities over which control could in principle be maintained by the institutional organization of space and language and suggested how in fact control was ignored or bypassed. People walk their own way through the grid of city streets, zigzagging, slowing down, preferring streets with certain names, making turns and detours, their own 'walking rhetoric'. People read in ways that escape the social hierarchy and 'imposed system' of written texts: they read in all kinds of places from libraries to toilets. They read with their own rhythms and interruptions, thinking or daydreaming; they read making gestures and sounds, stretching, 'a wild orchestration of the body', and end up with their own ideas about the book. These procedures and ruses . . . compose the network of an antidiscipline.[23]

Query: How contrive not to waste one's time?

Answer: By being fully aware of it all the while.

Ways in which this can be done: By spending one's days in an uneasy chair in a dentist's waiting room; by remaining on one's balcony all Sunday afternoon; by listening to lectures in a language one doesn't know; by travelling by the longest and least convenient train routes, and of course standing all the way; by queuing at the box-office of theatres and then not booking a seat. And so forth.[24]

As we had acknowledged at the very beginning of this book, in the opening pages of our Prologue, there is a problem that resides at the very interface of human volition and moral responsibility; it is a problem that is most tellingly

---

[23] Zemon Davis, N. The quest of Michel de Certeau. *New York Review of Books*, May 15 2008, 57–60 (citation from p. 59).

[24] Albert Camus. *The Plague* (translated by S. Gilbert). London: Hamish Hamilton, 1973: 27. (First published in French 1947).

exposed by the findings of Benjamin Libet's classic EEG experiments concerning the immediate antecedents of human voluntary acts. For, if we take his findings at face value (supplemented by the incisive clarifications offered by the work of Patrick Haggard and his colleagues; reviewed in Chapter 3), then we have to accept the empirical fact that we humans become aware of our voluntary acts only *after* they have been 'set in motion', only *after* the neural antecedents of such acts have become discernible on the putative actor's EEG. Conscious intentions arise relatively 'late' in the volitional process; consciousness is not 'causal'; to an arch-determinist (a radical reductionist), there is no difference between an action and an accident; intentions do not matter. There is no 'freedom'. Murder equals manslaughter: there is a killing just the same.

Is this in any way acceptable to a thinking human being? Is this in any way compatible with the phenomenological evidence offered to us by our senses?

Well, trying to fully articulate this problem and to seek its resolution has provided much of the drive for writing this book; yet, it is clear that we have failed to resolve the central issue. For, on the one hand, we appear to know of our acts only after they have commenced; yet, on the other hand, we have the very strong impression that we (and others) know what we (and they) are doing.

My impression is that we have paid far too little attention to the 'purpose' of consciousness, and indeed, to the role of others in 'open' human communications. Yes, we may have hinted at the role of consciousness in deception (for deceivers do, by definition, utilize the consciousness of their acts, knowledge of their subterfuge, ahead of events, *before* they attempt to dupe their victim; Chapter 8). And yes, we have connected with the very real influence exerted upon agents by other people, through the ways in which the latter might bias subjective agency, as when we assayed the medical literature concerning hysteria (conversion disorder; Chapter 7), where the presence of others might literally change an actor's acts. However, when we use the tools of modern neuroscience, we tend to study individuals as single, isolated organisms (objects); we sometimes overlook the gaps in our awareness (e.g. that we cannot 'know' the subject's consciousness); we sometimes forget that we live as social beings; material entities yes, but embedded within a nexus of other people's minds (and subject to their varying influences on us).

Hence, this Epilogue represents my attempt to provide something of an antidote to these omissions. As we have concluded in Chapter 10, human freedom, if it exists, is a finite, limited resource: we are 'hemmed in' on all 'sides' by our genes, our environment, the habits of our thoughts, our cognitive 'stamina'. Yet, there may be grounds for defending a small, 'narrow' freedom, in the immediate, lived present (the kind of freedom that the improviser pursues, albeit with varying success).

The problem

Since Libet and his colleagues (1983) demonstrated that electrical activity predictive of voluntary behaviour arises from within the brain not only prior to manifest movement but also prior to the *conscious intention* to move, it has seemed that 'free will' is radically undermined at precisely that moment when it might have been most likely to effect change—in those hundreds of milliseconds immediately prior to spontaneous voluntary acts. *Post*-Libet, how can we defend 'free will' without resorting to the speculation that freedom must be enacted *unconsciously*, that is, before its 'author' is aware of his (or her) own 'authorship' (Spence, 1996)?

On the other hand, much of day-to-day life, social interaction, and our ideas of responsibility and culpability hinge upon our notions of what people can reasonably be said to have 'known' that they were doing and, by inference, what they might reasonably have *prevented* themselves from doing. For, although certain legal problems might simply 'go away' if we wished solely to identify the organism that had performed a certain behaviour at a certain time in a certain place, usually this is not good enough: what we really want to know is whether that organism was 'acting' as an 'agent', that is, whether he 'intended' to do what he did (Macmurray, 1991).

Our problem, then, is to reconcile our current recognition of curtailed agency at the point of action with our strong intuition, and phenomenological experience, that we (and others) are free. In order to try to address this problem, we proceed to illuminate it from a variety of angles. Are there any *other* ways of seeing this issue, ways that might shed light upon our current difficulties? Here, we attempt to assay several contrasting perspectives.

Responsibility without power

Consider this statement taken from the Christian New Testament:

> You have heard that it was said, 'You shall not commit adultery.' But I say to you that every one who looks at a woman lustfully has already committed adultery with her in his heart.
>
> (*Matthew*, 5, 27–28)

Does this judgement seem unfair or unreasonable? Well, maybe it does if we understand Jesus to be critiquing automatic responses, automatic thoughts, and temptations, ideas that 'simply' appear in the mind unbidden. For, if (*post*-Libet) we cannot claim authorship of our physical acts, then are we really any more likely to 'own' the thoughts arising in our heads? Can I help what I am thinking? My thoughts seem to just 'appear' most of the time; I may inhabit them, 'identify with them' or adopt a certain distance from them, but generally they follow their own 'flow'. How can I be 'responsible' for them?

Well, one might compromise and suggest that the thoughts referred to by Jesus are most likely to be those that are 'intentionally' ruminated upon, the fantasies occasionally entertained by the human mind, so that any inner conflict that arises in response to such a 'teaching' is actually akin to that occurring within the mind of a patient who suffers from obsessive compulsive disorder (OCD). A man with OCD experiences recurrent intrusive thoughts or images ('obsessions'), which he knows to have originated from within his own mind, yet he rejects their 'content'. They may disgust or frighten him; they may concern matters that he holds to be immoral. His struggle is to resist them, to keep them at bay, to keep them *out* of his consciousness. If they compel him towards an act (a 'compulsion'), then he will resist its performance, but he might also eventually 'give in'. So, if his obsessions concern contamination, then his compulsion may be to wash his hands repeatedly, scrubbing them until they bleed. This man is resisting his own thoughts, not 'entertaining' them (as might the hedonist or pervert, who likes to think of sex and dirt together). The obsessive is trying *not* to think of certain thoughts that strike him as morally unacceptable. Hence, by his very existence (and his reported experience), our obsessive patient actually informs us of the 'normal state' of human affairs in several important ways:

1. Almost by default, it must be possible for the 'rest of us' as humans to 'control' our thoughts, because this is what seems to 'go wrong' in the mind of the obsessive: the patient cannot control the frequency with which certain thoughts 'surface', he cannot control their 'content'; he is suffering for want of ('normal') cognitive control.

2. He seems also to implicitly acknowledge (and identify) an attribute that is common to us all: we have to be *conscious* in order to be immoral. Consciousness is instrumental to each of those states of mind associated with what the religious person might call 'sin' or the moral person 'wrong'; it is hard to imagine that an unconscious automaton or a zombie (so beloved of philosophers of mind) could be guilty of lust, jealousy, pride, or avarice; we seem to 'require' consciousness to be 'able' to 'sin'. 'Sinning' is rendered nonsensical if the sinner himself or herself is unconscious.

Without consciousness, we cease to be moral agents.

Therefore, as is sometimes the case in psychiatry, the existence of an abnormal state of mind tells us something crucial about those states of mind that we regard (and perhaps 'take for granted') as 'normal'. The man with OCD shows us (albeit vicariously) that 'normal' thinking can be controlled and that the control of consciousness, the manipulation of its contents, is what drives human behaviour, human action. For, to offer a rather basic observation, there would be no pornography if the consumer of pornography did not experience conscious pleasure from its consumption. There would be no 'experience' of lust if there were no substrate for its experience (i.e. human consciousness). There would be no musical composition if humans did not experience music aesthetically, consciously. There would be no visual art if we did not experience visual aesthetics. Consciousness is the substrate for our experience; it is the prerequisite for much of what drives human conduct and ingenuity. A scientist might create a machine that could 'paint', but it is highly unlikely that the machine would 'feel' motivated or driven by the 'need' to 'create'.

Conscious experiences are what drive human actors.

So, although consciousness may not initiate acts in the immediate future (it does not constitute the biological 'button' that is 'pressed' before we move our fingers), it nevertheless provides the venue, the medium for the 'goals' that we pursue (See figure 103). If we were not conscious, there would be nothing to attain (for there would be no experience of its attainment).

Respecting our automatisms

Therefore, if we cannot claim 'authorship' of our acts in the immediate short term, over the milliseconds prior to action, might we nevertheless retain some other form of responsibility, some rather more custodial stewardship over those things that *might* be done in a given, future situation? Should we be able

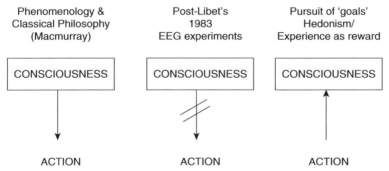

Fig. 103 Schematic demonstrating different understandings of the relationship between consciousness and action. In classical philosophy (left), conscious thought is posited to lead to action, whereas this has been shown to be flawed by the experiments of Benjamin Libet and others (centre). Nevertheless, consciousness is relevant to action because actions are often directed towards producing specific states of consciousness (right).

to 'see things coming' before they happen? Should we experience 'foresight'? If so, should we be anticipating future difficulties, rehearsing what we might do and thereby protecting ourselves from our own precipitated 'automatisms' (I use the term loosely here, to describe all reflexes, habitual responses, and repetitive patterns of behaviour that we might exhibit and to acknowledge what 'actions' would become if we applied Libet's findings universally, and reductively)? Our new problem would be one of 'meta-responsibility': moral accountability for *future* situations and behaviours (Mitchell, 1999; Spence, 2008).

Consider what happens if we ignore this problem:

1. A drunken driver had not wished (consciously) to veer across the road, drive across the pavement, and kill the young child who was walking there, but might he not have anticipated that being inebriated at the wheel of a car would precipitate some form of mishap?

2. The youths who were intoxicated on Saturday night had not planned to assault the boy they met as they emerged from the club, but might they not have anticipated some sort of trouble through their use of disinhibiting substances and their choice of companions when they went out that evening? (In forensic settings, there tends to be a lesser penalty afforded such 'reactive', or even 'provoked', violence than that applied to violence that is 'premeditated' or 'instrumental' [Chapter 9]: society places a premium on conscious awareness and planning, *ahead of the event*.)

Furthermore, don't we all, routinely, experience and exhibit some element of awareness of 'what we are like'? The future is not totally unknown or unpredictable to us (thanks in part, perhaps, to BA 10; see Paul Burgess's work reviewed in Chapter 2). Would we go to the bakery if we did not anticipate buying bread? Would we go to the cinema if we thought the main feature would be dull?

Nevertheless, there may be some occasions when we do, genuinely, surprise ourselves:

> I did not know I loved you till I heard myself telling you so—for one instant I thought, 'Good God, what have I said?' and then I knew it was the truth.

> (Bertrand Russell, in Dennett [1991, p. 246])

Such is his distance from his agency that when Russell tells his friend that he loves her, we might (again) resort to using many inverted commas: 'he' said that 'he' loved her, but 'he' seems to be saying that 'he' didn't realize that 'he' was about to say what 'he' said; 'he' (interpreted as his conscious mind) identifies the utterance as some form of unconscious product, but 'he' also identifies *with* it

('I knew [that] it was the truth.') Hence, at least in Russell, some form of conscious 'self' identifies with and accepts what its own unconsciousness seems to be 'saying'; then, he abides by it. There is a kind of symmetry between his statements (his speech acts) and his beliefs.

The point is that although we may not 'author' actions in the conscious way that we experience them phenomenologically (because action initiation has occurred prior to our awareness of it), we nevertheless live in a longer-term relationship with our behaviours and propensities, and if we are mindful of ourselves, we recognize certain patterns emerging.

However, it might still be argued that there is something rather 'unfair' at work here: for, we are the performers of actions that contribute towards our fates, yet (*post*-Libet) 'we' cannot claim to have consciously authored them (in the very short term, at least). 'We' have to live with the consequences of such unthought, unplanned, unconsciously initiated behaviours. So, are 'we' really victims after all? No, because our consciousness grants us knowledge of the future; though we may not 'author' immediate, contingent acts, we do experience some conscious awareness of 'where we are going'; the qualities that we retain in consciousness, our feelings for and about our behaviours, *influence* what we will do: 'I knew [that] it was the truth.'

Blaming people and passing judgement

It is concluded that cerebral initiation of a spontaneous, freely voluntary act can begin unconsciously, that is, before there is any (at least recallable) subjective awareness that a 'decision' to act has already been initiated cerebrally. This introduces certain constraints on the potentiality for conscious initiation and control of voluntary acts.

(Libet et al. [1983, p. 623], concerning the emergence of the
Bereitschaftspotential prior to conscious intention)

As we have seen, the impact of Libet's work has been to radically subvert the short-term authorship of voluntary action: the 'agent' performs an act that began prior to 'her' awareness of its authorship. Yet, the EEG signal that Libet identified as constitutive of that moment of generation of movement prior to awareness (the *Bereitschaftspotential*) has elsewhere been seen as a potentially incriminating factor among those patients who exhibit hysterical, 'psychogenic' movement disorders:

Terada et al. demonstrated that in five out of six patients with [hysterical] myoclonus, a *Bereitschaftspotential*, indicative of voluntary causation, preceded abnormal movements. Therefore, it is most likely that the jerks in these patients were generated through the mechanisms common to those underlying voluntary movement.

(Spence [2006a, p. 227], citing Terada et al. [1995])

So, even though the 'voluntariness' evinced by the presence of a *Bereitschaftspotential* is a voluntariness that arises post-action initiation, there is still the feeling among neurologists that there is 'enough' voluntary involvement evidenced in the act to imply something meaningful with regard to the genesis of hysterical or psychogenic movement disorders. Even though 'normal' actors become aware of their own intentions some time after the emergence of the *Bereitschaftspotential* (and in specific relation to the timing of its 'late' component; see Chapter 3), we are still faced with the conclusion that its occurrence in the hysterical agent makes their motor behaviour look more 'voluntary' than 'unconscious'.

As we had rehearsed in Chapter 7, such patients present the doctor with the quasi-psychic task of determining whether they are 'unconsciously' generating 'hysterical' symptoms or 'consciously' malingering, 'acting' them (Spence, 1999). It is hard to justify such a distinction on purely phenomenological grounds (they would both 'look' the same externally, and one can't 'know' what a patient is 'thinking', internally); however, if one takes Libet's findings seriously, then the task becomes even more problematic. For, if we accept that the 'healthy' subject who moves his (or her) limb exhibits a *Bereitschaftspotential*, which emerges *before* the 'intention to act', then what significance may we attribute to the discovery that many patients performing hysterical movements evince the same signal? What is the significance of this *Bereitschaftspotential*, which serves to subvert the agency of the healthy subject (*post*-Libet) while also implicating the voluntary involvement of the 'hysteric' in their symptom (Terada et al., 1995)? How can 'proof' of unconscious agency in one context constitute 'proof' of voluntary agency in another? (If nothing else, this suggests that we should be very careful in drawing causal inferences and attributing blame to others.) Painstaking work is required to adequately resolve this problem.

Furthermore, what can any person be said to 'know' of the actions that they perform? We cannot articulate an awareness of motor units in our motor cortices or neuronal signals within our spines. We are always speaking 'at a distance' from the raw mechanics of our own activity (and at a temporal 'delay'). Yet, in the 'hysterical' patient, we seem to be looking for just such a form of awareness:

> [T]he difference between the malingerer and the [hysterical] patient who sincerely acts the illness role may be less a matter of the latter's relative honesty than his relative lack of insight.

> (Wenegrat, 2001, p. 226)

It is as if Wenegrat would really, ideally, like the hysteric to 'own' their symptom, to 'admit' to its authorship. It is subjective awareness (or lack of it) that implicates the patient, not their EEG signal.

The psychiatric defence

Now consider a problem that confronts psychiatrists working in the forensic arena: an organism (a person) is acknowledged to have performed an awful deed (e.g. a killing), but two questions have arisen:

1. Did it (the organism) know what it was doing (i.e. was it acting as an 'agent' at the time)?

2. Did it (the organism) know that what it was doing was wrong (i.e. was it acting as a '*moral* agent')?

Such are the questions that guide the psychiatric defence, as laid out in the McNaughten rules (utilized in the United Kingdom):

> To establish a defence on the grounds of insanity, it must be clearly proved that, at the time of the committing of the act, the . . . accused was labouring under such a defect of reason, from disease of the mind, as not to know the nature and quality of the act he was doing or, if he did know it, he did not know he was doing what was wrong.

> (Gooderson, 2005, p. 254)

So it is that forensic psychiatrists are often called upon to estimate the intentional stance of an agent, usually at some remove from the events described. Did the deluded man really believe the victim was the 'devil' and, if he did, did he think it was permissible to stab him in the eye? There are shades of grey here: we may intuit that the subject was mistaken and thereby absolve him of guilt for 'his' actions, but are we not (again) attempting to label or attribute significance to an act that might well have 'behaved' normally, neurologically, rather like any of those described by Libet? As the killer raised his knife, did he exhibit a *Bereitschaftspotential* and does it matter? (Although a 'truly' automatic, involuntary movement directing the knife towards the victim might have been associated with an abnormal *Bereitschaftspotential*, thereby 'exonerating' the perpetrator [see Chapter 3], on most occasions this will not have been the case; the 'act' will have been voluntary, but it is the *reason* for the act that will come to vex us: 'He did not know he was doing what was wrong.')

Hence, in both the 'hysterical' patient and the psychiatric 'offender', what we seem to value is *awareness*, and it is an awareness of the *consequences of actions*. This suggests that the emphasis in our judgement and the location of what we value most in human responsibility is *not* that instant (those hundreds of milliseconds) immediately prior to the 'voluntary act' (after all, a *Bereitschaftspotential* is neither moral nor immoral). It is instead more of a subjective stance towards the world, an attitude which the subject adopts, and a consideration of consequences, for others and for their own future 'selves', that matters. Hence, the drunken driver and the brutal gang are guilty not only for what they *did* but also for not *minding what they might do*: for being reckless with their own future selves.

In navigating the world, 'we' may not consciously initiate the electrical signals that trigger 'our' actions, but there is a sense in which our very real phenomenological awareness, our consciousness, provides a field, a context, both a goal and a source for such action. If we do not care for others and we do not care for ourselves, then we will not care for those actions executed by components of ourselves (and our future selves) and we will come to constitute a certain kind of agent—an antisocial person (see Table 21, Chapter 9).

Saying sorry

However, if we try to make reparation, then there is another apparent disconnection, for we are making amends for self-states which preceded 'us' (as we are 'now'), for which we might retain little current sympathy. Nevertheless, we must simply accept that 'we' (as our current conscious selves) are indeed answerable for all the rest: the habits, mannerisms, losses of control, distractions, and failures of planning, the things that we did that we may now believe to have been wrong. This might seem unfair, but then life is hardly fair.

Saintliness presupposes free will—a conscious choice.

(Yuli Schreider, in Luxmoore [2000, p. 709])

So, what Schreider has to say about saintliness seems to constitute the mirror image of these antisocial states of responsibility (the good 'field' displacing the bad; see Fig. 94; Chapter 9), for similarly, the saint must walk into some very bad circumstance, fully aware that her current behaviours will have negative consequences for her future selves. However, unlike the drunken driver or the gang member, these consequences are acknowledged, and accepted, for some better 'higher' purpose, which is nevertheless regarded as 'worth dying for' although it might cost the self its life. Again, we are not so much concerned with the *Bereitschaftspotentials* preceding her 'voluntary' acts as we are with the knowledge that the 'saint' seems to have accepted their likely *consequences*: if she speaks truth unto power, she will probably pay dearly for it, but she does so anyway.

Raising a fist

So, in accordance with this conclusion, if we should encounter a man raising his fist, and we make the assumption that he has just exhibited a *Bereitschaftspotential* (albeit an invisible one, because we have not applied our EEG electrodes to his skull), would we thereby have 'explained' his action? Is it enough to know that the fist has been raised 'voluntarily', that the intention to act was itself preceded by trains of electrical activity within his cerebrum? Is that all there is to it? Well, consider Fig. 104–105. Both these images show men raising their arms. They may look quite different, but they are all raising their right arms. Do they simply 'equal' each other? If you could see a *Bereitschaftspotential* emerging prior to each act, would you have acquired full 'knowledge' of that act and its meaning? Would the subject's intentions be 'known' to you? No, I think that they would not.

The action engaged in by Adolf Hitler (Fig. 104) has a particular meaning, within a particular time and context; indeed, to our eyes now, it probably evinces a rather sinister purpose, to do with power and tyranny. Many people saluted Hitler with the very same gesture, evoking the same themes; however, these days when the German artist Anselm Kiefer performs a very similar salute: this time the purpose is one of apparent parody. He is 'commenting' in an artistic sense upon the recent past of his country. So, the tyrant's gesture is stolen from him; it is reappropriated. It is the same act, involving the same nerves and muscle groupings, yet it is also a different act. It means something different, in a different time and place. Unfortunately we have been unable to obtain permission to reproduce any of Kiefer's work.

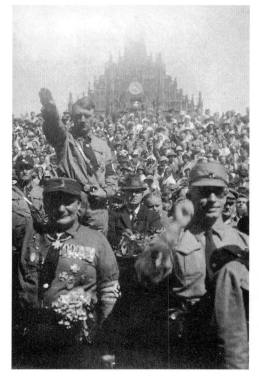

Fig. 104 Adolf Hitler and others engaging in the Nazi salute.

(This image is believed to be in the public domain and is from the National Archives.)

So, then consider Tommi Smith's gesture on the podium at the 1968 Olympics in Mexico City (Fig. 105). He wears a black glove but otherwise his gesture is very similar (albeit made using a clenched fist rather than an out-stretched hand). What does it mean? It seems to mean that now the gesture of the tyrant has actually been stolen not for the purposes of parody but instead to symbolize the power of the oppressed. The meaning of the symbol has been radically inverted. Though he probably uses many of the same muscles and nerve groupings as Hitler, the 'message' is one of subversion not suppression. I am condensing some very powerful gestures into some very brief descriptive sentences, but the point is this: there is more to an action than the presence (or absence) of a *Bereitschaftspotential*.

Human acts occur in a context that is both external and internal. How well we know the person determines the limits of our understanding of them (and their act). However, even the actor himself and those close to him experience only a 'surface' awareness of his volition and its aims. We do not

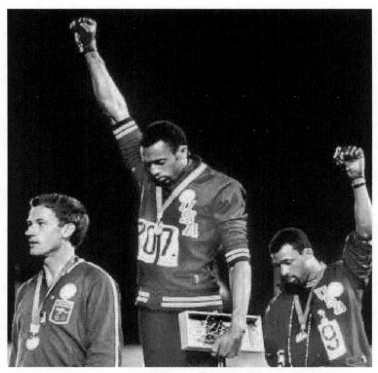

Fig. 105 Tommi Smith giving a black power salute in the context of the 1968 Olympics in Mexico City.

know everything about ourselves, nor do we know everything about anyone else. A complex organism resists interpretation (and so, we return to the 'it' of Bernhard Schlink, cited in the Prologue).

Trying to do the right thing

What we focus on when considering 'responsible' volition is the planning that arises over relatively long periods of time, while the agent is fully conscious, aware of his (or her) situation in the world and of the likely outcomes of events in his (or her) future. In other words, it matters that a person can inhabit a mental, virtual space of potential consequences (and that such a space is 'conscious' because, again, a man who walks into the firing line without thinking is not saintly, merely reckless).

However, although brain centres that are superordinate in the executive hierarchy (e.g. dorsolateral prefrontal cortex [DLPFC]) can be shown to project to 'lower' centres, and to modulate their outputs (e.g. Ganesan et al., 2005), the contents of phenomenological awareness exert an influence that seems less straightforward, more extended, in time. An agent may choose, over very longer timescales indeed (months, years), to rehearse certain behaviours in preference to others: 'Men become builders by building and lyre-players by playing the lyre; so too we become just by doing just acts, temperate by doing temperate acts, brave by doing brave acts' (Aristotle, 1998, p. 29). These, rehearsed, behaviours can become the attribute that best defines their host (e.g. he was a 'great swimmer', a 'fine acrobat', a 'serial adulterer'). However, the contents of consciousness are themselves the products of neural activity, so that although their role in our futures seems obvious (I go to the cinema to see the film of which I have been thinking), such thinking is nevertheless the product of an earlier, unconscious, stream of events. There is something in my experience, the quality of what it feels like to have the thoughts that I have in my head, that then affects my future plans: if I didn't like the thought of the film, I wouldn't go to the cinema; if something better intervened, I'd 'change my mind'. So, consciousness does not cause action in the (hundreds of milliseconds) short term, but its quality certainly affects the course of my longerterm cycle of acts (Spence, 2006b; see Fig. 103).

Becoming 'ourselves'

What comes out of a man is what defiles a man. For from within, out of the heart of man, come evil thoughts, fornication, theft, murder, adultery, coveting, wickedness, deceit, licentiousness, envy, slander, pride, foolishness. All these evil things come from within, and they defile a man.

(*Mark*, 7: 20–23)

In the long run, it is our actions that will define us and, neurobiologically, 'create us' (the circuits of our future behaviours are sculpted by our current habits; yes, we have wandered into the domain of brain imaging studies, which demonstrate experiential changes arising in the brains of London taxi drivers and classical musicians; e.g. Maguire et al., 2000; Gaser and Schlaug, 2003). However, consideration of this statement, in all its ramifications, also prompts another realization: we are dependent for our future formation upon our early carers, those who were in a position to dictate or facilitate our early experiences and activities, those activities that later contributed towards and constitute our characters. In the brain of the musician, it wasn't solely the hours of practice and tuition that mattered, in sculpting his (or her) motor circuits; there was someone who sent him (or her) to study (rather than allowing him [or her] to play outside!). That person's influence is also evinced through those motor circuit changes. Similarly, in the life of any moral being, there are beliefs acquired from those who were important to her (or him), whose examples she (or he) witnessed, whose words she (or he) may remember. As unfortunate 'wolf children' bear witness (albeit counterfactually), we are reliant upon other humans for our future development as agents.

The unknowing altruism of others

We don't choose our genes or our families and we only gradually learn about our 'selves': certain lessons we might only learn in certain environments (I don't know how I may treat people from other cultures unless I meet them); we are dependent upon others revealing to us who we are. They also, perhaps unwittingly, hold us in check. When people, consciously or unconsciously, set limits on our behaviour, they may be helping or hindering us.

When I give a presentation, the motor behaviours that I exhibit might easily be conceptualized statistically (I am temporarily afforded a relatively constrained 'human response space'; Chapter 10): for instance, though it is highly probable that I shall stand near the podium, speak towards the microphone, and point towards the screen, it is statistically highly improbable that I shall dance, sing, or recount my desire to acquire each of Jackie McLean's *Blue Note* recordings from the 1960s (the latter would be highly inappropriate, even incomprehensible to some). Nevertheless, as if to prove that we carry statistical presuppositions, one may attend lectures where the conduct of the speaker is such that he makes people in the audience rather uneasy. Does he wander too near to the people in the front row? If he walks along an aisle, is he going to make an example of someone? If he were to cry, what should we do? Our presence to each other holds us all in some kind of equilibrium, and that may be good or bad.

One emerging theme in the biology of psychopathy and antisocial personality disorder is the extent to which genetic endowment and early environment may interact, how certain individuals may fail to learn from punishment or conditioning (because of a proposed absence of feeling, possibly implicating their amygdalae), and how the presence of at least one 'good' relationship may be important in preventing an even worse future trajectory (I am drawing, here, on the work of many authors [see Chapter 9].) Indeed, one of the violent men I visit in the 'community', who has suffered extreme things and done extreme things to others, remarked spontaneously to me one day: 'I didn't choose to become what I've become.' One way of understanding his problem, which invokes both biology (genetics) and early environment (abuse and genealogical uncertainty), is to say that through the absence of positive influences (that he was capable of assimilating) he has arrived at the end of some very bad decisions, so that now it is difficult for him to go back (the product of former bad choices is often a situation wherein it is very difficult to find a 'right' choice now, in the present.) Without a 'good-enough' carer to 'mirror' our behaviour (to provide our moral socialization), and the good-enough neurology to assimilate such feedback, we may be deprived of ethical development (a thought developed in Mullen [1992]). To progress, we need help from others and we need help from within: do we have the 'moral luck' to meet the 'right' people, the 'biological luck', the good fortune, to possess the requisite brain systems (Nagel, 1982)?

Doing things in front of others

> Strange things were said about [Charcot's] hold on the Salpetriere's hysterical young women and about happenings there . . . [D]uring a patient's ball . . . a gong was inadvertently sounded, whereupon many hysterical women instantaneously fell into catalepsy and kept [the] plastic poses in which they found themselves when the gong was sounded.

> (Ellenberger, 1994, p. 95)

We have encountered this quotation before (in Chapter 7), and if we return now to considering 'hysterical' movement disorders, then part of the problem in interpreting Charcot's contribution is our uncertainty regarding the influence of this man's personality on others; did he 'train' his patients to be dysfunctional, and were patients (and indeed, their physicians) 'merely' playing roles? This is Wenegrat's (2001) contention (earlier in this chapter). However, this may be too harsh and it may be quite unfair to single out Charcot in this way. For, in the daily assessment of people exhibiting 'functional' and 'personality' disorders, much is made of whether their behaviours change in certain contexts: social influence is ubiquitous (it is not confined to the Salpêtrière).

Does a tremor get worse when the doctor is passing by? Is an 'overdose' consumed in full view of the nurses? Does the patient anticipate their spouse's arrival as they hoist the noose? Whether or not we describe events in such terms, much of neurological, psychiatric, and forensic practice involves implicit judgements regarding the contextual modulation of conduct by the presence of other human beings.

Of course, social context may inhibit bad behaviour as much as good: loss of 'normal' feedback (and restraint) can isolate leaders and allow them to become tyrants (consider Owen's [2007] recent concern with our own political leaders' 'hubris syndrome'); footballers and rock stars can become grotesques in the absence of someone who will say 'enough is enough'.

Just as we might conceive of our own behaviours through the representation of statistical probabilities (see the preceding section), so we might conceive of others' influence on us as capable of statistical impact: one group of friends might encourage me towards finer acts, and another might facilitate 'lesser' parts of me (see Spence [2008]). In other words, my friends and enemies, my colleagues and rivals, my lovers and acquaintances, all impact the borders of my 'human response space': they encourage certain behaviours and sanction others; they tolerate certain habits and proscribe others; if I am fortunate, they may tell me 'who I am'.

A very physical redemption

So, what may we conclude from all that has gone before?

Well, first, we might accept that the agency that we exert, in the short term, over individual physical acts is indeed rather restricted following the discovery that our actions are initiated prior to our awareness of our own (immediate) intentions. So, this is a problem if we had really wished to 'own' the typing movements that we make at a keyboard or the strokes of a pen when we sign our name. Much of what we do is (thankfully) automated, allowing us to be 'free' from the constant monitoring of procedural events (i.e. movements). However, we have also seen that when we are really called upon to consider what it is that is important to us, when we have to answer for what we have done, it is not the muscular deformations of hands or tongues that constitute guilt. We are much more concerned with what we knew, what we believed, and what we cared about, over relatively long periods of time.

Hence, we see that the contents of consciousness *influence* our behaviours, even if they do not initiate them (see Fig. 103). Consciousness is required to sin and to imitate saints. It is awareness and feelings that matter.

Furthermore, besides the limits constraining our short-term agency, we have other reasons to be humble, for not only is our agency less than it might have seemed (in the milliseconds preceding voluntary action), but also any sincere consideration of our characters and those of others reveals multiple constraints, exerted by our psychobiological environment: we are formed as a consequence of what others do for us (for good or ill) and what we can appreciate them doing for us (depending upon our biological 'luck'). We are social beings. We exist at the interface of nature and nurture.

In psychiatry, we encounter the human consequences of a range of social, psychological, and biological perturbations, which have impacted upon the human beings with whom we meet. As with the concept of capacity, there is likely to be a spectrum of 'freedom', variously constrained in different contexts and companies. The man with debilitating negative symptoms of schizophrenia (e.g. 'avolition') may have very limited freedom to express; the manic women may find her behavioural parameters extended, episodically, in dangerous and distressing ways. And although we cannot predict whether the violent man will be provoked on a Saturday or a Sunday morning by a chance encounter on the street, or on the stairwell, we nevertheless intermittently share a space, a conscious present with the people that we see as patients: a moment for understanding, elucidation of past and future selves, a time to learn what they (and we, ourselves) care about. These are the moments when we contribute to the other's future, to what it is that they might become (and they contribute to ours). We only gather this if we are really fully 'in the room' and if we are really fully present 'for the patient'.

> Because the doctors cared, and because one of them still believed in me when I believed in nothing, I have survived to tell the tale. It is not only the doctors who perform hazardous operations or give life-saving drugs in obvious emergencies who hold the scales at times between life and death. To sit quietly in a consulting room and talk to someone would not appear to the general public as a heroic or dramatic thing to do. In medicine, there are many different ways of saving lives. This is one of them.
>
> (Coate, 1964)

In the right circumstances, and in the right company, conscious awareness is potentially redemptive; it tells us about ourselves, and it may tell us where we are going. It is not the instant of the act but its context that seems to matter.

References

Prologue

Gilden L, Vaughan HG, Costa LD. Summated human EEG potentials with voluntary movement. *Electroencephalography and Clinical Neurophysiology* 1966; 20: 433–438.

Kornhuber HH, Deecke L. Hirnpotentialanderungen bei Willkurbewegungen und passiven Bewegungen des Menschen: Bereitschaftspotential und reafferente Potentiale. *Pflugers Arch ges Physiol* 1965; 284: 1–17.

Libet B. *Mind Time: The temporal factor in consciousness.* Cambridge, Massachusetts: Harvard University Press, 2004.

Libet B, Alberts WW, Wright EW, Delattre LD, Levin G, Feinstein B. Production of threshold levels of conscious sensation by electrical stimulation of human somatosensory cortex. *Journal of Neurophysiology* 1964; 27: 546–578.

Libet B, Gleason CA, Wright EW, Pearl DK. Time of conscious intention to act in relation to onset of cerebral activity (readiness-potential). *Brain* 1983; 106: 623–642.

Libet B, Wright EW, Feinstein B, Pearl DK. Subjective referral of the timing for a conscious sensory experience: A functional role for the somatosensory specific projection system in man. *Brain* 1979; 102: 193–224.

Libet B, Wright EW, Gleason CA. Readiness potentials preceding unrestricted 'spontaneous' vs. pre-planned voluntary acts. *Electroencephalography and clinical Neurophysiology* 1982; 54: 322–335.

Macmurray J. *The self as agent.* London: Faber and Faber, 1991, first published 1957.

Schlink B. *The reader.* London: Phoenix, 1998 (first published 1997; translated by C. Brown Janeway).

Spence SA. Free will in the light of neuropsychiatry. *Philosophy, Psychiatry & Psychology* 1996; 3: 75–90.

Spence SA. The cycle of action: A commentary on Garry Young (2006). *Journal of Consciousness Studies* 2006; 13: 69–72.

Walter WG, Cooper R, Aldridge VJ, McCallum WC, Winter AL. Contingent negative variation: An electric sign of sensorimotor association and expectancy in the human brain. *Nature* 1964; 203: 380–384.

Young G. Preserving the role of conscious decision making in the *initiation* of intentional action. *Journal of Consciousness Studies* 2006; 13: 51–68.

Chapter 1 – Moving a finger

The neuroanatomy described in this chapter has been compiled using a variety of sources, often for cross-verification. Where sources disagree I have attempted to represent the most prevalent view in the text (though I also mention where there are marked variations between authors). The sources used are the following:

Aitken JT, Causey G, Joseph J, Young JZ. *A manual of human anatomy, volume III: The upper and lower limbs.* Edinburgh: Churchill Livingstone, 1976 (3rd edition).

Amunts K, Schlaug G, Schleicher A, Steinmetz H, Dabringhaus A, Roland PF, Zilles K. Asymmetry in the human motor cortex and handedness. *NeuroImage* 1996; 4: 216–222.

Barker RA, Barasi S. *Neuroscience at a glance.* Oxford: Blackwell, 1999 (1st edition) and 2003 (2nd edition).

Buxton RB. *Introduction to functional magnetic resonance imaging: Principles and techniques.* Cambridge: Cambridge University Press, 2002.

Filley CM. *The behavioural neurology of white matter.* Oxford: Oxford University Press, 2001.

Fitzgerald MJT. *Neuroanatomy: Basic and clinical.* London: Bailliere Tindall, 1992 (2nd edition).

Ganong WF. *Review of medical physiology.* Los Altos, California: Lange Medical Publications, 1979 (9th edition).

Georgopoulos A. Motor cortex and cognitive processing. In '*The cognitive neurosciences*' (ed. M.S. Gazzaniga). Cambridge, Massachusetts: Bradford MIT press 1995, 507–517.

Jeannerod M. *The cognitive neuroscience of action.* Oxford: Blackwell, 1997.

Kalat JW. *Biological psychology.* Belmont, CA: Wadsworth/Thomson Learning, 2004 (8th edition).

Medical Research Council (memorandum no. 45). *Aids to the examination of the peripheral nervous system.* London: Her Majesty's Stationery Office, 1976 (3rd impression, 1981).

Mitchell GAG, Mayor D. *The essentials of neuroanatomy.* Edinburgh: Churchill Livingstone, 1977 (3rd edition).

Mountcastle VB. The columnar organization of the neocortex. *Brain* 1997; 120: 701–722.

Passingham R. *The frontal lobes and voluntary action.* Oxford: Oxford University Press, 1993 (reprinted 1995).

Preuss TM. What's Human about the Human brain? In '*The cognitive neurosciences*' (ed. M.S. Gazzaniga). Cambridge, Massachusetts: Bradford MIT press, 1995, 1219–1234.

Semenderefi, Damasio KH, Frank R, Van Hoesen GW. The evolution of the frontal lobes: A volumetric analysis based on three-dimensional reconstructions of magnetic resonance image scans of human and ape brains. *Journal of Human Evolution* 1997; 32: 375–388.

Standring S. (Ed.) *Gray's Anatomy: The anatomical basis of clinical practice.* Edinburgh: Elsevier, Churchill Livingstone, 2005 (39th edition).

Volkmann J, Schnitzler A, Witte OW, Freund H-J. Handedness and asymmetry of hand representation in human motor cortex. *Journal of Neurophysiology* 1998; 79: 2149–2154.

Williams PL, Warwick R. (Ed.) *Gray's Anatomy.* Edinburgh: Churchill Livingstone, 1980 (36th edition).

Woolsey TA, Hanaway J, Gado MH. *The brain atlas: A visual guide to the human central nervous system.* Hoboken, New Jersey: Wiley, 2008 (3rd edition).

Discussion of the hand is informed by several interesting texts devoted to its anatomy, evolution and cultural significance:

Leakey R. *The origins of humankind*. London: Phoenix, 1995 (first published 1994).

McManus C. *Right hand, left hand: The origins of asymmetry in brains, bodies, atoms and cultures*. London: Weidenfeld & Nicolson, 2002.

Napier J. *Hands*. Revised by RH Tuttle. Princeton, New Jersey: Princeton University Press, 1993 (original first published 1980).

Oakley A. *Fracture: Adventures of a broken body*. Bristol: The Policy Press, 2007.

Wilson FR. *The hand: How its use shapes the brain, language, and human culture*. New York: Pantheon Books, 1998.

More recent data concerning the evolution of humans and their differentiation from other primates can be found in the following journal articles:

Carroll SB. Genetics and the making of Homo sapiens. *Nature* 2003; 422: 849–857.

Pollard KS, Salama SR, King B, Kern AD, Dreszer T, Katzman S, Siepel A, Pedersen JS, Bejerano G, Baertsch R, Rosenbloom KR, Kent J, Haussler D. Forces shaping the fastest evolving regions in the Human genome. *PLOS Genetics* 2006; 2: e168 (1–13).

The sketches of neurological diseases contained in Table 4 are taken from respective chapters of the 4th edition of the Oxford Textbook of Medicine (Oxford University Press, 2005), edited by DA Warrell, TM Cox and JD Firth:

Compston A. Chapter 24.13.13 (multiple sclerosis). OTM, volume 3: 1158–1163. 2005.

Donaghy M. Chapter 24.16 (motor neurone diseases). OTM, volume 3: 1075–1079. 2005.

Hilton-Jones D, Palace J. Chapter 24.17 (myaesthenia gravis). OTM, volume 3: 1167–1172.

Chapter 2 – Assembling a 'Will'

As in the first chapter, much of the basic anatomy described here is sourced from several anatomical texts and verified accordingly:

Jeannerod M. *The cognitive neuroscience of action*. Oxford: Blackwell, 1997.

Kalat JW. *Biological psychology*. Belmont, CA: Wadsworth/Thomson Learning, 2004 (8th edition).

Mitchell GAG, Mayor D. *The essentials of neuroanatomy*. Edinburgh: Churchill Livingstone, 1977 (3rd edition).

Passingham R. *The frontal lobes and voluntary action*. Oxford: Oxford University Press, 1993 (reprinted 1995).

Standring S. (Ed.) *Gray's Anatomy: The anatomical basis of clinical practice*. Edinburgh: Elsevier, Churchill Livingstone, 2005 (39th edition).

Williams PL, Warwick R. (Ed.) *Gray's Anatomy*. Edinburgh: Churchill Livingstone, 1980 (36th edition).

Woolsey TA, Hanaway J, Gado MH. *The brain atlas: A visual guide to the human central nervous system*. Hoboken, New Jersey: Wiley, 2008 (3rd edition).

In addition, the following publications are cited in the course of the chapter:

Arnold K, Zuberbuhler K. Meaningful call combinations in a non-human primate. *Current Biology* 2008; 18: R202–203.

Baddeley AD. The capacity for generating information by randomisation. *Quarterly Journal of Experimental Psychology* 1966; 18: 119–129.

Baddeley AD. *Working memory*. Oxford: Clarendon Press, 1986.

Baddeley AD. Recent developments in working memory. *Current Opinion in Neurobiology* 1998; 8: 234–238.

Baddeley AD, Della Sala S. Working memory and executive control. *Proceedings of the Royal Society of London [Biol]* 1996; 351: 1397–1404.

Bench CJ, Frith CD, Grasby PM, Friston KJ, Paulesu E, Frackowiak RS, Dolan RJ. Investigations of the functional anatomy of attention using the Stroop test. *Neuropsychologia* 1993; 31: 907–922.

Benson DF, Geschwind N. Aphasia and related disorders: a clinical approach. In *'Principles of behavioural neurology'* (ed. M.M. Mesulam). Philadelphia: Davis, 1985: 193–238.

Berrios GE, Gili M. Will and its disorders: A conceptual history. *History of Psychiatry* 1995; vi: 87–104.

Brown P, Marsden CD. What do the basal ganglia do? *Lancet* 1998; 351: 1801–1804.

Brunia CHM, Van Boxtel GJM. Motor preparation. In *Handbook of Physiology* (2nd edition; ed. JT Cacioppo, LG Tassinary & GG Berntson). Cambridge: Cambridge University Press, 2000: 507–532.

Burgess PW, Gilbert SJ, Dumontheil I. Function and localization within rostral prefrontal cortex (area 10). *Philosophical Transactions of the Royal Society of London, series B* 2007; 362: 887–899.

Bush G, Luu P, Posner MI. Cognitive and emotional influences in anterior cinculate cortex. *Trends in Cognitive Neuroscience* 2000; 4: 215–222.

Buzsaki G. *Rhythms of the brain*. Oxford: Oxford University Press, 2006.

Chambers. *Chambers concise dictionary*. Edinburgh: Chambers Harrap, 1997.

Cunnington R, Windischberger C, Moser E. Premovement activity of the pre-supplementary motor area and the readiness for action: Studies of time-resolved event-related functional MRI. *Human Movement Science* 2005; 24: 644–656.

Damasio AR. *Descartes' error*. New York: Putnam, 1994.

Damasio AR, Van Hoesen GW. Focal lesions of the limbic frontal lobe. In *'Neuropsychology of human emotion'* (ed. KM Heilman, P Satz). New York: Guilford Press,1983: 85–110.

Damasio AR, Tranel D, Damasio H. Individuals with sociopathic behaviour caused by frontal damage fail to respond autonomically to social stimuli. *Behavioural Brain Research* 1990; 41: 81–94.

Deiber M-P, Passingham RE, Colebatch JG, Friston KF, Nixon PD, Frackowiak RSJ. Cortical areas and the selection of movement: A study with positron emission tomography. *Experimental Brain Research* 1991; 84: 393–402.

Devinsky O, Morrell MJ, Vogt BA. Contributions of anterior cingulate cortex to behaviour. *Brain* 1995; 118: 279–306.

Dilman I. *Free will: An historical and philosophical introduction*. London: Routledge, 1999.

Dolan RJ. Keynote address: Revaluing the orbital prefrontal cortex. *Annals of the New York Academy of Sciences* 2007; 1121: 1–9.

Elliott R, Dolan RJ, Frith CD. Dissociable functions in the medial and lateral orbitofrontal cortex: Evidence from human neuroimaging studies. *Cerebral Cortex* 2000; 10: 308–317.

Fox PT, Parsons LM, Lancaster JL. Beyond the single study: function/location metanalysis in cognitive neuroimaging. *Current Opinion in Neurobiology* 1998; 8: 178–187.

Freedman M, Alexander MP, Naeser MA. Anatomic basis of transcortical motor aphasia. *Neurology* 1984; 34: 409–417.

Fried I. Electrical stimulation of the supplementary motor area. *Advances in Neurology* 1996; 70: 177–185.

Fried I, Katz A, McCarthy G, Sass KJ, Williamson P, Spencer SS, Spencer DD. Functional organization of human supplementary motor cortex studied by electrical stimulation. *Journal of Neuroscience* 1991; 11: 3656–3666.

Frith CD. The positive and negative symptoms of schizophrenia reflect impairment in the perception and initiation of action. *Psychological Medicine* 1987; 17: 631–648.

Frith CD, Friston KJ, Liddle PF, Frackowiak RSJ. A PET study of word finding. *Neuropsychologia* 1991a; 29: 1137–1148.

Frith CD, Friston K, Liddle PF, Frackowiak RSJ. Willed action and the prefrontal cortex in man: a study with PET. *Proceedings of the Royal Society of London [Biol]* 1991b; 244: 241–246.

Fuster JM. *The prefrontal cortex.* New York: Raven, 1980.

Gallese V, Fadiga L, Fogassi L, Rizzolatti G. Action recognition in the premotor cortex. *Brain* 1996; 119: 593–609.

Goldberg G. Supplementary motor area structure and function: Review and hypotheses. *Behavioural Brain Research* 1985; 8: 567–588.

Goldberg TE, Berman KF, Fleming K, Ostrem J, Van Horn JD, Esposito G, Mattay VS, Gold JM, Weinberger DR. Uncoupling cognitive workload and prefrontal cortical physiology: A PET rCBF study. *NeuroImage* 1998; 7: 296–303.

Goldman-Rakic PS. Motor control function of the prefrontal cortex. In *'Motor areas of the cerebral cortex'* (Ciba Foundation Symposium 132). Chichester: Wiley, 1987: 187–200.

Goldman-Rakic PS. The prefrontal landscape: Implications of functional architecture for understanding human mentation and the central executive. *Philosophical Transactions of the Royal Society of London [Biol]* 1996; 351: 1445–1462.

Goldman-Rakic PS, Bates JF, Chafee MV. The prefrontal cortex and internally generated motor acts. *Current Opinion in Neurobiology* 1992; 2: 830–835.

Goldman-Rakic PS, Selemon LD. Functional and anatomical aspects of prefrontal pathology in schizophrenia. *Schizophrenia Bulletin* 1997; 23: 437–458.

Hagoort P. The memory, unification, and control (MUC) model of language. In *'Automaticity and control in language processing'* (ed. AS Meyer, LR Wheeldon & A Krott). Hove, Sussex: Psychology Press, 2007: 243–270.

Indefrey P, Levelt WJM. The neural correlates of language production. In *'The new cognitive neurosciences'* (ed. M Gazzaniga). Cambridge, Massachusetts: MIT Press, 2000: 845–865.

Ingvar DH. 'Memory of the future': An essay on the temporal organization of conscious awareness. *Human Neurobiology* 1985; 4: 127–136.

Jahanshahi M, Jenkins IH, Brown RG, Marsden CD, Passingham RE, Brooks DJ. Self-initiated versus externally triggered movements: I. an investigation using measurement of regional cerebral blood flow with PET and movement-related potentials in normal and Parkinson's disease subjects. *Brain* 1995; 118: 913–933.

Jahanshahi M, Profice P, Brown RG, Ridding MC, Dirnberger G, Rothwell JC. The effects of transcranial magnetic stimulation over the dorsolateral prefrontal cortex on suppression of habitual counting during random number generation. *Brain* 1998; 121: 1533–1544.

Jeannerod M. *The cognitive neuroscience of action.* Oxford: Blackwell, 1997.

Jeannerod M. *Motor cognition: What actions tell the self.* Oxford: Oxford University Press, 2006.

Jenkins IH, Brooks DJ, Nixon PD, Frackowiak RSJ, Passingham RE. Motor sequence learning: A study with positron emission tomography. *Journal of Neuroscience* 1994; 14: 3775–3790.

Jenkins IH, Fernandez W, Playford ED, Lees AJ, Frackowiak RSJ, Brooks DJ. Impaired activation of the supplementary motor area in Parkinson's disease is reversed when akinesia is treated with apomorphine. *Annals of Neurology* 1992; 32: 749–757.

Jonas S. The supplementary motor region and speech. In '*The frontal lobes revisited*' (ed. E Perecman). New York: IRBN Press, 1987: 241–250.

Koechlin E, Hyafil A. Anterior prefrontal function and the limits of human decision-making. *Science* 2007; 318: 594–598.

Koechlin E, Basso G, Pietrini P, Panzer S, Grafman J. The role of the anterior prefrontal cortex in human cognition. *Nature* 1999; 399: 148–151.

Krams M, Deiber M-P, Frackowiak RSJ, Passingham RE. Broca's area and mental preparation. *NeuroImage* 1996; 3(3): S392.

Lichteim L. On aphasia. *Brain* 1885; 7: 433–484.

Luppino G, Matelli M, Camarda R, Rizzolatti G. Corticocortical connections of area F3 (SMA-proper) and area F6 (pre-SMA) in the macaque monkey. Journal of *Comparative Neurology* 1993; 338: 114–140.

Macmillan M. *An odd kind of fame: Stories of Phineas Gage.* Cambridge, Massachusetts: MIT Press, 2000.

McGuire PK, Silbersweig DA, Murray RM, David AS, Frackowiak RS, Frith CD. Functional anatomy of inner speech and auditory verbal imagery. *Psychological Medicine* 1996; 26: 29–38.

McGuire PK, Robertson D, Thacker A, David AS, Kitson N, Frackowiak RS, Frith CD. Neural correlates of thinking in sign language. *NeuroReport* 1997; 8: 695–698.

McManus C. *Right hand, left hand: The origins of asymmetry in brains, bodies, atoms and cultures.* London: Weidenfeld & Nicolson, 2002.

Milner B. Effects of different brain lesions on card sorting. *Archives of Neurology* 1963; 9: 100–110.

Milner AD, Goodale MA. Visual pathways to perception and action. *Progress in Brain Research* 1993; 95: 317–337.

Morris ME, Iansek R, Matyas TA, Summers JJ. Stride length regulation in Parkinson's disease. *Brain* 1996; 119: 551–568.

Padoa-Schioppa C, Assad JA. Neurons in the orbitofrontal cortex encode economic value. *Nature* 2006; 441: 223–226.

Pandya DN, Yeterian EH. Comparison of prefrontal architecture and connections. *Philosophical Transactions of the Royal Society of London [series B]* 1996; 351: 1423–1432.

Passingham RE. Attention to action. *Philosophical Transactions of the Royal Society of London [Biol]* 1996; 351: 1473–1479.

Passingham RE. Functional organization of the motor system. In '*Human brain function*' (eds. RSJ Frackowiak et al). San Diego: Academic Press, 1997: 243–274.

Paulesu E, Frith CD, Frackowiak RSJ. The neural correlates of the verbal components of working memory. *Nature* 1993; 362: 342–245.

Paus T. Location and function of the human frontal eye field: A selective review. *Neuropsychologia* 1996; 34: 475–483.

Paus T. Primate anterior cingulate cortex: Where motor control, drive and cognition interface. *Nature Reviews Neuroscience* 2001; 2: 417–424.

Petrides M. Specialised systems for the processing of mnemonic information within the primate prefrontal cortex. *Philosophical Transactions of the Royal Society of London [Biol]* 1996; 351: 1455–1462.

Petrides M, Mackey S. The orbitofrontal cortex: sulcal and gyral morphology and architecture. In '*The Orbitofrontal Cortex*' (ed. DH Zald & SL Rauch). Oxford: Oxford University Press, 2006: 19–37.

Petrides M, Milner B. Deficits on subject-ordered tasks after frontal and temporal-lobe lesions in man. *Neuropsychologia* 1982; 20: 249–262.

Playford ED, Jenkins IH, Passingham RE, Nutt J, Frackowiak RSJ, Brooks DJ. Impaired mesial frontal and putamen activation in Parkinson's disease: a PET study. *Annals of Neurology* 1992; 32: 151–161.

Rajkowska G, Goldman-Rakic PS. Cytoarchitectonic definition of prefrontal areas in the normal human cortex: II. Variability in location of areas 9 and 46 and relationship to the Talairach coordinate system. *Cerebral Cortex* 1995; 5: 323–337.

Rizzolatti G, Arbib MA. Language within our grasp. *Trends in Neurosciences* 1998; 21: 188–194.

Rizzolatti G, Fadiga L, Matelli M, Bettinardi V, Paulesu E, Perani D, Fazio F. Localization of grasp representations in humans by PET: I. Observation versus execution. *Experimental Brain Research* 1996; 112: 103–111.

Roland PE. *Brain activation*. New York: Wiley-Liss, 1993.

Rolls ET. The orbitofrontal cortex. *Philosophical Transactions of the Royal Society of London [Biol]* 1996; 351: 1433–1444.

Rudebeck PH, Walton ME, Smyth AN, Bannerman DM, Rushworth MFS. Separate neural pathways process different decision costs. *Nature Neuroscience* 2006; 9: 1161–1168.

Shallice T, Burgess PW, Schon F, Baxter DM. The origins of utilization behaviour. *Brain* 1989; 112: 1587–1598.

Spence SA, Brooks DJ, Hirsch SR, Liddle PF, Meehan J, Grasby PM. A PET study of voluntary movement in schizophrenic patients experiencing passivity phenomena (delusions of alien control). *Brain* 1997; 120: 1997–2011.

Spence SA, Frith CD. Towards a functional anatomy of volition. *Journal of Consciousness Studies* 1999; 6: 11–29.

Spence SA, Hirsch SR, Brooks DJ, Grasby PM. Prefrontal cortex activity in people with schizophrenia and control subjects. Evidence from positron emission tomography for remission of 'hypofrontality' with recovery from acute schizophrenia. *British Journal of Psychiatry* 1998; 172: 316–323.

Spence SA, Hughes CJ, Cooley L, Green RD, Wilkinson ID, Parks RW, Hunter MD. Towards a cognitive neurobiological account of free association. *Neuro-Psychoanalysis*, in press (to be published 2009).

Spence SA, Liddle PF, Stefan MD, Hellewell JS, Sharma T, Friston KJ, Hirsch SR, Frith CD, Murray RM, Deakin JF, Grasby PM. Functional anatomy of verbal fluency in people with schizophrenia and those at genetic risk. Focal dysfunction and distributed disconnectivity reappraised. *British Journal of Psychiatry* 2000; 176: 52–60.

Stephan KM, Fink GR, Passingham RE, Silbersweig D, Ceballos-Baumann AO, Frith CD, Frackowiak RS. I. Functional anatomy of the mental representation of upper extremity movements in healthy subjects. *Journal of Neurophysiology* 1995; 73: 373–386.

Ungerleider L, Mishkin M. Two cortical visual systems. In *'Analysis of visual behaviour'* (eds DJ Ingle et al). Cambridge, Massachusetts: MIT Press, 1982: 549–586.

Warren JD, Warren JE, Fox NC, Warrington EK. Nothing to say, something to sing: Primary progressive dynamic aphasia. *Neurocase* 2003; 9: 140–155.

Wise RJS, Greene J, Buchel C, Scott SK. Brain regions involved in articulation. *Lancet* 1999; 353: 1057–1061.

Chapter 3 – The timing of intentions

Baars BJ, McGovern K. Cognitive views of consciousness. What are the facts? How can we explain them? In *'The science of consciousness: Psychological, neuropsychological and clinical reviews'* (ed. M. Velmans). London: Routledge, 1996: 63–95.

Brass M, Haggard P. To do or not to do: The neural signature of self-control. *Journal of Neuroscience* 2007; 27: 9141–9145.

Brunia CHM, Van Boxtel GJM. Motor preparation. In *Handbook of Physiology* (2nd edition; editors: JT Cacioppo, LG Tassinary & GG Berntson). Cambridge: Cambridge University Press, 2000: 507–532.

Cunnington R, Windischberger C, Moser E. Premovement activity of the pre-supplementary motor area and the readiness for action: Studies of time-resolved event-related functional MRI. *Human Movement Science* 2005; 24: 644–656.

Farmer SF. Mirror movements in neurology. *Journal of Neurology, Neurosurgery and Psychiatry* 2005; 76: 1330.

Haggard P, Clark S, Kalogeras J. Voluntary action and conscious awareness. *Nature Neuroscience* 2002; 5: 382–385.

Haggard P, Eimer M. On the relation between brain potentials and the awareness of voluntary movements. *Experimental Brain Research* 1999; 126: 128–133.

Haggard P, Magno E. Localising awareness of action with transcranial magnetic stimulation. *Experimental Brain Research* 1999; 127: 102–107.

Haggard P, Newman C, Magno E. On the perceived time of voluntary actions. *British Journal of Psychology* 1999; 90: 291–303.

Libet B, Alberts WW, Wright EW, Delattre LD, Levin G, Feinstein B. Production of threshold levels of conscious sensation by electrical stimulation of human somatosensory cortex. *Journal of Neurophysiology* 1964; 27: 546–578.

Libet B, Gleason CA, Wright EW, Pearl DK. Time of conscious intention to act in relation to onset of cerebral activity (readiness-potential). *Brain* 1983; 106: 623–642.

Maegaki Y, Seki A, Suzaki I, Sugihara S, Ogawa T, Amisaki T, Fukuda C, Koeda T. Congenital mirror movement: A study of functional MRI and transcranial magnetic stimulation. Developmental Medical and Childhood Neurology 2002; 44: 838–843.

Passingham R. *The frontal lobes and voluntary action.* Oxford: Oxford University Press, 1993 (reprinted 1995).

Serrien DJ, Ivry RB, Swinnen SP. Dynamics of hemispheric specialization and integration in the context of motor control. *Nature Reviews Neuroscience* 2006; 7: 160–167.

Shibasaki H, Hallett M. What is the Bereitschaftspotential? *Clinical Neurophysiology* 2006; 117: 2341–2356.

Spence SA. Free will in the light of neuropsychiatry. *Philosophy, Psychiatry & Psychology* 1996; 3: 75–90.

Sternberg S, Monsell S, Knoll RL, Wright CE. The latency and duration of rapid movement sequences: Comparisons of speech and typewriting. In GE Stelmach (Ed.) *Information processing in motor control and learning.* Amsterdam: North-Holland, 1978, 117–152.

Vidal F, Grapperon J, Bonnet M, Hasbroucq T. The nature of unilateral motor commands in between-hand choice tasks as revealed by surface Laplacian estimation. *Psychophysiology* 2003; 40: 796–805.

Chapter 4 – Volitional architectures

In common with Chapters 1 and 2, much of the neuroanatomy, and neurochemistry, of this chapter has been verified from a variety of sources, and the following were central:

Anderson IM, Reid IC. (Ed.) *Fundamentals of clinical psychopharmacology.* Oxon: Informa, 2006 (3rd edition).

Bianchi L. *The mechanism of the brain and the function of the frontal lobes.* Edinburgh: Livingstone, 1922.

Cooper JR, Bloom FE, Roth RH. *The biochemical basis of neuropharmacology.* Oxford: Oxford University Press, 1996 (7th edition).

Fitzgerald MJT. *Neuroanatomy: Basic and clinical.* London: Bailliere Tindall, 1992 (2nd edition).

Kapur S. Lecrubier Y. (Ed.) *Dopamine in the pathophysiology and treatment of schizophrenia: New findings.* London: Martin Dunitz, 2003.

Stahl SM. *Essential psychopharmacology: Neuroscientific basis and practical applications.* Cambridge: Cambridge University Press, 1996.

Standring S. (Ed.) *Gray's Anatomy: The anatomical basis of clinical practice.* Edinburgh: Elsevier, Churchill Livingstone, 2005 (39th edition).

Stuss DT, Knight RT. (Ed.) *Principles of frontal lobe function.* Oxford: Oxford University Press, 2002.

Williams PL, Warwick R. (Ed.) *Gray's Anatomy.* Edinburgh: Churchill Livingstone, 1980 (36th edition).

Woolsey TA, Hanaway J, Gado MH. *The brain atlas: A visual guide to the human central nervous system.* Hoboken, New Jersey: Wiley, 2008 (3rd edition).

In addition, the following publications are cited:

Alexander GE, DeLong MR, Strick PL. Parallel organization of functionally segregated circuits linking basal ganglia and cortex. *Annual Review of Neuroscience* 1986; 9: 357–381.

Arnsten AFT, Robbins TW. Neurochemical modulation of prefrontal cortical function in humans and animals. In '*Principles of frontal lobe function*' (ed. DT Stuss & RT Knight). Oxford: Oxford University Press, 2002: 51–84.

Asberg M, Traskman L, Thoren P. 5-HIAA in the cerebrospinal fluid – a biochemical suicide predictor? *Archives of General Psychiatry* 1976; 33: 1193–1197.

Barnes TRE, Spence SA. Movement disorders associated with antipsychotic drugs: Clinical and biological implications. In '*The psychopharmacology of schizophrenia*' (ed. MA Reveley & JFW Deakin). London: Arnold, 2000: 178–210.

Bonkalo A. Impulsive acts and confusional states during incomplete arousal from sleep: Criminological and forensic implications. *Psychiatric Quarterly* 1974; 48: 400–409.

Brown GL, Ebert MH, Goyer PF, Jimerson DC, Klein WJ, Bunney WE, Goodwin FK. Aggression, suicide and serotonin: Relationships to CSF metabolites. *American Journal of Psychiatry* 1982; 139: 741–746.

Brown GL, Goodwin FK, Ballenger JC, Goyer PF, Major LF. Aggression in humans correlates with cerebrospinal fluid metabolites. *Psychiatry Research* 1979; 1: 131–139.

Brown P, Marsden CD. What do the basal ganglia do? *Lancet* 1998; 351: 1801–1804.

Courtney C, Farrell D, Gray R, Hills R, Lynch L, Sellwood E, Edwards S, Hardyman W, Raftery J, Crome P, Lendon C, Shaw H, Bentham P, AD2000 Collaborative Group. Long-term donepezil treatment in 565 patients with Alzheimer's disease (AD2000): Randomised double-blind trial. *Lancet* 2004; 363: 2105–2115.

Creese I, Burt DR, Snyder SH. Dopamine receptor binding predicts clinical and pharmacological potencies of antischizophrenic drugs. *Science* 1976; 192: 481–483.

Das SK, Fox J, Elsdon D, Hammond P. A flexible architecture for autonomous agents. *Journal of Experimental and Theoretical Artifical Intelligence* 1997; 9: 407–440.

Deutch AY, Roth RH. Neurochemical systems in the central nervous system. In 'Neurobiology of mental illness' (ed. DS Charney, EJ Nestler, BS Bunney). Oxford: Oxford University Press, 1999: 10–25.

Doble A, Martin IL, Nutt D. *Calming the brain: Benzodiazepines and related drugs from laboratory to clinic.* London: Martin Dunitz, 2004.

Egan MF, Goldberg TE, Kolachana BS, Callicott JH, Mazzanti CM, Straub RE, Goldman D, Weinberger DR. Effects of COMT Val [108/158] Met genotype on frontal lobe function and risk of schizophrenia. *Proceedings of the National Academy of Sciences* USA 2001; 98: 6917–6922.

Fink M, Taylor MA. *Catatonia: A clinician's guide to diagnosis and treatment.* Cambridge: Cambridge University Press, 2003.

Freud S, Breuer J. *Studies on hysteria.* London: Penguin, 1991 (first published in English translation by James and Alix Strachey, in 1955; originally published in German 1895).

Gartside SE, Marsden CA. Neuropharmacology and drug action. In 'Fundamentals of clinical psychopharmacology' (ed. IM Anderson & IC Reid). Oxon: Informa, 2006: 1–24.

Grant DA, Berg EA. A behavioural analysis of degree of reinforcement and ease of shifting to new responses in a Weigl-type card-sorting problem. *Journal of Experimental Psychology* 1948; 38: 404–411.

Hosak L. Role of the COMT gene Val158Met polymorphism in mental disorders: A review. *European Psychiatry* 2007; 276–281.

Jenkins IH, Fernandez W, Playford ED, Lees AJ, Frackowiak RSJ, Brooks DJ. Impaired activation of the supplementary motor area in Parkinson's disease is reversed when akinesia is treated with apomorphine. *Annals of Neurology* 1992; 32: 749–757.

Jueptner M, Frith CD, Brooks DJ, Frackowiak RS, Passingham RE. Anatomy of motor learning. II. Subcortical structures and learning by trial and error. *Journal of Neurophysiology* 1997b; 77: 1325–1337.

Jueptner M, Stephan KM, Frith CD, Brooks DJ, Frackowiak RS, Passingham RE. Anatomy of motor learning. I. Frontal cortex and attention to action. *Journal of Neurophysiology* 1997a; 77: 1313–1324.

Kramer P. *Listening to Prozac*. New York: Penguin Books, 1993.

Linnoila M, Charney DS. The neurobiology of aggression. In '*Neurobiology of mental illness*' (ed. DS Charney, EJ Nestler, BS Bunney). Oxford: Oxford University Press, 1999: 855–871.

Linnoila M, Virkkunen M, Scheinin M, Nuutila A, Rimon R, Goodwin FK. Low cerebrospinal fluid 5 hydroxyindoleacetic acid concentration differentiates impulsive from nonimpulsive violent behaviour. *Life Sciences* 1983; 33: 2609–2614.

Litvan I, Paulsen JS, Mega MS, Cummings JL. Neuropsychiatric assessment of patients with hyperkinetic and hypokinetic movement disorders. *Archives of Neurology* 1998; 55: 1313–1319.

Ludwig AM. Hysteria: A neurobiological theory. *Archives of General Psychiatry* 1972; 27: 771–777.

Milner B. Effects of different brain lesions on card-sorting. *Archives of Neurology* 1963; 9: 90–100.

Olson EJ, Boeve BF, Silber MH. Rapid eye movement sleep behaviour disorder: Demographic, clinical and laboratory findings in 93 cases. *Brain* 2000; 123: 331–339.

Pereira EAC, Aziz TZ. Surgical insights into Parkinson's disease. *Journal of the Royal Society of Medicine* 2006; 99: 238–244.

Playford ED, Jenkins IH, Passingham RE, Nutt J, Frackowiak RSJ, Brooks DJ. Impaired mesial frontal and putamen activation in Parkinson's disease: a PET study. *Annals of Neurology* 1992; 32: 151–161.

Raleigh MJ, McGuire MT, Brammer GL, Pollack DB, Yuwiler A. Serotonergic mechanisms promote dominance acquisition in adult vervet monkeys. *Brain Research* 1991; 559: 181–190.

Raleigh MJ, McGuire MT, Brammer GL, Yuwiler A. Social and environmental influences on blood serotonin concentrations in monkeys. *Archives of General Psychiatry* 1984; 41: 405–410.

Rogers H, Spector R, Trounce J. *An introduction to mechanisms in pharmacology and therapeutics*. London: Heinemann, 1976.

Schenck CH, Bundlie SR, Ettinger MG, Mahowald MW. Chronic behavioural disorders of human REM sleep: A new category of parasomnia. *Sleep* 1986; 9: 293–308.

Seeman P, Lee T. Antipsychotic drugs: Direct correlation between clinical potency and presynaptic action on dopamine neurons. *Science* 1975; 188: 1217–1219.

Shallice T. *From neuropsychology to mental structure*. Cambridge: Cambridge University Press, 1988.

Shallice T. Fractionation of the supervisory system. In '*Principles of frontal lobe function*' (ed. DT Stuss & RT Knight). Oxford: Oxford University Press, 2002: 261–277.

Spence SA. Hysterical paralyses as disorders of action. *Cognitive Neuropsychiatry* 1999; 4: 203–226.

Stahl SM. *Psychopharmacology of antipsychotics*. London: Martin Dunitz, 1999.

Stradling JR. Sleep-related disorders of breathing. In '*Oxford textbook of medicine*' (ed. DA Warrell, TM Cox, JD Firth). Oxford: Oxford University Press, 2005 (4th edition); volume 2: 1409–1420.

Thomas P, Rascle C, Mastain B, Maron M, Vaiva G. Test for catatonia with zolpidem. *Lancet* 1997; 349: 702.

Yin HH, Knowlton BJ. The role of the basal ganglia in habit formation. *Nature Reviews Neuroscience* 2006; 7: 464–476.

Wilkinson RG. *The impact of inequality: How to make sick societies better*. London: Routledge, 2005.

Zeman A. *Consciousness: A user's guide*. New Haven: Yale University Press, 2002.

Chapter 5 – Losing control

Angyal A. The experience of the body-self in schizophrenia. *Archives of Neurology & Psychiatry* 1936; 35: 1029–1053.

Banks G, Short P, Martinez J, Latchaw R, Ratcliff G, Boller F. The alien hand syndrome: clinical and post mortem findings. *Archives of Neurology* 1989; 46: 456–459.

Bisiach E, Rusconi ML, Vallar G. Remission of somatoparaphrenic delusion through vestibular stimulation. *Neuropsychologia* 1991; 29: 1029–1031.

Blakemore S-J, Smith J, Steel R, Johnstone CE, Frith CD. The perception of self-produced sensory stimuli in patients with auditory hallucinations and passivity experiences: evidence for a breakdown in self-monitoring. *Psychological Medicine* 2000; 30: 1131 – 1139.

Bottini G, Karnath HO, Vallar G, Sterzi R, Frith CD, Frackowiak RS, Paulesu E. Cerebral representations for egocentric space: Functional-anatomical evidence from caloric vestibular stimulation and neck vibration. *Brain* 2001; 124: 1182–1196.

Brion S, Jedynak CP. Troubles du transfert interhemispherique. A propos de trios observations de tumeurs du corps calleux. Le signe de la main etrangere. *Revue Neurologique (Paris)* 1972; 126: 257–266.

Critchley M. *The parietal lobes*. New York: Hafner Press, 1953.

Della Sala S, Marchetti C, Spinnler H. Right-sided anarchic (alien) hand: A longitudinal study. *Neuropsychologia* 1991; 29: 1113–1127.

Denny-Brown D. The nature of apraxia. *Journal of Nervous & Mental Disease* 1958; 126: 9–32.

Farmer SF. Mirror movements in neurology. *Journal of Neurology, Neurosurgery and Psychiatry* 2005; 76: 1330.

Feinberg TE, Schindler RJ, Flanagan NG, Haber LD. Two alien hand syndromes. *Neurology* 1992; 42: 19–24.

Frith CD. *The cognitive neuropsychology of schizophrenia*. Hove: Lawrence Erlbaum, 1992.

Frith CD, Done DJ. Experiences of alien control in schizophrenia reflect a disorder of the central monitoring of action. *Psychological Medicine* 1989; 13: 779–786.

Ganesan V, Green RD, Hunter MD, Wilkinson ID, Spence SA. Expanding the response space in chronic schizophrenia: the relevance of left prefrontal cortex. *NeuroImage* 2005; 25: 952–957.

Ganesan V, Hunter MD, Spence SA. Schneiderian first rank symptoms are associated with right parietal hyperactivity: a replication utilising fMRI. *American Journal of Psychiatry* 2005; 162: 1545.

Giovanetti T, Buxbaum LJ, Biran I, Chatterjee A. Reduced endogenous control in alien hand syndrome: evidence from naturalistic action. *Neuropsychologia* 2005; 43: 75–88.

Goldberg G, Bloom KK. The alien hand sign: localization, lateralization and recovery. *American Journal of Physical Medicine & Rehabilitation* 1990; 69: 228–238.

Goldberg G, Mayer NH, Toglia JU. Medial frontal cortex and the alien hand sign. *Archives of Neurology* 1981; 38: 683–686.

Goldman-Rakic PS. Motor control function of the prefrontal cortex. In *Motor areas of the cerebral cortex*, Ciba Foundation Symposium 132. Chichester: Wiley.

Jaspers, K. *General Psychopathology*. Engl. Translation (J Hoenig & MW Hamilton). Manchester: Manchester University Press, 1963.

Kikkert MA, Ribbers GM, Koudstaal PJ. Alien hand syndrome in stroke: a report of 2 cases and review of the literature. *Archives of Physical Medicine Rehabilitation* 2006; 87: 728–732.

Leiguarda R, Starkstein S, Nogues M, Berthier M, Arbelaiz R. Paroxysmal alien hand syndrome. *Journal of Neurology Neurosurgery & Psychiatry* 1993; 56: 788–792.

Libet B, Gleason CA, Wright EW, Pearl DK. Time of conscious intention to act in relation to onset of cerebral activity (readiness potential). The unconscious initiation of a freely voluntary act. *Brain* 1983; 106: 623–642.

Macmurray J. *The self as agent*. London: Faber and Faber, 1991 (first published 1957).

Maruff P, Wood SJ, Velakoulis D, Smith DJ, Soulsby B, Suckling J, Bullmore ET, Pantelis C. Reduced volume of parietal and frontal association areas in patients with schizophrenia characterized by passivity delusions. *Psychological Medicine* 2005; 35: 783–789.

Matsui M, Yoneyama E, Sumiyoshi T, Noguchi K, Nohara S, Susuki M, Kawasaki Y, Seto H, Kurachi M. Lack of self-control as assessed by a personality inventory is related to reduced volume of supplementary motor area. *Psychiatry Research: Neuroimaging* 2002; 116: 53–61.

Mellor, C.S. First rank symptoms of Schizophrenia. 1. The frequency in schizophrenics on admission to hospital. 2. Differences between individual first rank symptoms. *British Journal of Psychiatry* 1970; 117: 15–23.

Mortimer A, Spence S. *Managing negative symptoms of schizophrenia*. London: Science Press, 2001.

Mullins S, Spence SA. Re-examining thought insertion: Semi-structured literature review and conceptual analysis. *British Journal of Psychiatry* 2003; 182: 293–298.

Nightingale S. Somatoparaphrenia: a case report. *Cortex* 1982; 18: 463–467.

Passingham RE. Functional organisation of the motor system. In *'Human brain function'* (ed. RSJ Frackowiak et al). San Diego: Academic Press, 1997: 243–274.

Scepkowski LA, Cronin-Golomb A. The alien hand: Cases, categorizations, and anatomical correlates. *Behavioural and Cognitive Neuroscience Reviews* 2003; 2: 261–277.

Schneider K. Primary and secondary symptoms in schizophrenia. In *'Themes and variations in European psychiatry'* (ed. SR Hirsch & M Shepherd). Bristol: John Wright, 1974: 40–46. (First published in 1957.)

Shallice T. *From neuropsychology to mental structure*. Cambridge: Cambridge University Press, 1988.

Shallice T, Burgess PW. The domain of supervisory processes and temporal organization of behaviour. *Philosophical Transactions of the Royal Society of London [Biol]* 1996; 351: 1405–1412.

Spence SA. Free will in the light of neuropsychiatry. *Philosophy Psychiatry & Psychology* 1996; 3: 75–90.

Spence SA. The screaming man. *BMJ* 1999; 319: 489.

Spence SA. Disorders of willed action. In *Contemporary approaches to the study of hysteria* (ed. Halligan, PW, Bass C, Marshall JC), pp. 235–250. Oxford: Oxford University Press, 2001.

Spence SA. Alien control: from phenomenology to cognitive neurobiology. *Philosophy Psychiatry & Psychology* 2002; 8 (2–3): 163–172.

Spence SA, Frith CD. Towards a functional anatomy of volition. *Journal of Consciousness Studies* 1999; 6: 11–29.

Spence SA, Brooks DJ, Hirsch SR, Liddle PF, Meehan J, Grasby PM. A PET study of voluntary movement in schizophrenic patients experiencing passivity phenomena (delusions of alien control). *Brain* 1997; 120: 1997–2011.

Trojano L, Crisci C, Lanzillo B, Elefante R, Caruso G. How many alien hand syndromes? Follow up of a case. *Neurology* 1993; 43: 2710–2712.

Yamaguchi S, Yamagata S, Bokura H, Toyoda G, Nagai A, Takahashi K, Kobayashi S. Somatosensory disinhibition and frontal alien hand signs following medial frontal damage. *Journal of Clinical Neuroscience* 2006; 13: 279–282.

Chapter 6 – Failing to act

Abi-Dargham A. Evidence from brain imaging studies for dopaminergic alterations in schizophrenia. In *Dopamine in the pathophysiology and treatment of schizophrenia*, ed. S. Kapur & Y. Lecrubier. London: Martin Dunitz, 2003: 15–47.

Aron AR, Robbins TW, Poldrack RA. Inhibition and the right inferior frontal cortex. *Trends in Cognitive Sciences* 2004; 8: 170–177.

Barker RA, Dunnett SB. *Neural repair, transplantation and rehabilitation.* Hove: Psychology Press, 1999.

Barrett K. Treating organic abulia with bromocriptine and lisuride: four case studies. *Journal of Neurology, Neurosurgery and Psychiatry* 1991; 54: 718–721.

Blair RJR. The roles of orbital frontal cortex in the modulation of antisocial behaviour. *Brain & Cognition* 2004; 55: 198–208.

Blank SC, Scott SK, Murphy K, Warburton E, Wise RJ. Speech production: Wernicke, Broca and beyond. *Brain* 2002; 125: 1829–1838.

Bradshaw JL. *Developmental disorders of the frontostriatal system: Neuropsychological, neuropsychiatric and evolutionary perspectives.* Hove: Psychology Press, 2001.

Burgess PW, Quayle A, Frith CD. Brain regions involved in prospective memory as determined by positron emission tomography. *Neuropsychologia* 2001; 39: 545–555.

Carter CS, Braver TS, Barch DM, Botvinick MM, Noll D, Cohen JD. Anterior cingulate cortex, error detection, and the online monitoring of performance. *Science* 1998; 280: 747–749.

Chua SE, Wright IC, Poline J-B, Liddle PF, Murray RM, Frackowiak RSJ, Friston KJ, McGuire PK. Grey matter correlates of syndromes in schizophrenia: A semi-automated analysis of structural magnetic resonance images. *British Journal of Psychiatry* 1997; 170: 406–410.

Cummings JL. Frontal-subcortical circuits and human behaviour. *Archives of Neurology* 1993; 50: 873–880.

DeRosse P, Funke B, Burdick KE, Lencz T, Ekholm JM, Kane JM, Kucherlapati R, Malhorta AK. Dysbindin genotype and negative symptoms in schizophrenia. *American Journal of Psychiatry* 2006; 163: 532–534.

Desmond JE, Gabrieli JDE, Glover GH. Dissociation of frontal and cerebellar activity in a cognitive task: evidence for dissociation between selection and search. *NeuroImage* 1998; 7: 368–376.

De Zubicaray GI, Chalk JB, Rose SE, Semple J, Smith GA. Deficits on self ordered tasks associated with hyperostosis frontalis interna. *Journal of Neurology, Neurosurgery, and Psychiatry* 1997; 63: 309–314.

De Zubicaray GI, Williams SCR, Wilson SJ, Rose SE, Brammer MJ, Bullmore ET, Simmons A, Chalk JB, Semple J, Brown AP, Smith GA, Ashton R, Doddrell DM. Prefrontal cortex involvement in selective letter generation: a functional magnetic resonance imaging study. *Cortex* 1998; 34: 389–401.

Dolan RJ, Bench CJ, Liddle PF, Friston KJ, Frith CD, Grasby PM, Frackowiak RSJ. Dorsolateral prefrontal cortex dysfunction in the major psychoses: symptom or disease specificity? *Journal of Neurology, Neurosurgery and Psychiatry* 1993; 56: 1290–1294.

Egan MF, Goldberg TE, Kolachana BS, Callicott JH, Mazzanti CM, Straub RE, Goldman D, Weinberger DR. Effect of COMT Val108/158Met genotype on frontal lobe function and risk for schizophrenia. *Proceedings of the National Academy of Sciences of the United States of America* 2001; 98: 6917–6922.

Endelborghs S, Marien P, Pickut BA, Verstraeten S, De Deyn PP. Loss of psychic self-activation after paramedian bithalamic infarction. *Stroke* 2000; 31: 1762–1765.

Farrow TF, Zheng Y, Wilkinson ID, Spence SA, Deakin JF, Tarrier N, Griffiths PD, Woodruff PW. Investigating the functional anatomy of empathy and forgiveness. *NeuroReport* 2005; 12: 2433–2438.

Farrow TFD, Hunter MD, Haque R, Spence SA. Modafinil and unconstrained motor activity in schizophrenia: double-blind crossover placebo-controlled trial. *British Journal of Psychiatry* 2006; 189: 461–462.

Farrow TFD, Hunter MD, Wilkinson ID, Green RDJ, Spence SA. Structural brain correlates of unconstrained motor activity in people with schizophrenia. *British Journal of Psychiatry* 2005; 187: 481–482.

Fletcher PC, Shallice T, Dolan RJ. 'Sculpting the response space': an account of left prefrontal activation at encoding. *NeuroImage* 2000; 12: 404–417.

Frith CD, Friston KJ, Liddle PF, Frackowiak RSJ. A PET study of word finding. *Neuropsychologia* 1991a; 29: 1137–1148.

Frith CD, Friston KJ, Liddle PF, Frackowiak RSJ. Willed action and the prefrontal cortex in man: a study with PET. *Proceedings of the Royal Society of London [Series B]* 1991b; 244: 241–246.

Frith CD, Frith U. Interacting minds: a biological basis. *Science* 1999; 286: 1692–1695.

Ganesan V, Green RD, Hunter MD, Wilkinson ID, Spence SA. Temporal randomness in the spontaneous movements of people with schizophrenia: the role of left prefrontal cortex. *NeuroImage*, submitted.

Gaser C, Schlaug G. Brain structures differ between musicians and non-musicians. *Journal of Neuroscience* 2003; 23: 9240–9245.

Goldberg E. *The executive brain: frontal lobes and the civilized mind*. Oxford: Oxford University Press, 2001.

Goldman-Rakic PS. Motor control function of the prefrontal cortex. In *Motor areas of the cerebral cortex. Ciba Foundation Symposium 132*. Chichester: Wiley, 1987.

Goldman-Rakic PS, Bates JF, Chafee MV. The prefrontal cortex and internally generated motor acts. *Current Opinion in Neurobiology* 1992; 2: 830–835.

Grunsfeld AA, Login IS. Abulia following penetrating brain injury during endoscopic sinus surgery with disruption of the anterior cingulate circuit: case report. *BMC Neurology* 2006; 6: 4.

Gur RE, Cowell P, Turetsky BI, Gallacher F, Cannon T, Bilker W, Gur RC. A follow-up magnetic resonance imaging study of schizophrenia: relationship of neuroanatomical changes to clinical and neurobehavioural measures. *Archives of General Psychiatry* 1998; 55: 145–152.

Heckers S, Goff D, Schacter DL, Savage CR, Fischman AJ, Alpert NM, Rauch SL. Functional imaging of memory retrieval in deficit vs nondeficit schizophrenia. *Archives of General Psychiatry* 1999; 56: 1117–1123.

Honey GD, Bullmore ET, Soni W, Varatheesan M, Williams SCR, Sharma T. Differences in frontal cortical activation by a working memory task after substitution of risperidone for typical antipsychotic drugs in patients with schizophrenia. *Proceedings of the National Academy of Sciences* 1999; 96: 13432–13437.

Hunter MD, Farrow TFD, Papadakis N, Wilkinson ID, Woodruff PWR, Spence SA. Approaching an ecologically valid functional anatomy of spontaneous 'willed' action. *NeuroImage* 2003; 20: 1264–1269.

Hunter MD, Ganesan V, Wilkinson ID, Spence SA. Acute effects of modafinil on prefrontal function and cognitive control in chronic schizophrenia. *American Journal of Psychiatry* 2006; 163: 2184–2186.

Hunter MD, Green RDJ, Wilkinson ID, Spence SA. Spatial and temporal dissociation in prefrontal cortex during action execution. *NeuroImage* 2004; 23: 1186–1191.

Ingvar DH. The will of the brain: cerebral correlates of wilful acts. *Journal of Theoretical Biology* 1994; 171: 7–12.

Jahanshahi M, Dirnberger G, Fuller R, Frith CD. The role of dorsolateral prefrontal cortex in random number generation: a study with positron emission tomography. *NeuroImage* 2000; 12: 713–725.

Jahanshahi M, Profice P, Brown RG, Ridding MC, Dirnberger G, Rothwell JC. The effects of transcranial magnetic stimulation over the dorsolateral prefrontal cortex on suppression of habitual counting during random number generation. *Brain* 1998; 121: 1533–1544.

Jenkins IH, Brooks DJ, Nixon PD, Frackowiak RSJ. Motor sequence learning: a study with positron emission tomography. *Journal of Neuroscience* 1994; 14: 3775–3790.

Jenkins IH, Fernandez W, Playford ED, Lees AJ, Frackowiak RS, Passingham RE. Impaired activation of the supplementary motor area in Parkinson's disease is reversed when akinesia is treated with apomorphine. *Annals of Neurology* 1992; 32: 749–757.

Kolb B, Gibb R. Frontal lobe plasticity and behaviour. In *'Principles of frontal lobe function'*, ed. DT Stuss & RT Knight. Oxford: OUP, 2002, 541–556.

Libet B, Gleason CA, Wright EW, Pearl DK. Time of conscious intention to act in relation to onset of cerebral activity. *Brain* 1983; 106: 623–642.

Liddle PF, Friston KJ, Frith CD, Hirsch SR, Jones T, Frackowiak RSJ. Patterns of cerebral blood flow in schizophrenia. *British Journal of Psychiatry* 1992; 160: 179–186.

Lipska BK, Kolb B, Halim N, Weinberger DR. Synaptic abnormalities in prefrontal cortex and nucleus accumbens of adult rats with neonatal hippocampal damage. *Schizophrenia Research* 2001; (suppl): 47.

Litvan I, Paulsen JS, Mega MS, Cummings JL. Neuropsychiatric assessment of patients with hyperkinetic and hypokinetic movement disorders. *Archives of Neurology* 1998; 55: 1313–1319.

Madsen AL, Karle A, Rubin P, Cortsen M, Andersen HS, Hemmingsen R. Progressive atrophy of frontal lobes in first-episode schizophrenia: interaction with clinical course and neuroleptic treatment. *Acta Psychiatrica Scandinavica* 1999; 100: 367–374.

Maguire EA, Gadian DG, Johnsrude IS, Good CD, Ashburner J, Frackowiak RSJ, Frith CD. Navigation-related structural change in the hippocampi of taxi drivers. *PNAS* 2000; 97: 4398–4403.

Marrin RS. Apathy: A neuropsychiatric syndrome. *Journal of Neuropsychiatry and Clinical Neurosciences* 1991; 3: 243–254.

McDowell S, Whyte J, D'Esposito M. Differential effect of a dopaminergic agonist on prefrontal function in traumatic brain injury patients. *Brain* 1998; 121: 1155–1164.

Milner B. Effects of difference brain lesions on card sorting. *Archives of Neurology* 1963; 9: 100–110.

Mortimer A, Spence S. *Managing negative symptoms of schizophrenia*. London: Science Press, 2001.

Nelson HE, O'Connell A. Dementia: the estimation of premorbid intelligence levels using the New Adult Reading Test. *Cortex* 1978; 14: 234–244.

Passingham R. *The frontal lobes and voluntary action*. Oxford: Oxford University Press, 1993.

Passingham RE. Attention to action. *Philosophical Transactions of the Royal Society of London [Series B]* 1996; 351: 1473–1479.

Paus T. Primate anterior cingulate cortex: where motor control, drive and cognition interface. *Nature Reviews Neuroscience* 2001; 2: 417–424.

Perret E. The left frontal lobe of man and the suppression of habitual responses in verbal categorical behaviour. *Neuropsychologia* 1974; 12: 323–330.

Petrides M. Specialised systems for the procession of mnemonic information within the primate prefrontal cortex. *Philosophical Transactions of the Royal Society of London [Series B]* 1996; 351: 1455–1462.

Petrides M, Milner B. Deficits on subject-ordered tasks after frontal- and temporal-lobe lesions in man. *Neuropsychologia* 1982; 20: 249–262.

Rioult-Pedotti M-S, Donoghue JP. The nature and mechanisms of plasticity. In *'Plasticity in the Human nervous system'*, ed. S. Boniface & U. Ziemann. Cambridge: CUP, 2003, 1–25.

Rosen HJ, Allison SC, Schauer GF, Gorno-Tempini ML, Weiner MW, Miller BL. Neuroanatomical correlates of behavioural disorders in dementia. *Brain* 2005; 128: 2612–2625.

Roth RM, Flashman LA, Saykin AJ, McAllister TW, Vidaver R. Apathy in schizophrenia: reduced frontal lobe volume and neuropsychological deficits. *American Journal of Psychiatry* 2004; 161: 157–159.

Sallet PC, Elkis H, Alves TM, Oliveira JR, Sassi E, Campi-de-Castro C, Busatto GF, Gattaz WF. Rightward cerebral asymmetry in subtypes of schizophrenia according to Leonhard's classification and to DSM-IV: a structural MRI study. *Psychiatry Research, Neuroimaging* 2003; 123: 65–79.

Salokangas RKR, Cannon T, Van Erp T, Ilonen T, Taiminen T, Karlsson H, Lauerma H, Leinonen KM, Wallenius E, Kaljonen A, Syvaelahti E, Vilkman H, Alanen A, Hietala J. Structural magnetic resonance imaging in patients with first-episode schizophrenia, psychotic and severe non-psychotic depression and healthy controls. Results of the Schizophrenia and Affective Psychoses (SAP) project. *British Journal of Psychiatry* 2002; 181(Suppl 43): s58-s65.

Samuel M, Ceballos-Baumann AO, Turjanski N, Boecker H, Gorospe A, Linazasoro G, Holmes AP, DeLong MR, Vitek JL, Thomas DGT, Quinn NP, Obeso JA, Brooks DJ. Pallidotomy in Parkinson's disease increases supplementary motor area and prefrontal activation during performance of volitional movements. An $H_2{}^{15}O$ PET study. *Brain* 1997; 120: 1301–1313.

Shallice T. *From neuropsychology to mental structure*. Cambridge: Cambridge University Press, 1988.

Shallice T. Fractionation of the supervisory system. In *'Principles of frontal lobe function'*, ed. DT Stuss & RT Knight. Oxford: OUP, 2002, 261–277.

Spence SA. The cognitive executive is implicated in the maintenance of psychogenic movement disorders. In *'Psychogenic movement disorders'*, ed. M. Hallett et al. Philadelphia: American Academy of Neurology, 2006a: 222–229.

Spence SA. The cycle of action. *Journal of Consciousness Studies* 2006b; 13: 69–72.

Spence SA, Brooks DJ, Hirsch SR, Liddle PF, Meehan J, Grasby PM. A PET study of voluntary movement in schizophrenic patients experiencing passivity phenomena (delusions of alien control). *Brain* 1997; 120: 1997–2011.

Spence SA, Farrow TFD, Herford AE, Wilkinson ID, Zheng Y, Woodruff PWR. Behavioural and functional anatomical correlates of deception in humans. *NeuroReport* 2001; 12: 2849–2853.

Spence SA, Frith CD. Towards a functional anatomy of volition. *Journal of Consciousness Studies* 1999; 6: 11–29.

Spence SA, Green RDJ, Wilkinson ID, Hunter MD. Modafinil modulates anterior cingulate function in schizophrenia. *British Journal of Psychiatry* 2005; 187: 55–61.

Spence SA, Hirsch SR, Brooks JD, Grasby PM. Prefrontal cortical activity in people with schizophrenia and control subjects. Evidence from positron emission tomography for remission of 'hypofrontality' with recovery from acute schizophrenia. *British Journal of Psychiatry* 1998; 172: 316–323.

Spence SA, Hunter MD, Farrow TFD, Green RDJ, Leung DH, Hughes CJ, Ganesan V. A Cognitive neurobiological account of deception: evidence from functional neuroimaging. *Philosophical Transactions of the Royal Society of London [Series B]* 2004; 359: 1755–1762.

Spence SA, Hunter MD, Harpin G. Neuroscience and the will. *Current Opinion in Psychiatry* 2002; 15: 519–526.

Spence SA, Parry C. Schizophrenic avolition: implications from functional and structural neuroimaging. In *'Disorders of volition'* (ed. N. Sebanz & W. Prinz), Massachusetts: MIT Press, 2006: 207–232.

Starkstein SE, Merello M. *Psychiatric and cognitive disorders in Parkinson's disease*. Cambridge: Cambridge University Press, 2002.

Turner DC, Clark L, Pomarol-Clotet E, McKenna P, Robbins TW, Sahakian BJ. Modafinil improves cognition and attentional set shifting in patients with chronic schizophrenia. *Neuropsychopharmacology* 2004; 29: 1363–1373.

Van der Werf YD, Weerts JGE, Jolles J, Witter MP, Lindeboom J, Scheltens P. Neuropsychological correlates of a right unilateral lacunar thalamic infarction. *JNNP* 1999; 66: 36–42.

Wegner DM. *The illusion of conscious will.* Cambridge, Massachusetts: Bradford Books, MIT Press, 2002.

Wible CG, Anderson J, Shenton ME, Kricun A, Hirayasu Y, Tanaka S, Levitt JJ, O'Donnell BF, Kikinis R, Jolesz FA, McCarley RW. Prefrontal cortex, negative symptoms, and schizophrenia: an MRI study. *Psychiatry Research, Neuroimaging* 2001; 108: 65–78.

Wise RJS, Greene J, Buchel C, Scott SK. Brain regions involved in articulation. *Lancet* 1999; 353: 1057–1061.

Wolkin A, Choi SJ, Szilagyi S, Sanfilipo M, Rotrosen JP, Lim KO. Inferior frontal white matter anisotropy and negative symptoms of schizophrenia: A diffusion tensor imaging study. *American Journal of Psychiatry* 2003; 160: 572–574.

Youngren KD, Inglis FM, Pivirotto PJ, Jedema HP, Bradberry CW, Goldman-Rakic PS, Roth RH, Moghaddam B. Clozapine preferentially increases dopamine release in the rhesus monkey prefrontal cortex compared with the caudate nucleus. *Neuropsychopharmacology* 1999; 20: 403–412.

Chapter 7 – Hysterical agents

Adrian ED, Yealland LR. The treatment of some common war neuroses. *Lancet* 1917; I: 867–872.

American Psychiatric Association. *Diagnostic criteria from DSM IV*. Washington DC: American Psychiatric Association, 1994.

Baker JHE, Silver JR. Hysterical paraplegia. *Journal of Neurology, Neurosurgery & Psychiatry* 1987; 50: 375–382.

Campbell J. The shortest paper. *Neurology* 1979; 29: 1633.

Didi-Huberman G. *Invention of hysteria: Charcot and the photographic iconography of the Salpetriere.* Translated by A. Hartz. Cambridge, Massachusetts: MIT Press, 2003 (first published 1982).

Ellenberger H. *The discovery of the unconscious.* London: Fontana, 1994.

Fingarette H. *Self-deception.* Berkeley: University of California Press, 2000 (second edition, originally published 1969).

Freud S. The neuro-psychoses of defence. In *The complete psychological works*, vol. III (standard edn (1962, first published 1894) ed. Strachey, J.) pp. 45–61. London: Hogarth.

Frith CD, Friston KJ, Liddle PF, Frackowiak RSJ. A PET study of word finding. *Neuropsychologia* 1991a; 29: 1137–1148.

Frith CD, Friston K, Liddle PF, Frackowiak RSJ. Willed action and the prefrontal cortex in man: a study with PET. *Proceedings of the Royal Society of London [Biol]* 1991b; 244: 241–246.

Hallett, M., Fahn S., Jankovic J., Lang AE., Cloninger CR., Yudofsky SC(ed) *Psychogenic movement disorders: neurology and neuropsychiatry.*, Philadelphia: American Academy of Neurology Press, Lippincott Williams & Wilkins, 2006.

Halligan PW, Bass C, Marshall JC (ed.) *Contemporary approaches to the study of hysteria: Clinical and theoretical perspectives.* Oxford: Oxford University Press, 2001.

Jenkins IH, Fernandez W, Playford ED, Lees AJ, Frackowiak RS, Passingham RE. Impaired activation of the supplementary motor area in Parkinson's disease is reversed when akinesia is treated with apomorphine. *Annals of Neurology* 1992; 32: 749–757.

Lempert T, Brandt T, Dieterich M, Huppert D. How to identify psychogenic disorders of stance and gait: a video study in 37 patients. *Journal of Neurology* 1991; 238: 140–146.

Mailis-Gagnon, A., Giannoylis, I., Downar, J., *et al.* Altered central somatosensory processing in chronic pain patients with 'hysterical' anaesthesia. *Neurology* 2003; 60: 1501–1507.

Marshall JC, Halligan PW, Fink GR, Wade DT, Frackowiak RS. The functional anatomy of a hysterical paralysis. *Cognition* 1997; 64: B1–B8.

May C. Lord Moran's memoir: shell-shock and the pathology of fear. *Journal of the Royal Society of Medicine* 1998; 91: 95–100.

Merskey H. *The analysis of hysteria: understanding conversion and dissociation.* London: Gaskell, 1995.

Myers T. *Slavoj Zizek.* London: Routledge, 2003.

O'Suilleabhain PE, Matsumoto JY. Time-frequency analysis of tremors. *Brain* 1998; 121: 2127–2134.

Passingham RE. Attention to action. *Philosophical Transactions of the Royal Society of London [series B]* 1996; 351: 1473–1479.

Sanoo M. Abductor sign: a reliable new sign to detect unilateral non-organic paresis of the lower limb. *Journal of Neurology, Neurosurgery and Psychiatry* 2004; 75: 121–125.

Shallice T. *From neuropsychology to mental structure.* Cambridge: Cambridge University Press, 1988.

Shallice T., Burgess PW. The domain of supervisory processes and temporal organisation of behaviour. *Philosophical Transactions of the Royal Society of London [series B]* 1996; 351: 1405–1412.

Spence SA. Hysterical paralyses as disorders of action. *Cognitive Neuropsychiatry* 1999; 4: 203–226.

Spence SA. Disorders of willed action. In *Contemporary approaches to the study of hysteria* (ed. Halligan, PW, Bass C, Marshall JC), pp. 235–250. Oxford: Oxford University Press, 2001.

Spence SA. Hysteria: a new look. *Psychiatry* 2006a; 5(2): 56–60.

Spence SA. The cognitive executive is implicated in the maintenance of psychogenic movement disorders. In *Psychogenic movement disorders: neurology and neuropsychiatry* (ed. Hallett, M., Fahn S., Jankovic J., Lang AE., Cloninger CR., Yudofsky SC), pp 222–229. Philadelphia: American Academy of Neurology Press, Lippincott Williams & Wilkins, 2006b.

Spence SA. All in the mind? The neural correlates of unexplained physical symptoms. *Advances in Psychiatric Treatment* 2006c; 12: 349–358.

Spence SA. 'Others' and others: hysteria and the divided self. In *Cognitive neurology: a clinical textbook* (ed. S. Cappa, J. Abutalebi, J-F Demonet, P. Fletcher & P. Garrard), Oxford: Oxford University Press, 2008: 459–472.

Spence SA, Crimlisk HC, Cope H, Ron MA, Grasby PM. Discrete neurophysiological correlates in prefrontal cortex during hysterical and feigned disorder of movement. *Lancet* 2000; 356: 162–163.

Symonds C. Hysteria. In *The analysis of hysteria* (2nd edition, 1995) (ed. Merskey, H.) pp. 407–413. London: Gaskell, 1970.

Terada K, Ikeda A, Van Ness PC, Nagamine T, Kaji R, Kimura J, Shibasaki H. Presence of Bereitschaftspotential preceding psychogenic myoclonus: clinical application of jerk-locked back averaging. *Journal of Neurology, Neurosurgery and Psychiatry* 1995; 58: 745–747.

Tiihonen, J., Kuikka, J., Viinamaki, H., *et al.* Altered cerebral blood flow during hysterical paraesthesia. *Biological Psychiatry* 1995; 37: 134–135.

Vuilleumier, P., Chicherio, C., Assal, F., *et al.* Functional neuroanatomical correlates of hysterical sensorimotor loss. *Brain* 2001; 124: 1077–1090.

Wenegrat B. *Theatre of disorder: patients, doctors, and the construction of illness.* Oxford: Oxford University Press, 2001.

Werring, D.J., Weston, L., Bullmore, E.T., *et al.* Functional magnetic resonance imaging of the cerebral response to visual stimulation in medically unexplained visual loss. *Psychological Medicine* 2004; 34: 583–589.

Yazici, K.M., Kostakoglu, L. Cerebral blood from changes in patients with conversion disorder. *Psychiatry Research: Neuroimaging* 1998; 83: 163–168.

Zizek S. *Looking awry: an introduction to Jacques Lacan through popular culture.* Cambridge, Massachusetts: MIT Press, 1991.

Zizek S. *The art of the ridiculous sublime: on David Lynch's Lost Highway.* Washington, Seattle: Walter Chapin Simpson Centre for the Humanities, 2000.

Chapter 8 – Deceivers all

Abe N, Suzuki M, Mori E, Itoh M, Fujii T. Deceiving others: distinct neural responses of the prefrontal cortex and amygdala in simple fabrication and deception with social interactions. *Journal of Cognitive Neuroscience* 2007; 19: 287–295.

Abe N, Suzuki M, Tsukiura T, Mori E, Yamaguchi K, Itoh M, Fujii T. Dissociable roles of prefrontal and anterior cingulate cortices in deception. *Cerebral Cortex* 2006; 16: 192–199.

Aristotle. *The Nicomachean Ethics.* Translated by D. Ross (Revised by J.L. Ackrill & J.O. Urmson). Oxford: Oxford University Press, 1998 (first published 1980).

Bass C. Factitious disorders and malingering. In *Contemporary approaches to the study of hysteria: Clinical and theoretical perspectives* (ed. PW Halligan, C Bass, JC Marshall). Oxford: Oxford University Press, 2001: 126–142.

Beer JS, Heerey EA, Keltner D, Scabini D, Knight RT. The regulatory function of self-conscious emotion: Insights from patients with orbitofrontal damage. *Journal of Personality and Social Psychology* 2003; 85: 594–604.

Blumer D, Benson DF. Personality changes with frontal and temporal lobe lesions. In *Psychiatric aspects of neurologic disease* (ed. DF Benson & D Blumer). New York: Grune & Stratton, 1975: 151–170.

Bond CF, De Paulo BM. Accuracy of deception judgements. *Personality and Social Psychology Review* 2006; 10: 214–234.

Butters N, Butter C, Rosen J, Stein D. Behavioural effects of sequential and one-stage ablations of orbitofrontal prefrontal cortex in the monkey. *Experimental Neurology* 1973; 39: 204–214.

Byrne RW. Tracing the evolutionary path of cognition. In 'The Social Brain: Evolution and Pathology' (ed. M. Brune, H. Ribbert & W. Schiefenhovel). Chichester, West Sussex: Wiley & Sons, 2003: 43–60.

Chambers Concise Dictionary. Edinburgh: Chambers Harrap, 1997.

Byrne RW, Corp N. Neocortex size predicts deception rate in primates. *Proceedings of the Royal Society of London, series B* 2004; 271: 1693–1699.

Chambers. *Chambers concise dictionary.* Edinburgh: Chambers Harrap, 1997.

Davatzikos C, Ruparel K, Fan Y, Shen DG, Acharyya M, Loughead JW, Gur RC, Langleben DD. Classifying spatial patterns of brain activity with machine learning methods: application to lie detection. *NeuroImage* 2005; 28: 663–668.

Dunbar RIM. Why are good writers so rare? An evolutionary perspective on literature. *Journal of Cultural and Evolutionary Psychology* 2005; 3: 7–21.

Ekman P, O'Sullivan M. Who can catch a liar? *American Psychologist* 1991; 46: 913–920.

Fletcher PC, Happe F, Frith U, Baker SC, Dolan RJ, Frackowiak RSJ, Frith CD. Other minds in the brain: A functional imaging study of 'theory of mind' in story comprehension. *Cognition* 1995; 57: 109–128.

Ford CV, King BH, Hollender MH. Lies and liars: psychiatric aspects of prevarication. *American Journal of Psychiatry* 1988; 145: 554–562.

Galbraith JK. *The economics of innocent fraud.* London: Penguin, 2004.

Gamer M, Bauermann T, Stoeter P, Vossel G. Covariations among fMRI, skin conductance and behavioural data during processing of concealed information. *Human Brain Mapping* in press.

Ganis G, Kosslyn SM, Stose S, Thompson WL, Yurgelun-Todd DA. Neural correlates of different types of deception: an fMRI investigation. *Cerebral Cortex* 2003; 13: 830–836.

Giannetti E. *Lies we live by: The art of self-deception* (transl. J. Gledson). London: Bloomsbury, 2000.

Granhag PA, Stromwall LA. *The detection of deception in forensic contexts.* Cambridge: Cambridge University Press, 2004.

Happe F. *Autism: An introduction to psychological theory.* Hove: Psychology Press, 1994.

Hitchens C. *Letters to a Young Contrarian.* New York: Basic Books, 2001.

Hughes CJ, Farrow TFD, Hopwood A-C, Pratt A, Hunter MD, Spence SA. Recent developments in deception research. *Current Psychiatry Reviews* 2005; 1: 271–279.

Iversen SD, Mishkin M. Perseverative interference in monkeys following selective lesions of the inferior prefrontal convexity. *Experimental Brain Research* 1970; 11: 376–386.

Kozel FA, Revell LJ, Lorberbaum JP, Shastri A, Elhai JD, Horner MD, Smith A, Nahas Z, Bohning DE, George MS. A pilot study of functional magnetic resonance imaging brain correlates of deception in healthy young men. *Journal of Neuropsychiatry and Clinical Neurosciences* 2004a; 16: 295–305.

Kozel FA, Padgett TM, George MS. A replication study of the neural correlates of deception. *Behavioural Neuroscience* 2004b; 118: 852–856.

Kozel FA, Johnson KA, Mu Q, Grenesko EL, Laken SJ, George MS. Detecting deception using functional magnetic resonance imaging. *Biological Psychiatry* 2005; 58: 605–613.

Langleben DD, Loughead JW, Bilker WB, Ruparel K, Childress AR, Busch SI, Gur RC. Telling truth from lie in individual subjects with fast event-related fMRI. *Human Brain Mapping* 2005; 26: 262–272.

Langleben DD, Schroeder L, Maldjian JA, Gur RC, McDonald S, Ragland JD, O'Brien CP, Childress AR. Brain activity during simulated deception: an event-related functional magnetic resonance study. *NeuroImage* 2002; 15: 727–732.

Layard R. *Happiness: Lessons from a new science*. London: Allen Lane, 2005.

Lee TMC, Liu H-L, Chan CCH, Ng Y-B, Fox PT, Gao J-H. Neural correlates of feigned memory impairment. *NeuroImage* 2005; 28: 305–313.

Lee TMC, Liu H-L, Tan L-H, Chan CCH, Mahankali S, Feng C-M, Hou J, Fox PT, Gao J-H. Lie detection by functional magnetic resonance imaging. *Human Brain Mapping* 2002; 15: 157–164.

Machiavelli, N. *The Prince*. Translated by G. Bull. London: Penguin, 1999 (first published 1961.

Mealey L. The socio-biology of sociopathy: An integrated evolutionary model. *Behavioural and Brain Sciences* 1995; 18: 523–599.

Mohamed FB, Faro SH, Gordon NJ, Platek SM, Ahmad H, Williams JM. Brain mapping of deception and truth telling about an ecologically valid situation: functional MR imaging and polygraph investigation – initial experience. *Radiology* 2006; 238: 679–688.

Nunez JM, Casey BJ, Egner T, Hare T, Hirsch J. Intentional false responding shares neural substrates with response conflict and cognitive control. *NeuroImage* 2005; 25: 267–277.

Oborne P. *The use and abuse of terror: The construction of a false narrative on the domestic terror threat*. London: Centre for Policy Studies, 2006.

O'Connell S. *Mindreading: An investigation into how we learn to love and lie*. London: Arrow Books, 1998.

Phan KL, Magalhaes A, Ziemlewicz TJ, Fitzgerald DA, Green C, Smith W. Neural correlates of telling lies: a functional magnetic resonance imaging study at 4 Tesla. *Academic Radiology* 2005; 12: 164–172.

Roget's Thesaurus. London: Penguin, 2004 edition.

Shallice T. *From neuropsychology to mental structure*. Cambridge: Cambridge University Press, 1988.

Sokol DK. How the doctor's nose has shortened over time: a historical overview of the truth-telling debate in the doctor-patient relationship. *Journal of the Royal Society of Medicine* 2006; 99: 632–636.

Spence SA. The deceptive brain. *Journal of the Royal Society of Medicine* 2004; 97: 6–9.

Spence SA. Prefrontal white matter – the tissue of lies? Invited commentary on...
Prefrontal white matter in pathological liars. *British Journal of Psychiatry* 2005;
187: 326–327.

Spence SA. Playing Devil's Advocate: The case against fMRI lie detection. *Legal and
Criminological Psychology* 2008; 13: 11–25.

Spence SA, Hunter MD, Harper G. Neuroscience and the will. *Current Opinion in
Psychiatry* 2002; 15: 519–526.

Spence SA, Farrow TFD, Herford AE, Wilkinson ID, Zheng Y, Woodruff PWR.
Behavioural and functional anatomical correlates of deception in humans. *NeuroReport*
2001; 12: 2849–2853.

Spence SA, Hunter MD, Farrow TFD, Green RD, Leung DH, Hughes CJ, Ganesan V.
A cognitive neurobiological account of deception: evidence from functional neuroimaging. *Philosophical Transactions of the Royal Society of London series B* 2004; 359:
1755–1762.

Spence SA, Kaylor-Hughes CJ, Brook ML, Lankappa ST, Wilkinson ID. 'Munchausen's
syndrome by proxy' or a 'miscarriage of justice'? An initial application of functional
neuroimaging to the question of guilt versus innocence. *European Psychiatry* 2008; 23:
309–314.

Starkstein SE, Robinson RG. Mechanism of disinhibition after brain lesions. *Journal of
Nervous and Mental Diseases* 1997; 185: 108–114.

Vrij A. *Detecting lies and deceit: The psychology of lying and the implications for professional
practice.* Chichester: Wiley, 2000.

Vrij A, Mann S. Telling and detecting lies in a high-stake situation: the case of a convicted
murderer. *Applied Cognitive Psychology* 2001; 15: 187–203.

Wilkinson RG. *The impact of inequality: How to make sick societies healthier.* London:
Routledge, 2005.

Yang Y, Raine A, Lencz T, Bihrle S, LaCasse L, Colletti P. Prefrontal white matter in
pathological liars. *British Journal of Psychiatry* 2005; 187: 320–325.

Yang Y, Raine A, Narr KL, Lencz T, LaCasse L, Colletti P, Toga AW. Localisation of
increased prefrontal white matter in pathological liars. *British Journal of Psychiatry*
2007; 190: 174–175.

Chapter 9 – Harming others

American Psychiatric Association (APA). *Diagnostic criteria from DSM-IV.* Washington,
DC: American Psychiatric Association, 1994.

Amis M. *Koba the Dread: Laughter and the Twenty Million.* London: Jonathan Cape, 2002.

Anderson SW, Bechara A, Damasio H, et al. Impairment of social and moral behaviour
related to early damage to human prefrontal cortex. *Nature Neuroscience* 1999; 2:
1032–1037.

Blake P, Pincus JH, Buckner C. Neurologic abnormalities in murderers. *Neurology* 1995;
45: 1641–1647.

Blair RJR. Neurobiological basis of psychopathy. *British Journal of Psychiatry* 2003;
182: 5–7.

Blair RJR. The roles of orbitofrontal cortex in the modulation of antisocial behaviour.
Brain and Cognition 2004; 55: 198–208.

Blass T. *The man who shocked the world: The life and legacy of Stanley Milgram.* New York: Basic Books, 2004.

Brennan PA, Raine A, Schulsinger F, Kirkegaard-Sorensen L, Knop J, Hutchings B, Rosenberg R, Mednick SA. Psychophysiological protective factors for male subjects at high risk for criminal behaviour. *American Journal of Psychiatry* 1997; 154: 853–855.

Brower MC, Price BH. Neuropsychiatry of frontal lobe dysfunction in violent and criminal behaviour: a critical review. *Journal of Neurology, Neurosurgery & Psychiatry* 2001; 71: 720–726.

Brunner HG, Nelen M, Breakefield XO, Ropers HH, van Oost BA. Abnormal behaviour associated with a point mutation in the structural gene for monoamine oxidase A. *Science* 1993; 262: 578–580.

Caspi A, McClay J, Moffitt TE, Mill J, Martin J, Craig IW, Taylor A, Poulton R. Role of genotype in the cycle of violence in maltreated children. *Science* 2002; 297: 851–854.

Farrington DP. The Twelfth Jack Tizard Memorial Lecture: The development of offending and antisocial behaviour from childhood: Key findings from the Cambridge study in delinquent development. *Journal of Child Psychology and Psychiatry* 1995; 360: 929–964.

Grafman J, Schwab, Warden D et al. Frontal lobe injuries, violence, and aggression: a report of the Vietnam head injury study. *Neurology* 1996; 46: 1231–1238.

Gur RC, Gunning-Dixon F, Bilker WB, Gur RE. Sex differences in temporo-limbic and frontal brain volumes of healthy adults. *Cerebral Cortex* 2002; 12: 998–1003.

Hare RD. *Without conscience: The disturbing world of the psychopaths among us.* New York: Guilford Press, 1993.

Ishikawa SS, Raine A, Lencz T, Bihrle S, LaCasse L. Increased height and bulk in antisocial personality disorder and its subtypes. *Psychiatry Research* 2001; 105: 211–219.

Jaffee SR, Caspi A, Moffitt TE, Taylor A. Physical maltreatment victim to antisocial child: Evidence of an environmentally mediated process. *Journal of Abnormal Psychology* 2004; 113: 44–55.

Jaffe SR, Moffitt TE, Caspi A, Taylor A. Life with (or without) father: The benefits of living with two biological parents depend on the father's antisocial behaviour. *Child Development* 2003; 74: 109–126.

Kiehl KA, Smith AM, Hare RD, Mendrek A, Forster BB, Brink J, Liddle PF. Limbic abnormalities inn affective processing by criminal psychopaths as revealed by functional magnetic resonance imaging. *Biological Psychiatry* 2001; 50: 677–684.

Komar DA. Variables influencing victim selection in genocide. *Journal of Forensic Science* 2008; 53: 172–177.

Lewis DO, Pincus JH, Bard B, Richardson E, Prichep LS, Feldman M, Yeager C. Neuropsychiatric, psychoeducational, and family characteristics of 14 juveniles condemned to death in the United States. *American Journal of Psychiatry* 1988; 145: 584–589.

Lilla M. *The Reckless Mind: Intellectuals in Politics.* New York: New York Review Books, 2001.

Liu J, Raine A, Venables PH, Mednick SA. Malnutrition at age 3 years and externalising behaviour problems at ages 8, 11, and 17 years. *American Journal of Psychiatry* 2004; 161: 2005–2013.

Luntz BK, Widom CS. Antisocial personality disorder in abused and neglected children grown up. *American Journal of Psychiatry* 1994; 151: 670–674.

Meyer-Lindberg A, Buckholtz JW, Kolachana BR, Hariri A, Pezawas L, Blasi G, Wabnitz A, Honea R, Verchinski B, Callicott JH, Egan M, Mattay V, Weinberger DR. Neural mechanisms of genetic risk for impulsivity and violence in humans. *Proceedings of the National Academy of Sciences of the United States of America* 2006; 103: 6269–6274.

Milgram S. Behavioural study of obedience. *Journal of Abnormal and Social Psychology* 1963; 67: 371–378.

Mitchell EW. Madness and meta-responsibility: the culpable causation of mental disorder and the insanity defence. *Journal of Forensic Psychiatry* 1999; 10: 597–622.

Moosajee M. Violence – a noxious cocktail of genes and the environment. *Journal of the Royal Society of Medicine* 2003; 96: 211–214.

Mullen PE. Psychopathy: A developmental disorder of ethical action. *Criminal Behaviour and Mental Health* 1992; 2: 234–244.

Neiman S. *Evil in modern thought: An alternative history of philosophy.* Princeton: Princeton University Press, 2002.

Nelson RJ, Trainor BC. Neural mechanisms of aggression. *Nature Reviews Neuroscience* 2007; 8: 536–546.

Pincus JH. *Base instincts: what makes killers kill.* New York: Norton & Company, 2001.

Raine A. Effect of early environment on electrodermal and cognitive correlates of schizotypy and psychopathy. *International Journal of Psychophysiology* 1987; 4: 277–287.

Raine A. *The psychopathology of crime: Criminal behaviour as a clinical disorder.* San Diego, California: Academic Press, Inc, 1993.

Raine A, Brennan P, Mednick SA. Interaction between birth complications and early maternal rejection in predisposing individuals to adult violence: specificity to serious, early-onset violence. *American Journal of Psychiatry* 1997a; 154:1265–1271.

Raine A, Buchsbaum M, LaCasse L. Brain abnormalities in murderers indicated by positron emission tomography. *Biological Psychiatry* 1997b; 42: 495–508.

Raine A, Buchsbaum MS, Stanley J, Lottenberg S, Abel L, Stoddard J. Selective reductions in prefrontal glucose metabolism in murderers. *Biological Psychiatry* 1994; 36: 365–373.

Raine A, Lencz T, Bihrle S, LaCasse L, Colletti P. Reduced prefrontal grey matter volume and reduced autonomic activity in antisocial personality disorder. *Archives of General Psychiatry* 2000; 57: 119–127.

Raine A, Venables PH. Tonic heart rate level, social class and antisocial behaviour in adolescents. *Biological Psychology* 1984; 18: 123–132.

Raine A, Venables PH, Williams M. Autonomic orienting responses in 15 year-old male subjects and criminal behaviour at age 24. *American Journal of Psychiatry* 1990; 147: 933–937.

Raine A, Venables PH, Williams M. High autonomic arousal and electrodermal orienting at age 15 years as protective factors against criminal behaviour at age 29 years. *American Journal of Psychiatry* 1995; 152: 1595–1600.

Raine A, Venables PH, Williams M. Better autonomic conditioning and faster electrodermal half-recovery time at age 15 years as possible protective factors against crime at age 29 years. *Developmental Psychology* 1996; 32: 624–630.

Relkin N, Plum F, Mattis S, Eidelberg D, Tranel D. Impulsive homicide associated with an arachnoid cyst and unilateral frontotemporal cerebral dysfunction. *Seminars in Clinical Neuropsychiatry* 1996; 1: 172–183.

Rose R. *The Nazi genocide of the Sinti and Roma*. Heidelberg, Germany: Documentary and Cultural Centre of German Sinti and Roma, 1995 (second revised edition).

Sampson RJ. Collective regulation of adolescent misbehaviour. *Journal of Adolescent Research* 1997; 12: 227–244.

Sampson RJ, Baudenbush SW, Earls F. Neighbourhoods and violent crime: a multilevel study of collective efficacy. *Science* 1997; 277: 918–924.

Struber D, Luck M, Roth G. Sex, aggression and impulse control: An integrative account. *Neurocase* 2008; 14: 93–121.

Tabucchi A. *The missing head of Damasceno Monteiro*. Translation by J.C. Patrick. London: Harvill Press, 2000 (originally published in 1997).

Tiihonen J, Hodgins S, Vaurio O, Laakso M, Repo E, Soininen H, Aronen HJ, Nieminen P, Savolainen L. Amygdaloid volume loss in psychopathy. *Society for Neuroscience Abstracts* 2000: 2017.

Treiman DM. Psychobiology of ictal aggression. In '*Advances in Neurology*', volume 55, edited by D. Trejman & M. Trimble. New York: Raven Press Ltd,1991: 341–355.

Vardy P. *The puzzle of evil*. London: Fount, 1992.

Viding E, Blair RJR, Moffitt TE, Plomin R. Evidence for substantial genetic risk for psychopathy in 7-year-olds. *Journal of Child Psychology and Psychiatry* 2005; 46: 592–597.

Waller J. *Becoming evil: How ordinary people commit genocide and mass killing*. Oxford: Oxford University Press, 2002.

WHO global consultation on violence and health. *Violence: A public health priority*. Geneva: World Health Organization, 1996.

Woodworth M, Porter S. In cold blood: Characteristics of criminal homicides as a function of psychopathy. *Journal of Abnormal Psychology* 2002; 111: 436–455.

Chapter 10 – Human response space

Adenzato M, Ardito RB. The role of theory of mind and deontic reasoning in the evolution of deception. In *Proceedings of the 21st Conference of the Cognitive Science Society* (ed. M. Hahn & SC Stoness). Mahwah, New Jersey: Erlbaum Associates, 1999: 7–12.

Ainslie G. *Breakdown of will*. Cambridge: Cambridge University Press, 2001.

Baddeley AD. The capacity for generating information by randomisation. Quarterly Journal of Experimental Psychology 1966; 18: 119–129.

Bailey D. *Improvisation: Its nature and practice in music*. New York: Da Capo Press, 1993.

Barrett K. Treating organic abulia with bromocriptine and lisuride: four case studies. *Journal of Neurology, Neurosurgery, and Psychiatry* 1991; 54: 718–721.

Bley P, Lee D. *Stopping time: Paul Bley and the transformation of jazz*. Quebec: Vehicule Press, 1999.

Farrow TFD, Hunter MD, Haque R, Spence SA. Modafinil and unconstrained motor activity in schizophrenia: double-blind crossover placebo-controlled trial. *British Journal of Psychiatry* 2006; 189: 461–462.

Hunter MD, Ganesan V, Wilkinson ID, Spence SA. Acute effects of modafinil on prefrontal function and cognitive control in chronic schizophrenia. *American Journal of Psychiatry* 2006; 163: 2184–2186.

Muraven M, Baumeister RF. Self-regulation and depletion of limited resources: Does self-control resemble a muscle? *Psychological Bulletin* 2000; 126: 247–259.

Owens T. *Bebop: The music and its players.* Oxford: Oxford University Press, 1995.

Sacks O. Awakenings. London: Picador, 1982 (revised edition), first published 1973.

Spence SA. Can pharmacology help enhance human morality? *British Journal of Psychiatry* 2008; 193: 179–180.

Turner DC, Sahakian BJ. Analysis of the cognitive enhancing effects of modafinil in schizophrenia. *Progress in Neurotherapeutics and Neuropsychopharmacology* 2006; 1: 133–147.

Vrij A. *Detecting lies and deceit: Pitfalls and opportunities* (second edition). Chichester, West Sussex: Wiley, 2008.

Vrij A, Mann S. Telling and detecting lies in a high-stake situation: The case of a convicted murderer. *Applied Cognitive Psychology* 2001; 15: 187–203.

Epilogue – Raising a fist

Anonymous. *Oxford Companion to the Mind* (2nd Ed.). Edited by RL Gregory. Oxford: Oxford University Press, 2005.

Aristotle. *The Nichomachean ethics.* Oxford: Oxford University Press, 1998.

Coate M. *Beyond all reason.* London: Constable, 1964.

Dennett DC. *Consciousness explained.* Boston: Little, Brown and Company, 1991.

Ellenberger HF. *The discovery of the unconscious.* London: Fontana, 1994.

Ganesan V, Green RD, Hunter MD, Wilkinson ID, Spence SA. Expanding the response space in chronic schizophrenia: the relevance of left prefrontal cortex. *NeuroImage* 2005; 25: 952–957.

Gaser C, Schlaug G. Brain structures differ between musicians and non-musicians. *Journal of Neuroscience* 2003; 23: 9240–9245.

Libet B. *Mind time: the temporal factor in consciousness.* Cambridge, Massachusetts: Harvard University Press, 2004.

Libet B, Gleason CA, Wright EW, Pearl DK. Time of conscious intention to act in relation to onset of cerebral activities (readiness-potential): the unconscious initiation of a freely voluntary act. *Brain* 1983; 106: 623–642.

Luxmoore J. The quiet saints of the gulag. *The Tablet* 27th May 2000: 708–709.

Macmurray J. *The self as agent.* London: Faber & Faber, 1991.

Maguire EA, Gadian DG, Johnsrude IS, Good CD, Ashburner J, Frackowiak RSJ, Frith CD. Navigation-related structural change in the hippocampi of taxi drivers. *PNAS* 2000; 97: 4398–4403.

Mitchell EW. Madness and meta-responsibility: the culpable causation of mental disorder and the insanity defence. *Journal of Forensic Psychiatry* 1999; 10: 597–622.

Mullen PE. Psychopathy: a developmental disorder of ethical action. *Criminal Behaviour and Mental Heath* 1992; 2: 234–244.

Nagel T. Moral luck. In *'Free will'* (Ed. G. Watson). Oxford: Oxford University Press, 1982: 174–186 (originally published 1979).

Owen D. *The hubris syndrome: Bush, Blair and the intoxication of power.* London: Politico's, 2007.

Spence SA. Free will in the light of neuropsychiatry. *Philosophy, Psychiatry & Psychology* 1996; 3: 75–90.

Spence SA. Hysterical paralyses as disorders of action. *Cognitive Neuropsychiatry* 1999; 4: 203–226.

Spence SA. The cognitive executive is implicated in the maintenance of psychogenic movement disorders. In *'Psychogenic movement disorders'*, ed. M. Hallett et al. Philadelphia: American Academy of Neurology, 2006a: 222–229.

Spence SA. The cycle of action. *Journal of Consciousness Studies* 2006b; 13: 69–72.

Spence SA. Can pharmacology help enhance human morality? *British Journal of Psychiatry* 2008; 193: 179–180.

Terada K, Ikeda A, Van Ness PC, Nagamine T, Kaji R, Kimura J, Shibasaki H. Presence of Bereitschaftspotential preceding psychogenic myoclonus: clinical application of jerk-locked back averaging. *Journal of Neurology, Neurosurgery and Psychiatry* 1995; 58: 745–747.

Waller J. *Becoming evil: how ordinary people commit genocide and mass killing.* Oxford: Oxford University Press, 2002.

Wenegrat B. *Theatre of disorder: patients, doctors, and the construction of illness.* Oxford: Oxford University Press, 2001.

Index

Printed and bound by CPI Group (UK) Ltd, Croydon, CR0 4YY